MW00416801

Statistical Analysis of Medical Data Using SAS

Geoff Der
University of Glasgow
Scotland
Brian S. Everitt
Institute of Psychiatry
King's College
London, UK

Chapman & Hall/CRC
Taylor & Francis Group
Boca Raton London New York

Dedication

To Rachel

Brian S. Everitt

To Helen and Freddie

Geoff Der

Published in 2006 by
Chapman & Hall/CRC
Taylor & Francis Group
6000 Broken Sound Parkway NW, Suite 300
Boca Raton, FL 33487-2742

Printed in the United States of America on acid-free paper
10 9 8 7 6 5 4 3 2 1

International Standard Book Number-10: 1-58488-469-X (Hardcover)
International Standard Book Number-13: 978-1-58488-469-9 (Hardcover)
Library of Congress Card Number 2005048547

Library of Congress Cataloging-in-Publication Data

Der, Geoff.
Statistical analysis of medical data using SAS / Geoff Der, Brian S. Everitt.
p. cm.
Includes bibliographical references and index.
ISBN 1-58488-469-X (alk. paper)
1. SAS (Computer file) 2. Medicine--Data processing. 3. Medical records--Data processing. I. Everitt, Brian. II. Title.

RA409.5.D465 2005
610'.285--dc22 2005048547

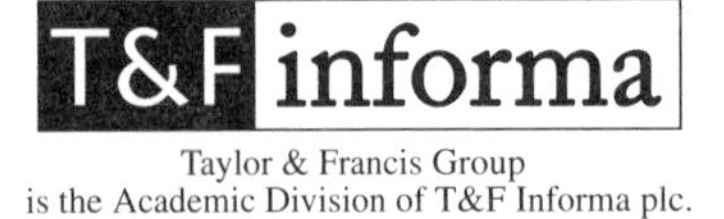

Taylor & Francis Group
is the Academic Division of T&F Informa plc.

Visit the Taylor & Francis Web site at
http://www.taylorandfrancis.com

and the CRC Press Web site at
http://www.crcpress.com

Preface

Statistical science plays an important role in medical research. Medical journals are full of statistical material and it is increasingly common to see statistical results from research papers quoted in promotional materials for drugs and other medical therapies. Indeed it is probably not overstating the case that the key to the progress of medicine has, in a considerable part, been due to the collection and valid interpretation of evidence, particularly quantitative evidence, provided by the application of statistical methods to medical investigations. In the last two decades, the field of medical statistics has grown rapidly and complex statistical procedures are now a routine part of medical research. But such methods can only be applied routinely with the aid of a statistical software package. In this book our aim is to combine brief accounts of the statistical methods most relevant to present day research in medicine, with details of how to apply these methods using SAS software. The emphasis is very much on the practical aspects of the methodology with the main theoretical details being confined to "Displays." In this way the reader who is already familiar with the theory, or wishes to see the practice before investing time in learning the details, can read the SAS code and results largely uninterrupted by the technical aspects of a method. In this way we hope the book will provide medical statisticians and applied researchers in medicine who are not primarily statisticians but do need to analyse data, with a self-contained means of doing this using SAS.

The SAS code and data sets are available on line at:
http://www.sas.com/service/library/onlinedoc/code.samples.html

Geoff Der and Brian S. Everitt
Glasgow and London 2005.

Contents

1

An Introduction to SAS

1.1 Introduction

The name SAS began as an acronym for Statistical Analysis System, reflecting the origins of the software and the company behind it. Today the software covers such a broad range of products that the acronym is no longer considered appropriate. The majority of these products comprise a set of modules that can be added to the basic system, known as BASE SAS. Here we concentrate on the SAS/STAT and SAS/GRAPH modules in addition to the main features of the base system. Any installation of SAS intended for statistical analysis should include these two modules at the very least. Where we use any features of SAS that require additional modules, this will be indicated in the text.

At the heart of SAS is a programming language made up of statements that specify how data are to be processed and analysed. The statements correspond to operations to be performed on the data or instructions about the analysis. A SAS program consists of a sequence of SAS statements grouped together into blocks, referred to as 'steps'. These fall into two types: data steps and procedure (proc) steps. A data step is used to prepare data for analysis. It creates a SAS data set and may reorganise the data and modify it in the process. A proc step is used to perform a particular type of analysis, or statistical test, on the data in a SAS data set.

A simple program might comprise a data step to read in some raw data followed by a series of proc steps analysing that data. If, in the course of the analysis, the data need to be modified, a second data step would be used to do this. Although the emphasis of this book is on the statistical analysis, one of the great strengths of SAS is the power and flexibility it gives the user to perform the data manipulation that is so often a large part of the overall task of analysing data.

The SAS system is available for a wide range of different computers and operating systems, and the way in which SAS programs are entered and run differs somewhat according to the computing environment. We describe the Microsoft Windows interface, as this is by far the most popular, although other windowing environments, such as X-windows, are quite similar.

At the time of writing, the latest version of SAS is version 9.1; all the examples have used version 9.1 running under Microsoft Windows XP.

1.2 The User Interface

Figure 1.1 shows how SAS version 9.1 appears running under Windows XP.

When SAS is started five main windows are open, namely the editor, log, output, results, and explorer windows. In Figure 1.1 the editor, log, and results windows are visible. The explorer window is hidden behind the results window, and the output window is hidden behind the program editor and log windows.

At the top are the SAS title bar, the menu bar, and the tool bar, with the command bar at its left end. The buttons of the tool bar change, depending on which window is active. The command bar allows less frequently used commands to be typed in. At the bottom, the status line comprises a message area with the current directory and editor cursor position at the right. Double clicking on the current directory allows it to be changed. Above the status line is a series of tabs, which allow a window to be selected when it is hidden behind other windows.

Briefly, the purpose of the main windows is as follows.

Editor. The editor window is for typing in programs, editing them, and running them. When a SAS program is run, two types of output, the log and the procedure output, are generated and are displayed in the log and output windows.

Log. The log shows the SAS statements that have been submitted, together with information about the execution of the program, including warning and error messages.

Output. This window shows the printed results of any procedures. It is here that the results of any statistical analyses are shown.

Results. Provides easy access to SAS output.

Explorer. Accesses files, SAS data sets, and libraries.

When graphical procedures are run, an additional window is opened to display the resulting graphs.

Managing the windows, e.g., moving between windows, resizing them, and rearranging them, can be done with the normal Windows controls, including the Windows menu, and the tabs at the bottom of the screen. If a window has been closed it can be reopened using the `View` menu.

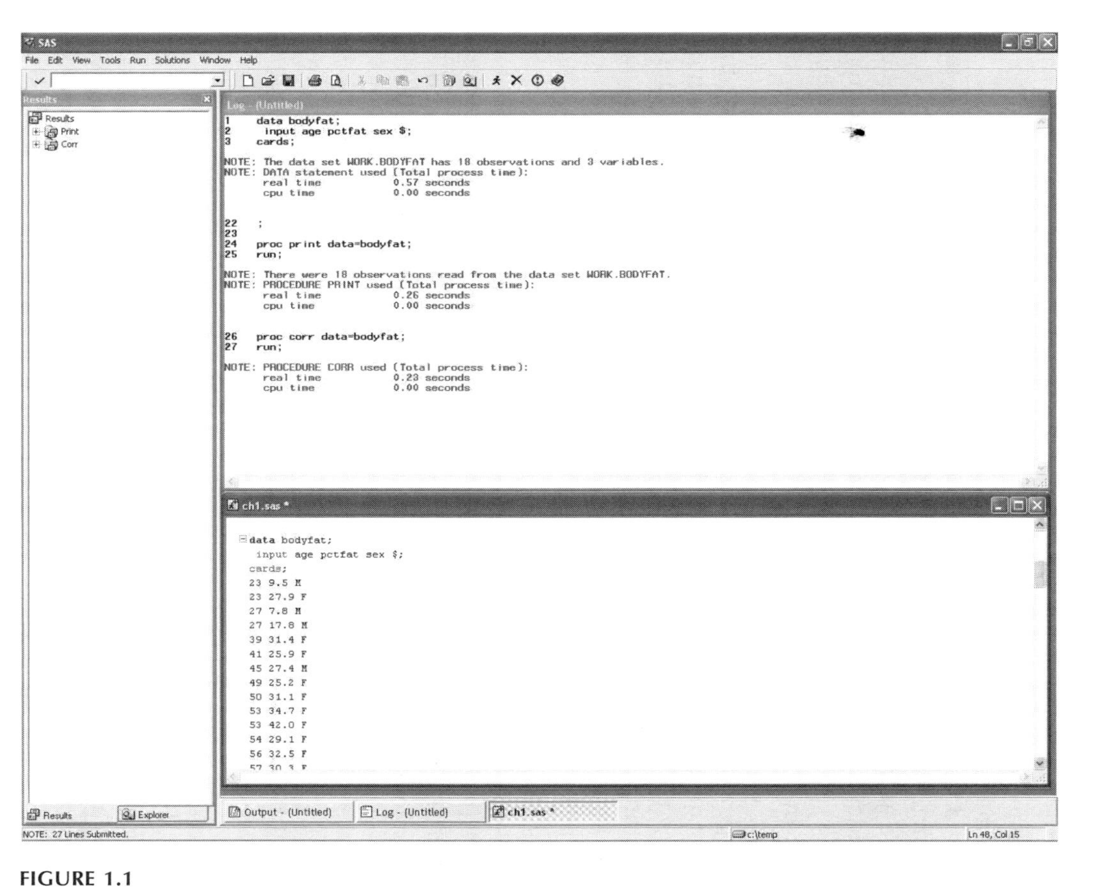

FIGURE 1.1
SAS version 9.1 running under Windows XP.

1.2.1 The Editor Window

SAS has two editors, a newer version introduced in version 8 and referred to as the enhanced editor, and an older version, known as the program editor. The program editor has been retained for reasons of compatibility but is not recommended. Here we describe the enhanced editor and may refer to it simply as 'the editor'. If SAS starts up using the program editor rather than the enhanced editor, then from the `Tools` menu select `Options; Preferences` then the `Edit` tab and select the `Use Enhanced Editor` box.

The editor is essentially a built in text editor specifically tailored to the SAS language and with additional facilities for running SAS programs.

Some aspects of the editor window will be familiar as standard features of Windows applications. The `File` menu allows programs to be read from a file; saved to a file; or printed. The `File` menu also contains the command to exit from SAS. The `Edit` menu contains the usual options for cutting, copying, and pasting text and those for finding and replacing text.

The program currently in the editor window may be run by choosing the `Submit` option from the `Run` menu. The `Run` menu is specific to the editor window and will not be available if another window is the active window. Submitting a program may remove it from the editor window. If so, it can be retrieved by choosing `Recall Last Submit` from the `Run` menu.

It is possible to run part of the program in the editor window by selecting the text and then choosing `Submit` from the `Run` menu. With this method the submitted text is not cleared from the editor window. When running parts of programs in this way, make sure that a full step has been submitted. The easiest way to do this is to include a `run` statement as the last statement.

The `Options` submenu within `Tools` allows the editor to be configured. When the enhanced editor window is the active window (`View, Enhanced Editor` will ensure that it is), `Tools; Options; Enhanced Editor` will open a window similar to that in Figure 1.2. This shows the setup we recommend, in particular, that the options for collapsible code sections and automatic indentation are selected; and that `clear text on submit` is not.

1.2.2 The Log Window

The log window is the main source of feedback to the user about the program or statements that have been submitted. It shows the statements themselves, together with notes, warnings, and error messages. Although it is tempting to assume that if some output is generated, the program has 'worked', this is by no means the case. It is a good discipline to check the log every time. While error messages and warnings obviously demand attention, the notes can also be important. For example, when a SAS dataset is created, a note in the log gives the number of observations and variables it contains and, if these are not as anticipated, there may be an error in the program.

The `Clear all` option in the `Edit` menu, or the `New` button on the toolbar, will empty the window. This is useful if a program has been run several times as errors were being corrected.

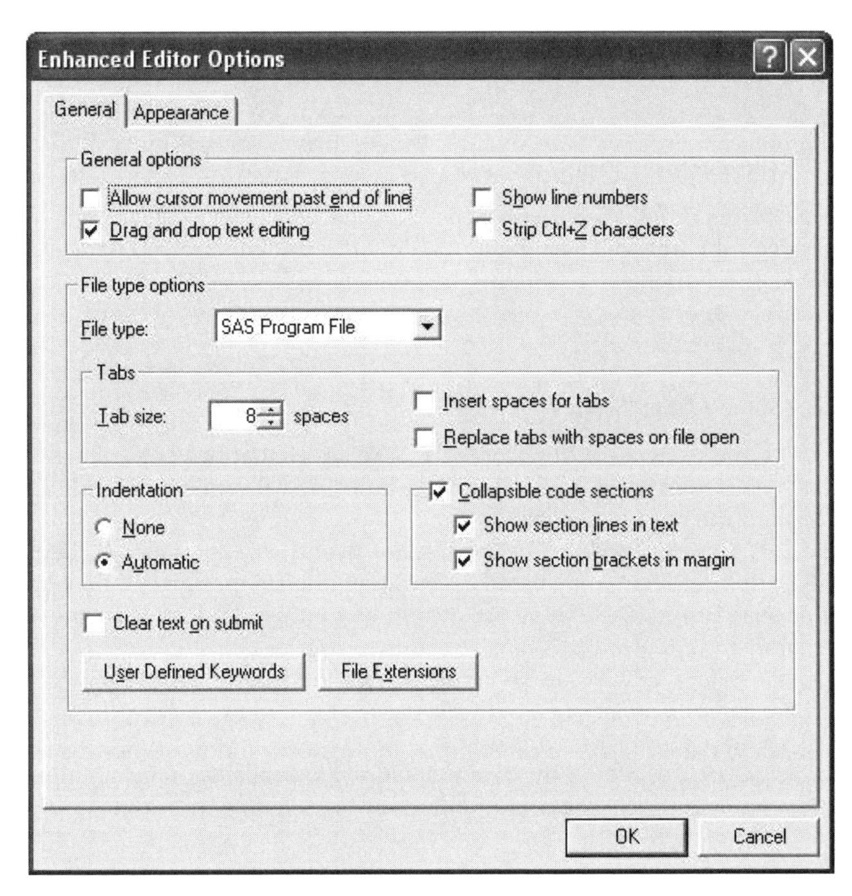

FIGURE 1.2
The Enhanced Editor Options window.

1.2.3 The Output Window

The output window works in tandem with the results window. The entire contents of the window can be cleared in the same way as the log window, or sections can be deleted via the results window.

1.2.4 The Results Window

This window provides a graphical index to the various procedure results, including the contents of the output window, the graph window, and any output in other formats, such as rich text tormat (rtf) or HTML, that may have been generated. It is useful for navigating around large amounts of output. Right-clicking on a procedure or section of output allows that portion of the output to be viewed, printed, deleted, or saved to file. Double-clicking on a section of output opens the appropriate window with that section of the output visible.

1.2.5 The Explorer Window

This performs much the same functions as the Windows explorer, but with the added advantage of being able to view the contents of SAS datasets or a list of the variables it contains (right-click `Open` and right-click `View Columns`, respectively).

1.2.6 Some Other Menus

The `View` menu is useful for reopening a window that has been closed.

The `Solutions` menu allows access to built-in SAS applications, but these are beyond the scope of this text.

The `Help` menu tends to become more useful as experience of SAS is gained, although there may be access to some tutorial materials if they have been licensed from SAS. There are also links to the main SAS Web site and the customer support Web site.

Context-sensitive help can be invoked with the F1 key. Within the editor, when the cursor is positioned over the name of a SAS procedure, the F1 key brings up the help for that procedure.

For version 9, pdf files of the documentation are available online at: http://support.sas.com/documentation/onlinedoc/

1.3 The SAS Language

Learning to use the SAS language is largely a question of learning the statements that are needed to do the analysis required and of knowing how to structure them into steps. Knowing a few general principles is useful.

Most SAS statements begin with a keyword that identifies the type of statement. (The most important exception is the assignment statement, which begins with a variable name.) The enhanced editor recognises keywords as they are typed and changes their colour to blue. If a word remains red, this indicates a problem. The word may have been mistyped or is invalid for some other reason.

All SAS statements must end with a semicolon.

The most common mistake for new users is to omit the semicolon, and the effect is to combine two statements into one. Sometimes, the result will be a valid statement, albeit one that has unintended results. If the result is not a valid statement, there will be an error message in the SAS log when the program is submitted. However, it may not be obvious that a semicolon has been omitted before the program is run, as the combined statement will usually begin with a valid keyword.

Statements may extend over more than one line, and there may be more than one statement per line. However, keeping to one statement per line, as far as possible, helps to avoid errors and to allow identification of those that do occur.

SAS statements fall into four broad categories according to where in a program they can be used. These are:

- Data step statements
- Proc step statements
- Statements that can be used in both data and proc steps
- Global statements, which apply to all following steps

Since the functions of the data and proc steps are so different, it is perhaps not surprising that many statements are only applicable to one type of step.

1.3.1 Program Steps

Data and proc steps begin with a `data` or `proc` statement, respectively, and end at the next `data` or `proc` statement or the next `run` statement. When a data step has the data included within it, the step ends after the data. Understanding where steps begin and end is important because SAS programs are executed in whole steps. If an incomplete step is submitted, it will not be executed. The statements that were submitted will be listed in the log, but SAS will appear to have stopped at that point without explanation. In fact, SAS will simply be waiting for the step to be completed before running it. For this reason it is good practice to explicitly mark the end of each step by inserting a `run` statement and especially important to include one as the last statement in the program.

The enhanced editor offers several visual indicators of the beginning and end of steps. The `data`, `proc`, and `run` keywords are colour-coded in navy blue rather than the standard blue used for other keywords. If the enhanced editor options for collapsible code sections have been selected as shown in Figure 1.2, each data and proc step will be separated by lines in the text and indicated by brackets in the margin. This gives the appearance of enclosing each data and proc step in its own box.

Data step statements must be within the relevant data step, i.e., after the `data` statement and before the end of the step. Likewise, proc step statements must be within the proc step.

Global statements may be placed anywhere. If they are placed within a step, they will apply to that step and all subsequent steps until reset. A simple example of a global statement is the `title` statement, which defines a title for procedure output and graphs. The title is then used until changed or reset.

1.3.2 Variable Names and Data Set Names

In writing a SAS program names must be given to variables and data sets. These may contain letters, numbers, and underline characters, and may be up to 32 characters long, but cannot begin with a number. (Prior to version 7 of SAS the maximum length was eight characters.) Variable names may be in upper or lower case, or a mixture, but differences in case are ignored. So `'Height'`, `'height'`, and `'HEIGHT'` would all refer to the same variable.

1.3.3 Variable Lists

When a list of variable names is needed in a SAS program, an abbreviated form can often be used. A variable list of the form `sex - - weight` refers to the variables `sex` and `weight` and all the variables positioned between them in the data set. A second form of variable list may be used where a set of variables have names of the form `score1, score2, ... score10`. That is, there are ten variables with the root, `score`, in common and ending in the digits 1 to 10. In this case, they can be referred to by the variable list `score1 - score10`, and do *not* need to be contiguous in the data set.

Before the SAS language is examined in more detail, the short example shown in Table 1.1 can be used to illustrate some of the preceding material. The data are adapted from Table 17 of *A Handbook of Small Data Sets (SDS)* and show the age, sex, and percentage of body fat for 18 subjects. The program consists of three steps: a data step followed by two proc steps. Submitting this program results in the log and procedure output shown in Table 1.2 and Table 1.3.

From the log we can see that the program has been split into steps and each step run separately. Notes on how the step ran follow the statements that comprise the step and in the case of the data step show that the `bodyfat` dataset contains the correct number of observations and variables.

The reason the log refers to the SAS data set as 'WORK.BODYFAT' rather than simply 'bodyfat' will be explained later.

1.4 Reading Data — The Data Step

Before data can be analysed in SAS they need to be read into a SAS data set. Creating a SAS data set for subsequent analysis is the primary function of the data step. The data may be 'raw' data or come from a previously created SAS data set. A data step is also used to manipulate or reorganise the data. This can range from relatively simple operations, like transforming variables, to more complex restructuring of the data. In many practical situations, organising and preprocessing the data take up a large proportion of the

TABLE 1.1

A Simple SAS Program

```
data bodyfat;
 input age pctfat sex $;
cards;
23   9.5 M
23  27.9 F
27   7.8 M
27  17.8 M
39  31.4 F
41  25.9 F
45  27.4 M
49  25.2 F
50  31.1 F
53  34.7 F
53  42.0 F
54  29.1 F
56  32.5 F
57  30.3 F
58  33.0 F
58  33.8 F
60  41.1 F
61  34.5 F
;
proc print data=bodyfat;
run;
proc corr data=bodyfat;
run;
```

overall time and effort. The power and flexibility of SAS for such data manipulation are among its great strengths.

We begin by describing how to create SAS data sets from raw data and store them on disk before turning to data manipulation. Each of the subsequent chapters includes the data step used to prepare the data for analysis, and several of them illustrate features not described in this chapter.

1.4.1 Creating SAS Data Sets from Raw Data*

Table 1.4 shows some hypothetical data on members of a slimming club, giving the membership number, team, starting weight, and current weight. The following data step could be used to create a SAS data set.

* A 'raw' data file may also be referred to as a text file or ASCII file. Such files only include the printable characters plus tabs, spaces, and end-of-line characters. The files produced by database programs, spreadsheets, and word processors are not normally 'raw' data, although such programs usually have the ability to 'export' their data to such a file.

TABLE 1.2

SAS Log after Submitting the Program in Table 1.1

```
27    data bodyfat;
28     input age pctfat sex $;
29    cards;

NOTE: The data set WORK.BODYFAT has 18 observations and 3 variables.
NOTE: DATA statement used (Total process time):
      real time           0.00 seconds
      cpu time            0.00 seconds

48    ;
49    proc print data=bodyfat;
50    run;

NOTE: There were 18 observations read from the data set WORK.BODYFAT.
NOTE: PROCEDURE PRINT used (Total process time):
      real time           0.00 seconds
      cpu time            0.00 seconds

51    proc corr data=bodyfat;
52    run;

NOTE: PROCEDURE CORR used (Total process time):
      real time           0.01 seconds
      cpu time            0.01 seconds
```

```
data SlimmingClub;
  infile 'c:\sasbook\data\slimmingclub.dat';
  input idno team $ startweight weightnow;
run;
```

1.4.2 The Data Statement

The `data` statement often takes this simple form, where it merely names the data set being created, in this case `SlimmingClub`.

1.4.3 The Infile Statement

The `infile` statement specifies the file where the raw data are stored. The full path name of the file is given. If the file is in the current directory, i.e., the one specified at the bottom right of the SAS window, the file name could have been specified simply as `'SlimmingClub.dat'`. The name of the raw data file must be in quotes. In many cases the `infile` statement will only need to specify the filename as in this example.

TABLE 1.3

Procedure Output of the Program in Table 1.1

Obs	age	pctfat	sex
1	23	9.5	M
2	23	27.9	F
3	27	7.8	M
4	27	17.8	M
5	39	31.4	F
6	41	25.9	F
7	45	27.4	M
8	49	25.2	F
9	50	31.1	F
10	53	34.7	F
11	53	42.0	F
12	54	29.1	F
13	56	32.5	F
14	57	30.3	F
15	58	33.0	F
16	58	33.8	F
17	60	41.1	F
18	61	34.5	F

The CORR Procedure

2 Variables: age pctfat

Simple Statistics

Variable	N	Mean	Std Dev	Sum	Minimum	Maximum
age	18	46.33333	13.21764	834.00000	23.00000	61.00000
pctfat	18	28.61111	9.14439	515.00000	7.80000	42.00000

Pearson Correlation Coefficients, N = 18
Prob > |r| under H0: Rho=0

	age	pctfat
age	1.00000	0.79209 <.0001
pctfat	0.79209 <.0001	1.00000

In some circumstances additional options on the `infile` statement will be needed. One such instance is where the values in the raw data file are not separated by spaces. Common alternatives are files where the data values are separated by tabs or commas. The `expandtabs` option changes tab characters into a number of spaces. The `delimiter` option can be used to specify a separator. For example, `delimiter=','` could be used for files where the data values are separated by commas. More than one delimiter can be specified. Tab- and comma-separated data are discussed in more detail below.

Another situation where additional options may be needed is to specify what happens when the program requests more data values than a line in the raw data file contains. This can happen for a number of reasons, particularly where character data are being read. Often the solution is to use the `pad` option, which adds spaces to the end of each data line as it is read.

TABLE 1.4

Hypothetical Data for a Slimming Club

```
1023 red    189 165
1049 yellow 145 124
1219 red    210 192
1246 yellow 194 177
1078 red    127 118
1221 yellow 220   .
1095 blue   135 127
1157 green  155 141
1331 blue   187 172
1067 green  135 122
1251 blue   181 166
1333 green  141 129
1192 yellow 152 139
1352 green  156 137
1262 blue   196 180
1087 red    148 135
1124 green  156 142
1197 red    138 125
1133 blue   180 167
1036 green  135 123
1057 yellow 146 132
1328 red    155 142
1243 blue   134 122
1177 red    141 130
1259 green  189 172
1017 blue   138 127
1099 yellow 148 132
1329 yellow 188 174
```

There is one situation where an `infile` statement is not needed. This is when the data are contained within the SAS program itself. This is referred to as 'instream' data. If data are instream an `infile` statement is only needed when additional options are required. When data are instream, SAS automatically expands tabs according to the tab size setting for the editor (see Figure 1.2), so the `expandtabs` option is not needed. Most of the examples in this book use instream data so that they can be easily run without modification. In practice, raw data are more commonly contained in an external file.

1.4.4 The Input Statement

The `input` statement in the example specifies that four variables are to be read in from the raw data file: `idno`, `team`, `startweight`, and `weightnow`, and the dollar sign after team indicates that it is a character variable. SAS only has two types of variables: numeric and character.

The function of the `input` statement is to name the variables, specify their type as numeric or character, and indicate where in the raw data the corresponding data values are. Where the data values are separated by spaces, as they are here, a simple form of the `input` statement is possible in which the variable names are merely listed in order and character variables are indicated by dollar signs after their names. This is the so called 'list' form of input. SAS has three main modes of input:

- List — for data separated by spaces
- Column — for data arranged in columns
- Formatted — for data in nonstandard formats

(There is a fourth form — named input — but data suitable for this form of input occur so rarely that its description can safely be omitted.)

List Input

In practice, there is often a choice of which mode of input to use, and it is a question of which mode is more convenient for the data at hand. As list input is the simplest, it is usually preferred for that reason. However, the requirement that the data values be separated by spaces has some important implications. The first is that missing values cannot be represented by spaces in the raw data; a period (.) should be used instead. In the example, the value of `weightnow` is missing for member number 1221. The second is that character values cannot contain spaces. With list input it is also important to bear in mind that the default length for character variables is eight.

When using list input *always* examine the SAS log. Check that the correct number of variables and observations have been read in. The message 'SAS went to a new line when INPUT statement reached past the end of a line' often indicates a problem in reading the data. If so, the `pad` option on the `infile` statement may be the answer.

With small datasets it is advisable to print them out with `proc print`, or open the dataset via the explorer window and check that the raw data have been read in correctly.

Column Input

If list input is problematic and the data are arranged in columns, column input may be simpler. Table 1.5 shows the slimming club data with members' names instead of their membership numbers. To read in the data in the column form of `input` statement would be:

```
input name $ 1-18 team $ 20-25 startweight 27-29
weightnow 31-33;
```

As can be seen, the difference between the two forms of input statement is simply that the columns containing the data values for each variable are specified after the variable name or after the dollar sign in the case of a character variable. The start and finish columns are separated by a hyphen,

TABLE 1.5

Hypothetical Slimming Data with Members' Names

David Shaw	red	189	165
Amelia Serrano	yellow	145	124
Alan Nance	red	210	192
Ravi Sinha	yellow	194	177
Ashley McKnight	red	127	118
Jim Brown	yellow	220	
Susan Stewart	blue	135	127
Rose Collins	green	155	141
Jason Schock	blue	187	172
Kanoko Nagasaka	green	135	122
Richard Rose	blue	181	166
Li-Hwa Lee	green	141	129
Charlene Armstrong	yellow	152	139
Bette Long	green	156	137
Yao Chen	blue	196	180
Kim Blackburn	red	148	135
Adrienne Fink	green	156	142
Lynne Overby	red	138	125
John VanMeter	blue	180	167
Becky Redding	green	135	123
Margie Vanhoy	yellow	146	132
Hisashi Ito	red	155	142
Deanna Hicks	blue	134	122
Holly Choate	red	141	130
Raoul Sanchez	green	189	172
Jennifer Brooks	blue	138	127
Asha Garg	yellow	148	132
Larry Goss	yellow	188	174

but for single-column variables it is only necessary to give the one column number. Note also that Jim Brown's current weight is missing, but the blanks in columns 31–33 are treated as a missing value, so the period is not needed as it would be with list input.

Formatted Input

With formatted input each variable is followed by its input format, referred to as its `informat`. Alternatively, a list of variables in parentheses is followed by a format list, also in parentheses. Formatted input is the most flexible, partly because a wide range of informats is available. To read the above data using formatted input, the following `input` statement could be used:

```
input name $19. team $7. startweight 4. weightnow 3.;
```

The informat for a character variable consists of a dollar sign, the number of columns occupied by the data values, and a period. The simplest form of informat for numeric data is simply the number of columns occupied by the data and a period. Note that the spaces separating the data values have been taken into account in the informat.

Formatted input must be used if the data are not in a standard numeric format. Such data are rare in practice. The most common use of special SAS informats is likely to be the date informats. When a date is read using a date informat, the resultant value is the number of days from January 1st 1960 to that date. The following data step illustrates the use of the `ddmmyyw.` informat. The width `w` may be from 6 to 32 columns. There is also the `mmddyyw.` informat for dates in American format. (There are also corresponding output formats, referred to simply as 'formats', to output dates in calendar form.)

```
data days;
input day ddmmyy8.;
cards;
020160
01/02/60
31 12 59
231019
231020
;
run;
proc print data=days;
run;
proc print data=days;
 format day ddmmyy10.;
run;
```

As the example illustrates, if the year is only given by its last two digits, values of 20 or above are assumed to be in the 20th century.

This data step is also an example of instream data. The data are contained between a `cards` statement (`datalines` is a synonym for `cards`) and a line with a single semicolon on it. The data must always be at the end of the data step.

Occasionally, data values will contain commas separating the thousands. These can be read with the comma format as follows:

```
data commas;
  input bignum comma6.;
cards;
 1,860
;
```

Another instance where formatted input may be needed is when numeric data contain an implied decimal point. In this case the informat has a second number after the period to indicate the number of digits to the right of the decimal point. For example, an informat of 5.2 would read five columns of numeric data and, in effect, move the decimal point two places to the left. Where the data contain an explicit decimal point this takes precedence over the informat.

```
data decimals;
 input realnum 5.2;
cards;
1234
 4567
123.4
  6789
;
proc print;
run;
```

Leading or trailing spaces, *within the field width*, as in lines 1 and 2, will not prevent the number from being read correctly. In the case of the last line, the final digit is outside the field width, i.e., in column 6, and so is not read as part of the number.

Formatted input can be much more concise than column input, particularly when consecutive data values have the same format. If the first 20 columns of the data line contain the single-digit responses to 20 questions, the data could be read as follows:

```
input (q1 - q20) (20*1.);
```

In this case using a numbered variable list makes the statement even more concise. The informats in the format list can be repeated by prefixing them with `n*`, where `n` is the number of times the format is to be repeated, 20 in this case. If the format list has fewer informats than there are variables in the variable list, the whole format list is reused. So the above input statement could be rewritten:

```
input (q1 - q20) (1.);
```

This feature is useful where the data contain repeating groups. If the answers to the 20 questions occupied one and two columns alternately, they could be read with

```
input (q1 - q20) (1. 2.);
```

The different forms of input may be mixed on the same input statement for maximum flexibility.

Multiple Lines per Observation

Where the data for an observation occupy several lines, the slash character (/), used as part of the input statement, indicates where to start reading data from the next line. Alternatively, a separate input statement could be written for each line of data, since SAS automatically goes on to the next line of data at the completion of each input statement.

Multiple Observations per Line

In some circumstances it is useful to be able to prevent SAS from automatically going on to the next line; this is done by adding an @ character to the end of the `input` statement. The usual reason for doing this is that there are data for more than one observation on the same line. These features of data input will be illustrated in later chapters.

Delimited Data

There are two commonly occurring forms of raw data that are worth commenting on specifically: tab-separated data and comma-separated data. Whilst list input is most commonly used for data separated by spaces, it can also be used to read data with other separators, referred to as 'delimiters'. One question which arises when delimiters other than spaces are used is how to treat two consecutive delimiters. With spaces as delimiters, list input by default treats consecutive spaces as a single delimiter. This is why spaces cannot be used for missing values. With comma-separated data it is more likely that two consecutive commas are intended to indicate that the value that would have been between them is missing. Tabs are more commonly treated like spaces but could be intended to be read either way. To change the default so that two consecutive delimiters are treated as having a missing value between them, use the `dsd` (delimiter-sensitive data) option on the `infile` statement.

Tab-Separated Data

The simplest way to read tab delimited data is to use list input with the `expandtabs` option on the `infile` statement. This substitutes a number of spaces for the tab character. If consecutive tabs indicate missing values the `delimiter=` and `dsd` options are needed, as follows:

```
Infile 'filename' delimiter='09'x dsd;
```

The value 09 is the hexadecimal code for the tab character in the ASCII character set.

Comma-Separated Data

Comma-delimited data files may also be referred to as comma separated value (CSV) files, with a file extension .csv, and many PC programs can produce files in this format. For most of these the `dsd` option on the `infile` statement will suffice, as it assumes the delimiter is a comma. Some comma-delimited files will have data values enclosed in quotes to avoid problems where data values include commas. The `dsd` option deals with this too by ignoring commas within quotes and removing the quotes from the data values. The `missover` option is also recommended for CSV files to prevent SAS going to a new line where the last value on a data line is missing. There is an example in Chapter 14. CSV files may also contain the names of the variables as the first line of the file. To skip this line when reading the data, use the `firstobs=2` option. So the recommended form of infile statement is:

```
infile 'filename' dsd missover;
```

or

```
infile 'filename' dsd missover firstobs=2;
```

where the variable names are on the first line.

1.4.5 Proc Import

For tab- and comma-delimited data, particularly where the first line contains the variable names, proc import is a useful alternative to reading in the data with a data step. For example, to read a tab-delimited file with the variable names in the first line, use:

```
Proc import datafile= 'filename' out=sasdataset dbms=tab
replace;
   getnames=yes;
run;
```

For comma-separated value files, substitute `dbms=csv`. Proc import does a good job of determining whether variables are numeric or character and their format, but the results need to be checked. If a numeric variable has any erroneous, nonnumeric values, proc import may make the variable a character variable. An alternative way of using proc import is via the import wizard. From the `file` menu, select `import data...`

1.4.6 Reading Data from Other Programs and Databases

SAS has a comprehensive set of modules enabling data held in proprietary databases to be read directly into SAS. This needs the appropriate SAS/

ACCESS module to be licensed and is beyond the scope of this book. In the PC context, however, it is worth mentioning that the SAS/ACCESS module for PC file formats will enable `proc import` to read data from Access, Excel, Dbase, and Lotus spreadsheets. The first screen of the import wizard will show which data sources have been licensed.

1.4.7 Temporary and Permanent SAS Data Sets — SAS Libraries

So far all the examples have shown temporary SAS data sets. They are temporary in the sense that they will be deleted when SAS is exited. To store SAS data sets permanently on disk, and to access such data sets, the `libname` statement is used, and the SAS data set referred to slightly differently.

```
libname db 'c:\sasbook\sasdata';
data db.SlimmingClub;
 set SlimmingClub;
run;
```

The `libname` statement specifies that the *libref* `db` refers to the directory `'c:\sasbook\sasdata'`. Thereafter, a SAS data set name prefixed with `'db.'` refers to a data set stored in that directory. When used on a data statement, the effect is to create a SAS data set in that directory. The data step reads data from the temporary SAS data set `SlimmingClub` and stores it in a permanent data set of the same name.

Since the `libname` statement is a global statement, the link between the libref `db` and the directory `'c:\sasbook\sasdata'` remains throughout the SAS session, or until reset. If SAS has been exited and restarted, the `libname` statement will need to be submitted again.

In Table 1.2 we saw that the temporary data set `bodyfat` was referred to in the log notes as `'WORK.BODYFAT'`. This is because `work` is the libref pointing to the directory where temporary SAS data sets are stored. SAS automatically sets up this directory and deletes the datasets in it when SAS is closed.

To use the SAS explorer window to examine the contents of a temporary dataset, or its variables, double-click on `libraries` in the explorer window, then double-click on `work`. To do the same for permanently stored datasets, after opening the libraries folder, double click on the libref (e.g., `db` in the above example).

1.4.8 Reading Data from an Existing SAS Data Set

To read data from a SAS data set, rather than from a raw data file, the `set` statement is used in place of the `infile` and `input` statements. For example, to retrieve a previously stored data set and continue working with a temporary copy:

```
libname db 'c:\sasbook\sasdata';
data SlimmingClub;
set db.SlimmingClub;
run;
```

creates a new, temporary, SAS data set `SlimmingClub`, reading in the data from the stored vesion of `SlimmingClub`.

1.5 Modifying SAS Data

As well as creating a SAS data set, the data step may also be used to modify the data in a variety of ways.

1.5.1 Creating and Modifying Variables

The assignment statement can be used both to create new variables and modify existing ones. The statement

```
weightloss=startweight-weightnow;
```

creates a new variable `weigtloss` and sets its value to the starting weight minus the current weight.

```
startweight=startweight * 0.4536;
```

will convert the starting weight from pounds to kilograms.

SAS has the normal set of arithmetic operators: +, -, / (divide), * (multiply), and ** (exponentiate), plus various arithmetic, mathematical, and statistical functions, some of which will be illustrated in later chapters.

Missing Values in Arithmetic Expressions

The result of an arithmetic operation performed on a missing value is itself a missing value. When this happens, a warning message is printed in the log. Missing values for numeric variables are represented by a period (.), and a numeric variable can be set to a missing value by an assignment statement such as:

```
age = . ;
```

With any arthimetical operation, it is worth considering what the effect of missing values will be. Say we want to calculate the mean of five variables, x1-x5. An assignment of the form xmean=(x1+x2+x3+x4+x5)/5; will result in a missing value if *any* of x1 to x5 are missing. On the other hand, xmean=mean(x1,x2,x3,x4,x5); will only result in a missing value if *all* of them are missing.

To assign a value to a character variable, the text string must be enclosed in quotes, e.g.,

```
team='green';
```

A missing value may be assigned to a character variable as follows:

```
Team='';
```

To modify the value of a variable for some observations and not others, or to make different modifications for different groups of observations, the assignment statement may be used within an if then statement.

```
reward=0;
if weightloss > 10 then reward=1;
```

If the condition weigtloss > 10 is true, then the assignment statement reward=1 is executed, otherwise the variable reward keeps its previously assigned value of 0. In cases like this an else statement could be used in conjunction with the if then statement.

```
if weightloss > 10 then reward=1;
   else reward=0;
```

The condition in the if then statement may be a simple comparison of two values. The form of comparison may be one of the following:

Operator		Meaning	Example
EQ	=	Equal to	a = b
NE	~=	Not equal to	a ne b
LT	<	Less than	a < b
GT	>	Greater than	a gt b
GE	>=	Greater than or equal to	a >= b
LE	<=	Less than or equal to	a le b

Comparisons can be combined into a more complex condition using and (&), or (|), and not.

```
if team='blue' and weightloss gt 10 then reward=1;
```

In more complex cases, it may be advisable to make the logic explicit by grouping conditions together with parentheses.

Some conditions involving a single variable can be simplified. For example, the following two statements are equivalent:

```
if age > 18 and age < 40 then agegroup = 1;
if 18 < age < 40 then agegroup = 1;
```

and conditions of the form:

```
x = 1 or x = 3 or x = 5
```

may be abbreviated to

```
x in(1, 3, 5)
```

using the `in` operator.

If the data contain missing values, it is important to allow for this when recoding.

In numeric comparisons, missing values are treated as smaller than any number.

For instance,

```
if age >= 18 then adult=1;
   else adult=0;
```

would assign the value 0 to `adult` if `age` was missing, whereas it may be more appropriate to assign a missing value. The missing function could be used do this, by following the `else` statement with:

```
if missing(age) then adult=.;
```

Care needs to be exercised when making comparisons involving character variables since these are case sensitive and sensitive to leading blanks.

A group of statements may be executed conditionally by placing them between a `do` statement and an `end` statement.

```
If weigtloss > 10 and weightnow < 140 then do;
target=1;
reward=1;
team ='blue';
end;
```

Every observation that satisfies the condition will have the values of `target`, `reward`, and `team` set as indicated. Otherwise, they will remain at their previous values.

Where the same operation is to be carried out on several variables, it is often convenient to use an array and an iterative do loop in combination. This is best illustrated with a simple example. Suppose we have 20 variables, q1 to q20, for which 'not applicable' has been coded –1, and we wish to set those to missing values, we might do it as follows:

```
array qall {20} q1-q20;
do i= 1 to 20;
  if qall{i}=-1 then qall{i}=.;
end;
```

The array statement defines an array by specifying the name of the array, qall here, the number of variables to be included in it in braces, and the list of variables to be included. All the variables in the array must be of the same type, that is all numeric or all character.

The iterative do loop repeats the statements between the do and the end a fixed number of times, with an index variable changing at each repetition. When used to process each of the variables in an array, the do loop should start with the index variable equal to 1 and end when it equals the number of variables in the array.

The array is a shorthand way of referring to a group of variables. In effect, it provides aliases for them so that each variable can be referred to by using the name of the array and its position within the array in braces. For example, q12 could be referred to as qall{12} or, when the variable i has the value 12, as qall{i}. However, the array only lasts for the duration of the data step in which it is defined.

1.5.2 Deleting Variables

Variables may be removed from the data set being created by using the drop or keep statements. The drop statement names a list of variables that are to be excluded from the data set, and the keep statement does the converse, that is it names a list of variables that are to be the only ones retained in the data set, all others being excluded. So the statement drop x y z; in a data step results in a data set that does not contain the variables x, y, and z, whereas keep x y z; results in a data set that contains only those three variables.

1.5.3 Deleting Observations

It may be necessary to delete observations from the data set either because they contain errors or because the analysis is to be carried out on a subset of the data. Deleting erroneous observations is best done by using the if then statement with the delete statement.

```
if weightloss > startweight then delete;
```

In a case such as this, it would also be useful to write out a message giving more information about the observation that contains the error.

```
if weightloss > startweight then do;
put 'Error in weight data' idno=  startweight= weightl
oss=;
delete;
end;
```

The put statement writes text (in quotes) and the values of variables to the log.

1.5.4 Subsetting Data Sets

If analysis of a subset of the data is needed, it is often convenient to create a new data set containing only the relevant observations. This can be achieved with either the subsetting if statement or the where statement. The subsetting if statement consists simply of the keyword if followed by a logical condition. Only observations for which the condition is true are included in the data set being created.

```
data women;
  set bodyfat;
  if sex='F';
run;
```

The statement where sex='F'; has the same form and could be used to the same effect. The difference between the subsetting if statement and the where statement will not concern most users, except that the where statement may also be used with proc steps as discussed below. More complex conditions may be specified on either statement in the same way as for an if then statement.

1.5.5 Concatenating and Merging Data Sets

Two or more data sets can be combined into one by specifying them on a single set statement.

```
data survey;
   set men women;
run;
```

This is also a simple way of adding new observations to an existing data set. First read the data for the new cases into a SAS data set; then combine this with the existing data set as follows.

```
data survey;
  set survey newcases;
run;
```

1.5.6 Merging Data Sets — Adding Variables

Data for a study may arise from more than one source, or at different times, and need to be combined. For instance, demographic details from a questionnaire may need to be combined with the results of laboratory tests. To deal with this situation, the data are read into separate SAS data sets and then combined using a merge with a unique subject identifier as a key. Assuming the data have been read into two data sets, `demographics` and `labtests`, and that both data sets contain the subject identifier `idnumber`, they can be combined as follows.

```
proc sort data=demographics;
  by idnumber;
proc sort data=labtests;
  by idnumber;
data combined;
  merge demographics (in=indem) labtest (in=inlab);
  by idnumber;
  if indem and inlab;
run;
```

First both data sets must be sorted by the matching variable, `idnumber`. This variable should be of the same type, numeric or character, and same length in both data sets. The `merge` statement in the data step specifies the data sets to be merged. The option in parentheses after the name creates a temporary variable that indicates whether that data set provided an observation for the merged data set. The `by` statement specifies the matching variable. The subsetting `if` statement specifies that only observations that have both the demographic data and the lab results should be included in the combined data set. Without this the combined data set may contain incomplete observations, i.e., those where there are demographic data but no lab results or vice versa. An alternative would be to print messages in the log in such instances as follows.

```
If not indem then put idnumber ' no demographics';
If not inlab then put idnumber ' no lab results';
```

This method of match merging is not confined to situations where a one-to-one correspondence exists between the observations in the data sets; it can be used for one-to-many or many-to-one relationships as well. A common practical application is in the use of look-up tables. For example, the research data set might contain the respondent's post code (or Zip code), and another file contain information on the characteristics of the area. Match merging the two data sets by post code would attach area information to the individual observations. A subsetting `if` statement would be used so that only observations from the research data were retained.

1.5.7 The Operation of the Data Step

In addition to learning the statements that may be used in a data step, it is useful to understand how the data step operates.

The statements that comprise the data step form a sequence according to the order in which they occur. The sequence begins with the data statement, finishes at the end of the data step, and is executed repeatedly until the source of data runs out. Starting from the data statement, a typical data step will read in some data with an `input` or `set` statement and use those data to construct an observation. The observation will then be used to execute the statements that follow. The data in the observation may be modified or added to in the process. At the end of the data step the observation will be written to the data set being created. The sequence will begin again from the data statement, reading the data for the next observation, processing it and writing it to the output data set. This continues until all the data have been read in and processed. The data step will then finish and the execution of the program will pass on to the next step.

In effect, then, the data step consists of a loop of instructions executed repeatedly until all the data are processed. The automatic SAS variable, `_n_`, records the iteration number but is not stored in the data set. Its use will be illustrated in later chapters.

The point at which SAS adds an observation to the data set can be controlled by the use of the `output` statement. When a data step includes one or more `output` statements, an observation is added to the data set each time an `output` statement is executed, but not at the end of the data step. In this way the data being read in can be used to construct several observations. This will be illustrated in later chapters.

1.6 The Proc Step

Once data have been read into a SAS data set, SAS procedures can be used to analyse the data. Roughly speaking, each SAS procedure performs a specific type of analysis. The proc step is a block of statements that specify the data set to be analysed, the procedure to be used, and any further details of the analysis. The step begins with a proc statement and ends with a run statement or when the next data or proc step starts. We recommend including a run statement for every proc step.

1.6.1 The Proc Statement

The proc statement names the procedure to be used and may also specify options for the analysis. The most important option is the data= option, which names the data set to be analysed. If the option is omitted, the procedure uses the most recently created data set. Although this is usually what is intended, it is safer to explicitly specify the data set.

Many of the statements that follow particular proc statements are specific to individual procedures and will be described in later chapters as they arise. A few, though, are more general and apply to a number of procedures.

1.6.2 The Var Statement

The var statement specifies the variables that are to be processed by the proc step. For example:

```
proc print data= SlimmingClub;
   var name team weightloss;
run;
```

restricts the printout to the three variables mentioned, whereas the default would be to print all variables.

1.6.3 The Where Statement

The where statement selects the observations to be processed. The keyword where is followed by a logical condition, and only those observations for which the condition is true are included in the analysis.

```
proc print data= SlimmingClub;
   where weightloss > 0;
run;
```

1.6.4 The By Statement

The by statement is used to process the data in groups. The observations are grouped according to the values of the variable named on the by statement, and a separate analysis is conducted for each group. In order to do this the data set must first be sorted on the by variable.

```
proc sort data= SlimmingClub;
   by team;
proc means;
   var weightloss;
   by team;
run;
```

1.6.5 The Class Statement

The class statement is used with many procedures to name variables that are to be used as classification variables, or factors. The variables named may be character or numeric variables and will typically contain a relatively small range of discreet values. There may be additional options on the class statement depending on the procedure.

1.7 Global Statements

Global statements may occur at any point in a SAS program and remain in effect until reset. The title statement is a global statement and provides a title that will appear on each page of printed output *and* each graph until reset. An example would be:

```
title 'Analysis of Slimming club data';
```

The text of the title must be enclosed in quotes. Multiple lines of titles can be specified with the title2 statement for the second line, title3 for the third line, and so on up to ten. The title statement is synonymous with title1. Titles are reset by a statement of the form:

```
title2;
```

This will reset line two of the titles and all lower lines, i.e., title3 etc.; title1; would reset all titles.

Comment statements are global statements in the sense that they can occur anywhere. There are two forms of comment statement. The first form begins with an asterisk and ends with a semicolon, for example:

```
* this is a comment;
```

The second form begins with `/*` and ends with `*/`.

```
/* this is also a
   comment
*/
```

Comments may appear on the same line as a SAS statement, e.g.,

```
bmi=weight/height**2;        /*  Body Mass Index */
```

The enhanced editor colour codes comments green, so it is easier to see if the `*/` has been omitted from the end or if the semicolon has been omitted in the first form of comment.

The first form of comment is useful for 'commenting out' individual statements, whereas the second is useful for commenting out one or more steps, since it can include semicolons.

1.7.1 Options

The `options` and `goptions` global statements are used to set SAS system options and graphics options, respectively. Most of the system options can be safely left at their default values. Some of those controlling the procedure output that may be considered useful are:

- `nocenter` aligns the output at the left, rather than centering it on the page — useful when the output linesize is wider than the screen.
- `nodate` suppresses printing of the date and time on the output.
- `ps=`*n* sets the output pagesize to *n* lines long.
- `ls=`*n* sets the output linesize to *n* characters.
- `pageno=`*n* sets the page number for the next page of output, e.g., `pageno=1` at the beginning of a program that is to be run repeatedly.

Several options can be set on a single options statement, e.g.,:

```
options nodate nocenter pagegno=1;
```

The `goptions` statement is analogous but sets graphical options. Some useful options are described below.

1.8 SAS Graphics

If the SAS/GRAPH module has been licensed, several of the statistical procedures can produce high-resolution graphics. Where the procedure does not have graphical capabilities built in, or different types of graphs are required, the general purpose graphical procedures within SAS/GRAPH may be used. The most important of these is the gplot procedure.

1.8.1 Proc Gplot

The simplest use of proc gplot is to produce a scatterplot of two variables, x and y for example.

```
proc gplot;
  plot y*x;
run;
```

A wide range of variations on this basic form of plot can be produced by varying the plot statement and using one or more symbol statements. The default plotting symbol is a plus sign. If no other plotting symbol has been explicitly defined, the default is used, and the result is a scatterplot with the data points marked by pluses. The symbol statement may be used to alter the plot character, but also to control other aspects of the plot. To produce a line plot rather than a scatter plot:

```
symbol1 i=join;
proc gplot;
   plot y * x;
run;
```

Here the symbol1 statement explicitly defines the plotting symbol and the i (interpolation) option specifies that the points are to be joined. The points will be plotted in the order in which they occur in the data set, so it is usually necessary to sort the data by the x axis variable first.

The data points will also be marked with pluses. The v= (value=) option on the symbol statement may be used to vary or remove the plot character. To change the above example so that only the line is plotted without the individual points being marked the symbol statement would be

```
symbol1 v=none i=join;
```

Other useful variations on the plot character are: x, star, square, diamond, triangle, hash, dot, and circle.

A variation of the plot statement uses a third variable to plot separate subgroups of the data.

```
symbol1 v=square i=join;
symbol2 v=triangle i=join;
```

```
proc gplot;
plot y * x = sex;
run;
```

will produce two lines with different plot characters (see Chapter 7 for an example). An alternative would be to remove the plot characters and use different types of line for the two subgroups. The `l=` (`linetype`) option of the symbol statement may be used to achieve this, e.g.,

```
symbol1 v=none i=join l=1;
symbol2 v=none i=join l=2;
proc gplot;
plot y * x = sex;
run;
```

Both of the above examples assume that two symbol definitions are being generated one by the `symbol1` statement and the other by `symbol2`. However, this is not the case when SAS is generating colour graphics. The reason is that SAS will use the symbol definition on the `symbol1` statement once for each colour currently defined before going on to use `symbol2`. If the final output is to be in black and white, then the simplest solution is to begin the program with

```
goptions colors=(black);
```

If the output is to be in colour, then it is simplest to use the `c= (color=)` option on the symbol statements themselves. For example:

```
symbol1 v=none i=join c=blue;
symbol2 v=none i=join c=red;
proc gplot;
plot y * x = sex;
run;
```

An alternative is to use the `repeat (r =)` option on the symbol statement with `r=1`. This is also used for the opposite situation, to force a symbol definition to be used repeatedly.

To plot means and standard deviations or standard errors, the `i=std` option can be used. This is explained with an example in Chapter 10.

Symbol statements are global statements and so remain in effect until reset. Moreover, all the options set on a symbol statement persist until reset. If a program contains the statement

```
symbol1 i=join v=diamond c=blue;
```

and a later symbol statement

```
symbol1 i=join;
```

the later plot will also have the diamond plot character as well as the line, and they will be coloured blue.

To reset a symbol1 statement and all its options, include

```
symbol1;
```

before the new `symbol1` statement.

To reset all the symbol definitions, include

```
goptions reset=symbol;
```

1.8.2 Overlaid Graphs

Overlaying two or more graphs is another technique that adds to the range of graphs that can be produced. The statement

```
plot y*x   z*x   / overlay;
```

will produce a graph where `y` and `z` are both plotted against `x` on the same graph (see Chapter 7 for an example). Without the `overlay` option two separate graphs would be produced. Note that it is not possible to overlay graphs of the form `y*x=z`.

Several other graphics procedures are illustrated in subsequent chapters: `proc boxplot` for box-and-whisker plots and `proc gchart`, for bar, block, pie, and star charts in Chapter 2; and `proc g3d`, for three-dimensional scatter plots and surface plots and `proc gcontour` for contour plots in Chapter 4.

1.8.3 Viewing and Printing Graphics

For any program that produces graphics, we recommend beginning the program with

```
goptions reset=all;
```

and then setting all the options required explicitly. Under Microsoft Windows a suitable set of graphics options might be:

```
goptions device=win target=winprtm rotate=landscape
ftext=swiss;
```

The device=win option specifies that the graphics are to be previewed on the screen. The target=winprtm option specifies that the hardcopy is to be produced on a monochrome printer set up in Windows, which can be configured from the File, Print Setup menu in SAS. For greyscale or colour printers, use target=winprtg or target=winprtc, respectively.*

The rotate option determines the orientation of the graphs. The alternative is rotate=portrait.

The ftext=swiss option specifies a sans-serif font for the text in the graphs.

When a goptions statement such as this is used, the graphs will be displayed one by one in the graph window, and the program will pause between them with the message "Press Forward to see next graph" in the status line. The Page Down and Page Up keys are used for Forward and Backward, respectively.

1.9 ODS — The Output Delivery System

The Output Delivery System is the facility within SAS for generating and saving output in different formats. Although it can be a complex subject to master, there are several basic uses well worth considering.

The first of these is the production of publication-quality results. Whether the results of a statistical analysis are destined to be published in a book, report, or scientific article or on the Web, ODS can simplify the process. Rather than saving output from the output window and then reformatting it, the output can be saved directly in HTML, pdf, or rtf files. Rtf (rich text format) files are particularly suitable for incorporating output in word processor documents. The output of one or more procedures can be saved in an rtf file by including ods rtf; beforehand and ods rtf close; afterwards.

```
ods rtf;
proc print data=bodyfat;
proc corr data=bodyfat;
run;
ods rtf close;
```

* Under X-windows the equivalent settings are device=xcolor and target=xprintm, xprintg, or xprintc.

The output appears in the output window as usual but is also saved in a file named `sasrtf.rtf` in the current directory. Since this file will be overwritten the next time rtf output is produced, it might be better to save the output to an explicitly named file with the `file='`*`filename`*`'` option on the `ods rtf` statement. ODS output can be formatted according to a number of built-in styles. The minimal style is a good starting point, so the `ods rtf` statement above would be replaced with

```
ods rtf style=minimal file='filename';
```

The names of other styles can be listed by submitting:

```
proc template;
  list styles;
run;
```

The rtf output may also appear in a results viewer window, and this may need to be closed before more rtf output is generated. The results viewer is switched on or off via `Tools`, `Options`, `Preferences`, `Results`, then `view results as they are generated`.

Another useful feature of ODS is the ability to save procedure output as SAS data sets. Prior to ODS, SAS procedures had could save output — parameter estimates, fitted values, residuals, etc. — in SAS data sets, via the `output` statement, or other procedure specific options. ODS extends this ability to the full range of procedure output. Each procedure's output is broken down into a set of tables and one of these may be saved to a SAS data set by including a statement of the form

```
ods output table = dataset;
```

within the `proc` step that generates the output.

Information on the tables created by each procedure is given in the "Details" section of the procedure's documentation. To find the variable names use the SAS explorer window, `proc contents data=`*`dataset`*`;` or even `proc print`, if the data set is small.

In version 9.1 of SAS, ODS graphics were introduced on an experimental basis. Using ODS graphics, many of the statistical procedures covered in this book can produce a selection of plots, either automatically or by specifying some graphing options.

The fact that these graphics are experimental means that they are liable to be changed in forthcoming versions. Nonetheless, they are an easy way of producing useful plots, some of which would be otherwise be difficult. As with the ODS tables, information on the ODS graphics that are available are given in the details section of the procedure's documentation. ODS graphics are switched on and off with the `ods graphics on;` and `ods graphics` `off;` statements. They also need an ODS destination to be open. The following example is given in Chapter 9.

```
ods html;
ods graphics on;
proc gam data=diabetes plots(clm commonaxes);
  model logpeptide=loess(age) loess(base) /
 method=gcv;
run;
ods graphics off;
ods html close;
```

We could also have used `ods rtf;` and there is another example in Chapter 9 that does. With rtf the graphs are included in the rtf document along with the tables. With html the graphs are each in a separate file. The html output and the graphs are put in the current directory by default, but different and separate directories can be specified by the `path=` and `gpath=` options on the `ods html` statement. The default format for the graphs is GIF, but JPEG and PNG are alternatives that can be set via the `imagefmt=` option on the `ods graphics` statement. In the example, we could use:

```
ods html gpath='c:\sasbook\graphs';
ods graphics on / imagefmt=jpeg;
```

to store a JPEG format graph in the named directory.

1.10 SAS Macros

SAS macros are general-purpose SAS programs. They are general purpose in the sense that they can be run repeatedly using different data sets, variables, or settings. Any SAS program can be adapted to use another data set and other variables by editing it and changing the names of the data sets and variables throughout. The advantage of a macro is that you supply the new names once, and SAS does all the necessary substitution. A simple example will help to illustrate this. First we write a macro definition:

```
%macro plotxy(data=,x=,y=);
proc gplot data=&data;
  plot &y*&x;
run;
%mend plotxy;
```

This is a macro to plot two variables. The definition begins with a `%macro` statement, which declares the name of the macro, `plotxy`, and then in parentheses the values it needs when it is used. These are called the macro's parameters. The body of the macro follows, along with the `%mend` statement to signal the end of the macro definition. The body of the macro consists of a proc gplot step, but with `&data`, `&y`, and `&x` in place of the data set and variable names.

```
options mprint;
```

will print in the log the statements that the macro creates when it is run. Before running the macro we must submit the macro definition. If the macro definition is stored in a file, this can be done by including it with, e.g., `%inc 'c:\sasbook\macros\plotxy.sas';`

The macro is run as follows:

```
%plotxy(data=bodyfat,x=age,y=pctfat);
```

and the log shows how the values provided have been substituted into the body of the macro:

```
MPRINT(PLOTXY):   proc gplot data=bodyfat;
MPRINT(PLOTXY):   plot pctfat*age;
MPRINT(PLOTXY):   run;
```

Macro parameters have two different forms. The form already illustrated is the so-called keyword form. The alternative is positional form. If the macro had been defined as follows:

```
%macro plotxy(data,x,y);
proc gplot data=&data;
  plot &y*&x;
run;
%mend plotxy;
```

it would have to be run with:

```
%plotxy(bodyfat,age,pctfat);
```

A few macros that we have written will be used in later chapters. There are also macros supplied by SAS and others available on the SAS Web site and elsewhere. Hence, it is useful to know how to use macros, even if one has no inclination to write any.

1.11 Some Tips for Preventing and Correcting Errors

When writing programs:

- One statement per line, where possible.
- End each step with a `run` statement.
- Indent each statement within a step, i.e., each statement between the `data` or `proc` statement and the `run` statement, by a couple of spaces. This is automated in the enhanced editor.
- Give the full path name for raw data files on the `infile` statement.
- Begin any programs that produce graphics with `goptions reset=all;` and then set the required options.

Before submitting a program:

- Check that each statement ends with a semicolon.
- Check that all opening and closing quotes match.

Use the enhanced editor colour coding to double check.

- Check any statement that does not begin with a keyword (blue or navy blue) or a variable name (black).
- Large blocks of purple may indicate a missing quotation mark.
- Large areas of green may indicate a missing */ from a comment.

'Collapse' the program to check its overall structure. Hold down the Ctrl and Alt keys and press the numeric keypad minus key. Only the `data`, `proc` statements, and global statements should be visible. To expand the program, press the numeric keypad plus key while holding down Ctrl and Alt.

After running a program:

- Examine the SAS log for warning and error messages.
- Check for the message: "SAS went to a new line when INPUT statement reached past the end of a line" when using list input.
- Verify that the number of observations and variables read in is correct.
- When reading raw data, check the number of lines read and the maximum and minimum line lengths reported.
- Print out small data sets to ensure that they have been read correctly.

If there is an error message for a statement that appears to be correct, check whether the semicolon was omitted from the previous statement.

The message that a variable is 'uninitialized' or 'not found' usually means it has been misspelled. If not, it might have been included in a `drop` statement or left out of a `keep` statement.

To correct a missing quote, submit: `'; run;` or `"; run;` then correct the program and resubmit it.

2

Describing and Summarizing Data

2.1 Introduction

The analysis of any data set generally involves a series of steps, the first of which is most often the calculation of a number of relevant summary statistics and the construction of a well-chosen graph. The aim of this step is to aid the researcher in understanding the general characteristics of the data and perhaps to identify any unusual observations or any 'patterns' in the data that may need to be considered later when more complex statistical procedures might be applied to the data. Which graphs and which summary statistics are most appropriate for a data set will depend to a great extent on the level of measurement of the observations. The main distinction will be between *continuous* (or quasi continuous) measurements and those that are *nominal* or *categorical* (see Altman, 1991, for a full discussion of scale types).

2.2 Graphing and Summarizing Continuous Data

Table 2.1 shows the heights of a sample of 351 elderly women randomly selected from the community in a study of osteoporosis. Table 2.2 gives the time intervals between successive pulses along a nerve fibre measured in seconds. Since there were 800 pulses observed, there are 799 recorded waiting times.

To begin let us get some information on the distribution of the heights in Table 2.1 and some statistics that summarize this distribution. In addition it will be helpful to look at some graphical displays that will allow us to judge the overall characteristics of the height distribution, in particular whether or not the distribution departs from normality. The data can be read into SAS as follows:

```
data heights;
 infile 'c:\sasbook\data\elderly.dat' expandtabs;
 input height @@;
run;
```

TABLE 2.1

Heights (cm) of 351 Elderly Women

156	163	169	161	154	156	163	164	156	166	177	158
150	164	159	157	166	163	153	161	170	159	170	157
156	156	153	178	161	164	158	158	162	160	150	162
155	161	158	163	158	162	163	152	173	159	154	155
164	163	164	157	152	154	173	154	162	163	163	165
160	162	155	160	151	163	160	165	166	178	153	160
156	151	165	169	157	152	164	166	160	165	163	158
153	162	163	162	164	155	155	161	162	156	169	159
159	159	158	160	165	152	157	149	169	154	146	156
157	163	166	165	155	151	157	156	160	170	158	165
167	162	153	156	163	157	147	163	161	161	153	155
166	159	157	152	159	166	160	157	153	159	156	152
151	171	162	158	152	157	162	168	155	155	155	161
157	158	153	155	161	160	160	170	163	153	159	169
155	161	156	153	156	158	164	160	157	158	157	156
160	161	167	162	158	163	147	153	155	159	156	161
158	164	163	155	155	158	165	176	158	155	150	154
164	145	153	169	160	159	159	163	148	171	158	158
157	158	168	161	165	167	158	158	161	160	163	163
169	163	164	150	154	165	158	161	156	171	163	170
154	158	162	164	158	165	158	156	162	160	164	165
157	167	142	166	163	163	151	163	153	157	159	152
169	154	155	167	164	170	174	155	157	170	159	170
155	168	152	165	158	162	173	154	167	158	159	152
158	167	164	170	164	166	170	160	148	168	151	153
150	165	165	147	162	165	158	145	150	164	161	157
163	166	162	163	160	162	153	168	163	160	165	156
158	155	168	160	153	163	161	145	161	166	154	147
161	155	158	161	163	157	156	152	156	165	159	170
160	152	153									

Using the `expandtabs` option on the `infile` statement is a simple way of reading tab-separated data. The trailing double `@` on the `input` statement holds the line for further values to be read, and this is one occasion when the message in the log about SAS going to a new line is not a cause for concern.

The summary statistics and graphs can be obtained from `proc univariate`.

```
proc univariate data=heights;
  var height;
  histogram height / normal;
  probplot height / normal;
run;
```

The `normal` option on the `histogram` statement specifies that a normal distribution is to be fitted to the data and the resulting curve overlaid on

TABLE 2.2

Nerve Impulse Times (Seconds)

0.21	0.03	0.05	0.11	0.59	0.06
0.18	0.55	0.37	0.09	0.14	0.19
0.02	0.14	0.09	0.05	0.15	0.23
0.15	0.08	0.24	0.16	0.06	0.11
0.15	0.09	0.03	0.21	0.02	0.14
0.24	0.29	0.16	0.07	0.07	0.04
0.02	0.15	0.12	0.26	0.15	0.33
0.06	0.51	0.11	0.28	0.36	0.14
0.55	0.28	0.04	0.01	0.94	0.73
0.05	0.07	0.11	0.38	0.21	0.49
0.38	0.38	0.01	0.06	0.13	0.06
0.01	0.16	0.05	0.10	0.16	0.06
0.06	0.06	0.06	0.11	0.44	0.05
0.09	0.04	0.27	0.50	0.25	0.25
0.08	0.01	0.70	0.04	0.08	0.16
0.38	0.08	0.32	0.39	0.58	0.56
0.74	0.15	0.07	0.26	0.25	0.01
0.17	0.64	0.61	0.15	0.26	0.03
0.05	0.34	0.07	0.10	0.09	0.02
0.30	0.07	0.12	0.01	0.16	0.14
0.49	0.07	0.11	0.35	1.21	0.17
0.01	0.35	0.45	0.07	0.93	0.04
0.96	0.14	1.38	0.15	0.01	0.05
0.23	0.31	0.05	0.05	0.29	0.01
0.74	0.30	0.09	0.02	0.19	0.47
0.01	0.51	0.12	0.12	0.43	0.32
0.09	0.20	0.03	0.05	0.13	0.15
0.05	0.08	0.04	0.09	0.10	0.10
0.26	0.07	0.68	0.15	0.01	0.27
0.05	0.03	0.40	0.04	0.21	0.29
0.24	0.08	0.23	0.10	0.19	0.20
0.26	0.06	0.40	0.51	0.15	1.10
0.16	0.78	0.04	0.27	0.35	0.71
0.15	0.29	0.04	0.01	0.28	0.21
0.09	0.17	0.09	0.17	0.15	0.62
0.50	0.07	0.39	0.28	0.20	0.34
0.16	0.65	0.04	0.67	0.10	0.51
0.26	0.07	0.71	0.11	0.47	0.02
0.38	0.04	0.43	0.11	0.23	0.14
0.08	1.12	0.50	0.25	0.18	0.12
0.02	0.15	0.12	0.08	0.38	0.22
0.16	0.04	0.58	0.05	0.07	0.28
0.27	0.24	0.07	0.02	0.27	0.27
0.16	0.05	0.34	0.10	0.02	0.04
0.10	0.22	0.24	0.04	0.28	0.10
0.23	0.03	0.34	0.21	0.41	0.15
0.05	0.17	0.53	0.30	0.15	0.19
0.07	0.83	0.04	0.04	0.14	0.34
0.10	0.15	0.05	0.04	0.05	0.65
0.16	0.32	0.87	0.07	0.17	0.10

TABLE 2.2 (continued)

Nerve Impulse Times (Seconds)

0.03	0.17	0.38	0.28	0.14	0.07
0.14	0.03	0.21	0.40	0.04	0.11
0.44	0.90	0.10	0.49	0.09	0.01
0.08	0.06	0.08	0.01	0.15	0.50
0.36	0.08	0.34	0.02	0.21	0.32
0.22	0.51	0.12	0.16	0.52	0.21
0.05	0.46	0.44	0.04	0.05	0.04
0.14	0.08	0.21	0.02	0.63	0.35
0.01	0.38	0.43	0.03	0.39	0.04
0.17	0.23	0.78	0.14	0.08	0.11
0.07	0.45	0.46	0.20	0.19	0.50
0.09	0.22	0.29	0.01	0.19	0.06
0.39	0.08	0.03	0.28	0.09	0.17
0.45	0.40	0.07	0.30	0.16	0.24
0.81	1.35	0.01	0.02	0.03	0.06
0.12	0.31	0.64	0.08	0.15	0.06
0.06	0.15	0.68	0.30	0.02	0.04
0.02	0.81	0.09	0.19	0.14	0.12
0.36	0.02	0.11	0.04	0.08	0.17
0.04	0.05	0.14	0.07	0.39	0.13
0.56	0.12	0.31	0.05	0.10	0.13
0.05	0.01	0.09	0.03	0.27	0.17
0.03	0.05	0.26	0.23	0.20	0.76
0.05	0.02	0.01	0.20	0.21	0.02
0.04	0.16	0.32	0.43	0.20	0.13
0.10	0.20	0.08	0.81	0.11	0.09
0.26	0.15	0.36	0.18	0.10	0.34
0.56	0.09	0.15	0.14	0.15	0.22
0.33	0.04	0.07	0.09	0.18	0.08
0.07	0.07	0.68	0.27	0.21	0.11
0.07	0.44	0.13	0.04	0.39	0.14
0.10	0.08	0.02	0.57	0.35	0.17
0.21	0.14	0.77	0.06	0.34	0.15
0.29	0.08	0.72	0.31	0.20	0.10
0.01	0.24	0.07	0.22	0.49	0.03
0.18	0.47	0.37	0.17	0.42	0.02
0.22	0.12	0.01	0.34	0.41	0.27
0.07	0.30	0.09	0.27	0.28	0.15
0.26	0.01	0.06	0.35	0.03	0.26
0.05	0.18	0.46	0.12	0.23	0.32
0.08	0.26	0.82	0.10	0.69	0.15
0.01	0.39	0.04	0.13	0.34	0.13
0.13	0.30	0.29	0.23	0.01	0.38
0.04	0.08	0.15	0.10	0.62	0.83
0.11	0.71	0.08	0.61	0.18	0.05
0.20	0.12	0.10	0.03	0.11	0.20
0.16	0.10	0.03	0.23	0.12	0.01
0.12	0.17	0.14	0.10	0.02	0.13
0.06	0.21	0.50	0.04	0.42	0.29
0.08	0.01	0.30	0.45	0.06	0.25
0.02	0.06	0.02	0.17	0.10	0.28
0.21	0.28	0.30	0.02	0.02	0.28

TABLE 2.2 (continued)

Nerve Impulse Times (Seconds)

0.09	0.71	0.06	0.12	0.29	0.05
0.27	0.25	0.10	0.16	0.08	0.52
0.44	0.19	0.72	0.12	0.30	0.14
0.45	0.42	0.09	0.07	0.62	0.51
0.50	0.47	0.28	0.04	0.66	0.08
0.11	0.03	0.32	0.16	0.11	0.26
0.05	0.07	0.04	0.22	0.08	0.08
0.01	0.06	0.05	0.05	0.16	0.05
0.13	0.42	0.21	0.36	0.05	0.01
0.44	0.14	0.14	0.14	0.08	0.51
0.18	0.02	0.51	0.06	0.22	0.01
0.09	0.22	0.59	0.03	0.71	0.14
0.02	0.51	0.03	0.41	0.17	0.37
0.39	0.82	0.81	0.24	0.52	0.40
0.24	0.06	0.73	0.27	0.18	0.01
0.17	0.02	0.11	0.26	0.13	0.68
0.13	0.08	0.71	0.04	0.11	0.13
0.17	0.34	0.23	0.08	0.26	0.03
0.21	0.45	0.40	0.03	0.16	0.06
0.29	0.43	0.03	0.10	0.10	0.31
0.27	0.27	0.33	0.14	0.09	0.27
0.14	0.09	0.08	0.06	0.16	0.02
0.07	0.19	0.11	0.10	0.17	0.24
0.01	0.13	0.21	0.03	0.39	0.01
0.27	0.19	0.02	0.21	0.04	0.10
0.06	0.48	0.12	0.15	0.12	0.52
0.48	0.29	0.57	0.22	0.01	0.44
0.05	0.49	0.10	0.19	0.44	0.02
0.72	0.09	0.04	0.02	0.02	0.06
0.22	0.53	0.18	0.10	0.10	0.03
0.08	0.15	0.05	0.13	0.02	0.10
0.51					

the histogram. Other distributions that can be specified include the beta, exponential, gamma, lognormal, and Weibull.

The numerical results are shown in Table 2.3 and the plots in Figure 2.1 and Figure 2.2. Much of the material in Table 2.3 is self-explanatory, and that which is not so obvious is explained briefly below:

Uncorrected SS — uncorrected sum of squares; simply the sum of squares of the observations

Corrected SS — corrected sum of squares; simply the sum of squares of the deviations of the observations from the sample mean

Coeff Variation — coefficient of variation; the standard deviation divided by mean and multiplied by 100

Std Error Mean — the standard deviation divided by the square root of the number of observations

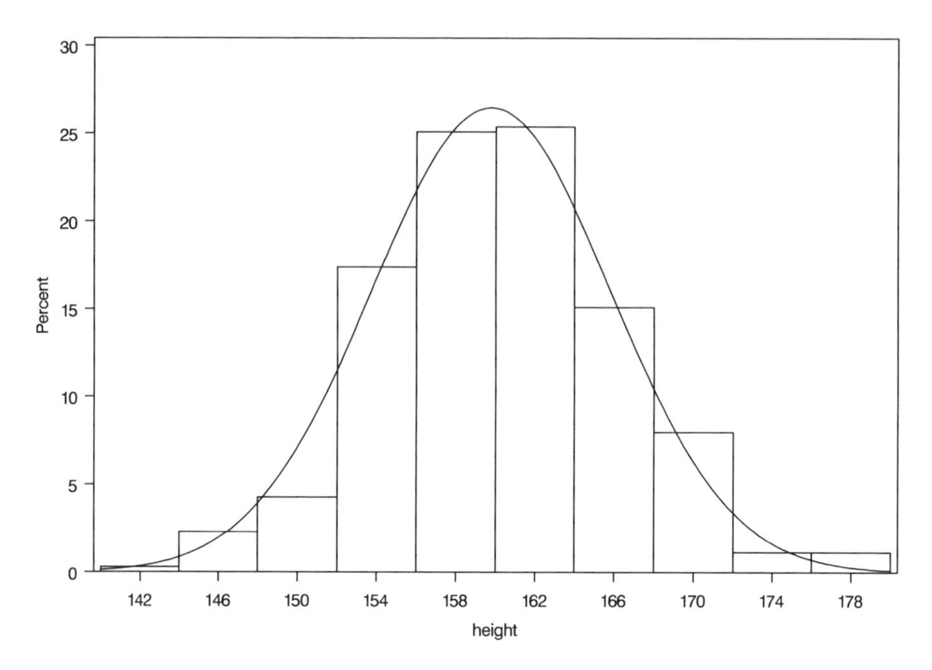

FIGURE 2.1
Histogram and fitted normal density for heights data.

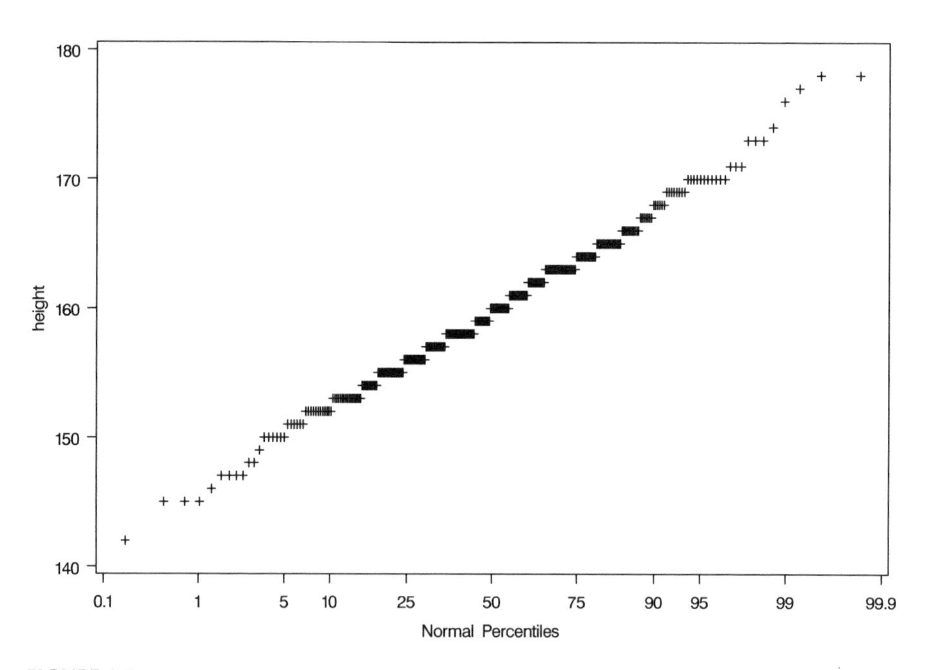

FIGURE 2.2
Normal probability plot for heights data.

Range — difference between largest and smallest observation in the sample

Interquartile Range — difference between 25 and 75% quantile (see values of quantiles given later in display to confirm)

Student's t — the Student's t-test value for testing that the population mean is zero

Pr > |*t*– the probability of a greater absolute value for the t-statistic

Sign Test – a nonparametric test statistic for testing whether the population median is zero

Pr > |*M*| — an approximation to the probability of a greater absolute value for the Sign test under the hypothesis that the population median is zero

Signed Rank — a nonparametric test statistic for testing whether the population mean is zero,

Pr > = |*S*| — an approximation to the probability of a greater absolute value for the Signed Rank statistic under the hypothesis that the population mean is zero

Shapiro-Wilk W — the Shapiro-Wilk statistic for assessing the normality of the data and the corresponding P-value (Shapiro and Wilk, 1965)

Kolmogorov-Smirnov D — the Kolmogorov-Smirnov statistic for assessing the normality of the data and the corresponding P-value (Fisher and Van Belle, 1993)

Cramer-von Mises W-sq — the Cramer-von Mises statistic for assessing the normality of the data and the associated P-value (Everitt, 2001)

Anderson-Darling A-sq — the Anderson-Darling statistic for assessing the normality of the data and the associated P-value (Everitt, 2001)

TABLE 2.3

Summary Statistics from SAS for Heights Data

Variable: height

Moments

N	351	Sum Weights	351
Mean	159.774929	Sum Observations	56081
Std Deviation	6.02974043	Variance	36.3577696
Skewness	0.12949157	Kurtosis	0.18019668
Uncorrected SS	8973063	Corrected SS	12725.2194
Coeff Variation	3.77389649	Std Error Mean	0.32184373

Basic Statistical Measures

Location		Variability	
Mean	159.7749	Std Deviation	6.02974
Median	160.0000	Variance	36.35777
Mode	158.0000	Range	36.00000
		Interquartile Range	8.00000

TABLE 2.3 (continued)

Summary Statistics from SAS for Heights Data

```
            Tests for Location: Mu0=0

Test              -Statistic-     -----p Value------

Student's t      t  496.4364      Pr > |t|     <.0001
Sign             M     175.5      Pr >= |M|    <.0001
Signed Rank      S     30888      Pr >= |S|    <.0001

Quantiles (Definition 5)

Quantile       Estimate

100% Max            178
99%                 176
95%                 170
90%                 168
75% Q3              164
50% Median          160
25% Q1              156
10%                 152
5%                  150
1%                  145

Variable:  height

Quantiles (Definition 5)

Quantile       Estimate

0% Min              142


               Extreme Observations

  ----Lowest----          ----Highest---

  Value       Obs          Value       Obs

    142       255            174       271
    145       332            176       200
    145       308            177        11
    145       206            178        28
    146       107            178        70
  Fitted Distribution for height

  Parameters for Normal Distribution

  Parameter    Symbol    Estimate

  Mean         Mu        159.7749
  Std Dev      Sigma      6.02974
```

TABLE 2.3 (continued)

Summary Statistics from SAS for Heights Data

```
         Goodness-of-Fit Tests for Normal Distribution

Test                  ---Statistic----     -----p Value-----

Kolmogorov-Smirnov    D      0.06020394    Pr > D       <0.010
Cramer-von Mises      W-Sq   0.12182358    Pr > W-Sq     0.059
Anderson-Darling      A-Sq   0.72182548    Pr > A-Sq     0.062


Quantiles for Normal Distribution

          ------Quantile------
Percent   Observed   Estimated

   1.0     145.000     145.748
   5.0     150.000     149.857
  10.0     152.000     152.048
  25.0     156.000     155.708
  50.0     160.000     159.775
  75.0     164.000     163.842
  90.0     168.000     167.502
  95.0     170.000     169.693
  99.0     176.000     173.802
```

The quantiles given in Table 2.3 provide information about the tails of the height distribution and also include what is sometimes termed the *five-number summary* of a data set, the five numbers in question being the minimum, lower quartile, median, upper quartile, and maximum value. For the heights, these values extracted from Table 2.3 are as follows;

Minimum	Lower Quartile	Median	Upper Quartile	Maximum
142	156	160	164	178

These five numbers can be used to construct a graphical display known as a *boxplot*, which is often very useful, particularly for comparing the distribution of a variable in different groups; we shall say more about how such displays are constructed from the five-number summary and give an example later in this section.

The fitted normal distribution shown at the end of Table 2.3 suggests that the height data do not depart to any great extent from a normal distribution, a point confirmed by Figure 2.1, showing both the histogram of the data and the fitted normal distribution.

Finally, Figure 2.2 shows a normal probability plot of the data (probability plots are briefly described in Display 2.1). The plot is approximately linear again, strongly suggesting that the data arise from a population with a normal distribution.

DISPLAY 2.1

Probability Plots

- Plots for comparing two probability distributions.
- There are two basic types, the *probability–probability plot* and the *quantile–quantile plot*. The diagram below may be used for describing each type.

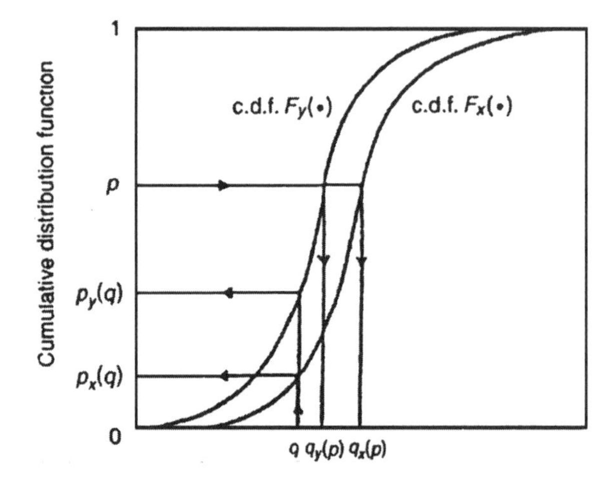

- A plot of points whose coordinates are the cumulative probabilities $\{p_x(q), p_y(q)\}$ for the different values of q is a probability–probability plot, whereas a plot of the points whose coordinates are the quantiles $\{q_x(p), q_y(p)\}$ for the different values of p is a quantile–quantile plot.
- As an example, a quantile–quantile plot for investigating the assumption that a set of data is from a normal distribution would involve plotting the ordered sample values $y_{(1)}, y_{(2)}, \ldots, y_{(n)}$ against the quantiles of a standard normal distribution, i.e.,

$$\Phi^{-1}\left[p_i\right]$$

where usually

$$p_i = \frac{i - \frac{1}{2}}{n} \text{ and } \Phi(x) = \int_{-\infty}^{x} \frac{1}{\sqrt{2\pi}} e^{-\frac{1}{2}u^2} du$$

This is usually known as a *normal probability plot*.

Now let us examine the results from using the previous SAS instructions, this time applied to the nerve fibre pulse times in Table 2.2. The output in this case is shown in Table 2.4 and in the plots in Figure 2.3 and Figure 2.4. The first thing to notice is that for these data the mean and the median are very different, a clear indicator of *skewness* in the data. For these data the tests of normality are all highly significant indicating that the distribution of the nerve pulse times cannot be assumed to be normal. The histogram/fitted normal diagram in Figure 2.3 also shows that a normal distribution is definitely not appropriate for these data, as does the clear departure from linearity of the probability plot in Figure 2.4.

A more suitable distribution for a skewed variable such as the waiting times between nerve pulses might be the exponential distribution with a single parameter, λ, and having the form

$$f\left(x\right)=\lambda e^{-\lambda x}$$

To fit this distribution and plot the fitted distribution onto the histogram we use the `exponential` option on the `histogram` statement.

```
proc univariate data=nerves noprint;
  var pulsetime;
  histogram pulsetime / exponential;
run;
```

The `noprint` option on the `proc` statement suppresses the main output, but the information on the fit of the exponential distribution is still included.

The resulting plot is shown in Figure 2.5. The exponential clearly provides a better description of the distribution of nerve pulse times than does a normal.

In many cases we may not be willing to assume a specific parametric form for the density function of a variable, but we would still like to find a more suitable estimate of this density than is provided by the simple histogram. In such cases we can use what is known as a *nonparametric density estimator.* Such estimators are explained in detail in Silverman (1986), and a brief description of how they work for univariate data is given in Display 2.2.

A variety of density estimates for the heights data, in which the bandwidth and kernel are varied, can be obtained using the following SAS instructions;

```
proc univariate data=heights;
  var height;
  histogram height / kernel;
  histogram height / kernel(k=n c=1 2 3 l=1 2 3) nobars;
  histogram height / kernel(k=t c=1 2 3 l=1 2 3) nobars;
  histogram height / kernel(k=q c=1 2 3 l=1 2 3) nobars;
run;
```

TABLE 2.4

Summary Statistics from SAS for Nerve Data

```
Variable:  pulsetime

                                 Moments

N                           799    Sum Weights                 799
Mean                 0.21857322    Sum Observations         174.64
Std Deviation        0.20918859    Variance             0.04375987
Skewness             1.76456297    Kurtosis             3.94706983
Uncorrected SS           73.092    Corrected SS         34.9203735
Coeff Variation      95.7064155    Std Error Mean       0.00740056


                      Basic Statistical Measures

            Location                    Variability

        Mean     0.218573     Std Deviation            0.20919
        Median   0.150000     Variance                 0.04376
        Mode     0.040000     Range                    1.37000
                              Interquartile Range      0.23000


                      Tests for Location: Mu0=0

           Test           -Statistic-    -----p Value------

           Student's t    t  29.53468    Pr > |t|    <.0001
           Sign           M     399.5    Pr >= |M|   <.0001
           Signed Rank    S    159800    Pr >= |S|   <.0001


                       Quantiles (Definition 5)

                        Quantile      Estimate

                        100% Max          1.38
                        99%               0.93
                        95%               0.68
                        90%               0.51
                        75% Q3            0.30
                        50% Median        0.15
                        25% Q1            0.07
                        10%               0.03
                        5%                0.02
                        1%                0.01
                        0% Min            0.01


                         Extreme Observations

                  ----Lowest----        ----Highest---

                  Value      Obs        Value      Obs

                   0.01      773         1.10      192
                   0.01      756         1.12      236
                   0.01      751         1.21      125
                   0.01      702         1.35      386
                   0.01      678         1.38      135
```

TABLE 2.4 (continued)

Summary Statistics from SAS for Nerve Data

```
                    Fitted Distribution for pulsetime

                    Parameters for Normal Distribution

                      Parameter    Symbol    Estimate

                      Mean         Mu        0.218573
                      Std Dev      Sigma     0.209189


             Goodness-of-Fit Tests for Normal Distribution

Test                  ---Statistic----    -----p Value-----

Kolmogorov-Smirnov    D       0.1600182   Pr > D      <0.010
Cramer-von Mises      W-Sq    6.6486773   Pr > W-Sq   <0.005
Anderson-Darling      A-Sq   38.4074546   Pr > A-Sq   <0.005


                     Quantiles for Normal Distribution

                               ------Quantile------
                      Percent    Observed   Estimated

                         1.0     0.01000    -0.26807
                         5.0     0.02000    -0.12551
                        10.0     0.03000    -0.04951
                        25.0     0.07000     0.07748
                        50.0     0.15000     0.21857
                        75.0     0.30000     0.35967
                        90.0     0.51000     0.48666
                        95.0     0.68000     0.56266
                        99.0     0.93000     0.70522
```

The first `histogram` statement produces a default kernel density estimate. This uses a normal kernel with the bandwidth determined by the approximate mean integrated square error (AMISE). The following three `histogram` statements vary the kernel type and bandwidth. The kernel type can be normal (`k=n`), triangular (`k=t`), or quadratic (`k=q`). The bandwidth is set by the standardized bandwidth parameter `c=`, which is related to the bandwidth by the formula

$$\lambda = cQn^{\frac{1}{5}}$$

with Q being the interquartile range. The bandwidth and AMISE are reported in the log. For this data set, values of c=1, 2, and 3 correspond to bandwidths of 2.5, 5, and 7.4, respectively. The `l=` option specifies different line types for the three curves, and the printing of the histogram bars is suppressed with the `nobars` option.

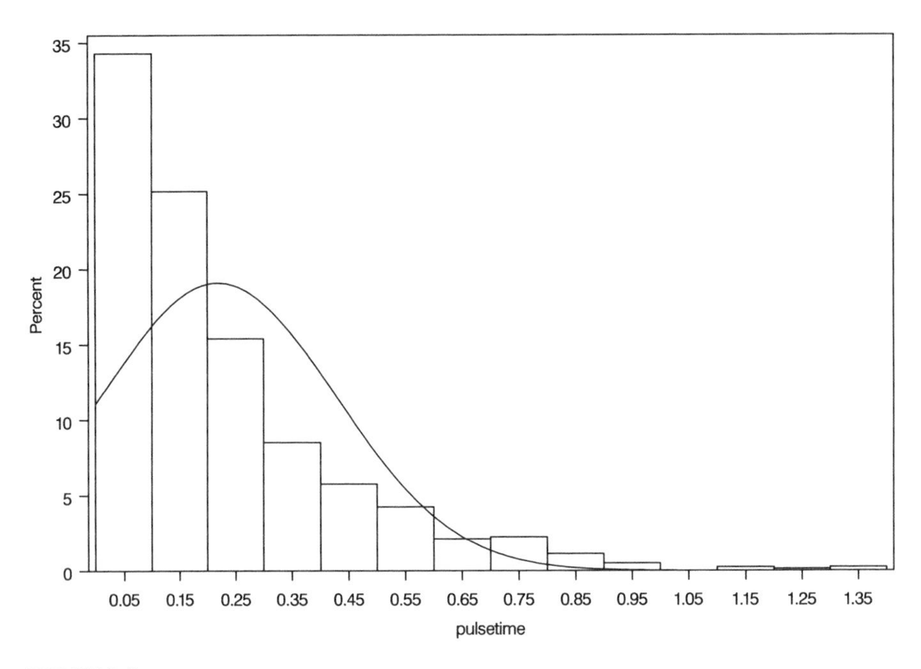

FIGURE 2.3
Histogram and fitted normal density for nerve impulse times.

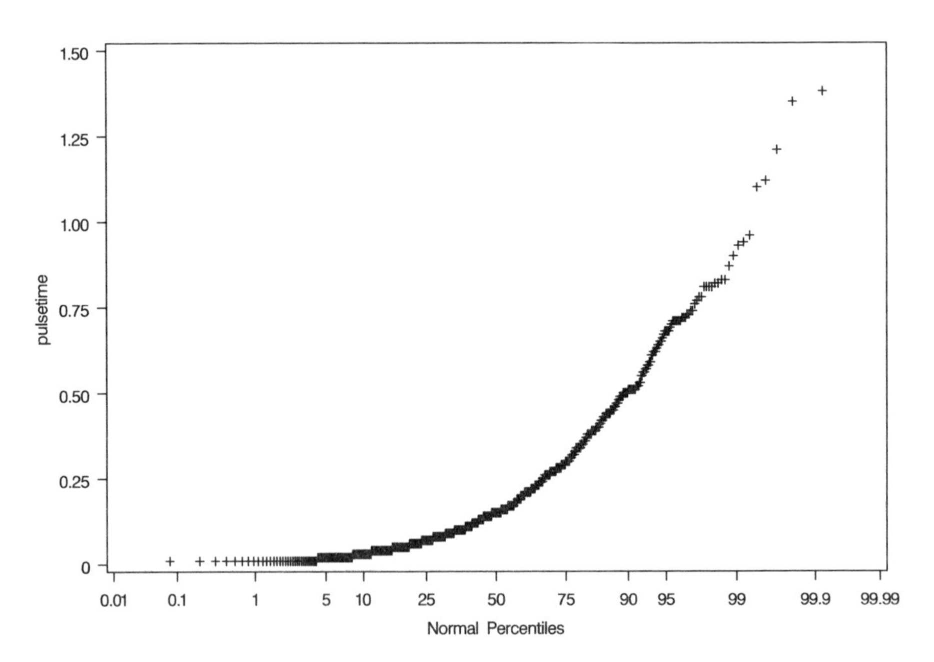

FIGURE 2.4
Normal probability plot for nerve impulse times.

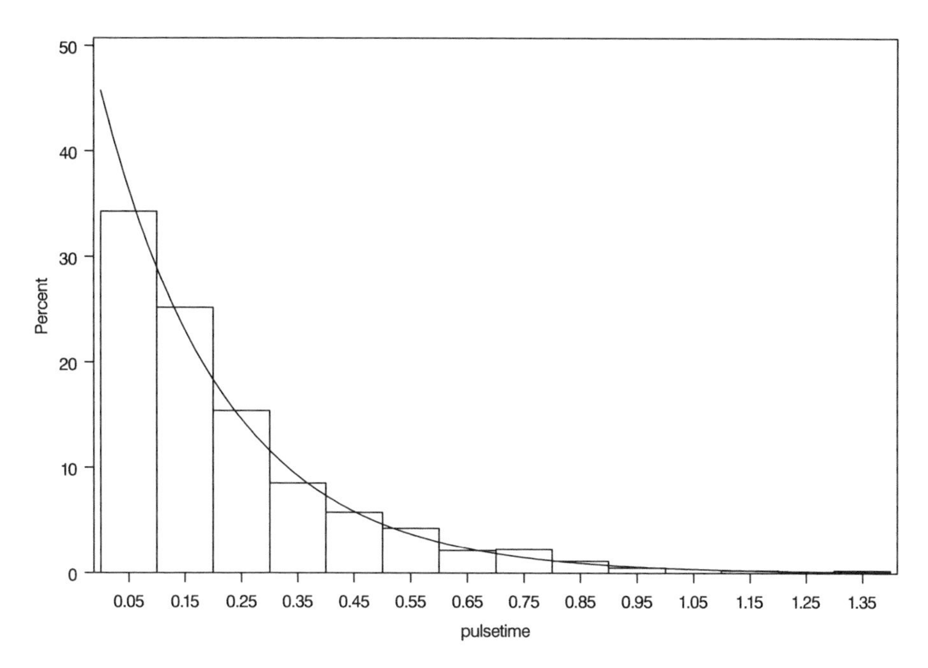

FIGURE 2.5
Histogram and fitted exponential distribution for nerve impulse times.

The resulting plots are shown in Figure 2.6, Figure 2.7, Figure 2.8, and Figure 2.9. Note how the kernel estimate changes as bandwidth and type of kernel are varied.

As mentioned previously, when comparing the distributions of a variable in different groups the boxplot is particularly useful. How a boxplot is constructed is shown in Display 2.3. To illustrate its use we will use the data shown in Table 2.5. These data have been collected from patients with advanced cancer of the stomach, bronchus, colon, ovary, or breast all treated with ascorbate. Interest lies in whether survival times differ with the organ affected. The data can be read in as follows;

```
data patient;
  do organ= 1 to 5;
   input days 6. @;
   if days~=. then output;
  end;
cards;
124   81    248   1234  1235
42    461   377   89    24
25    20    189   201   1581
45    450   1843  356   1166
```

DISPLAY 2.2

Nonparametric Density Estimation

- Methods for estimating a probability distribution without assuming a particular parametric form. The histogram is one example.
- Perhaps the most common class of density estimators is of the form

$$\hat{f}(x) = \frac{1}{nh}\sum_{i=1}^{n} K\left(\frac{x - X_i}{h}\right)$$

where h is known as *window width* or *bandwidth* and K is known as the *kernel function*, and is such that

$$\int_{-\infty}^{\infty} K(u)du = 1$$

- Essentially, such *kernel estimators* sum a series of 'bumps' placed at each of the observations. The kernel function determines the shape of the bumps, while h determines their width.
- Three widely used kernel functions are:

a. Gaussian

$$K(x) = \frac{1}{\sqrt{2\pi}} e^{-x^2/2}$$

b. Triangular

$$K(x) = 1 - |x|, |x| < 1$$

c. Rectangular

$$K(x) = \frac{1}{2}, |x| < 1$$

- A graphical representation of each kernel function is shown below.

DISPLAY 2.2 (continued)

Nonparametric Density Estimation

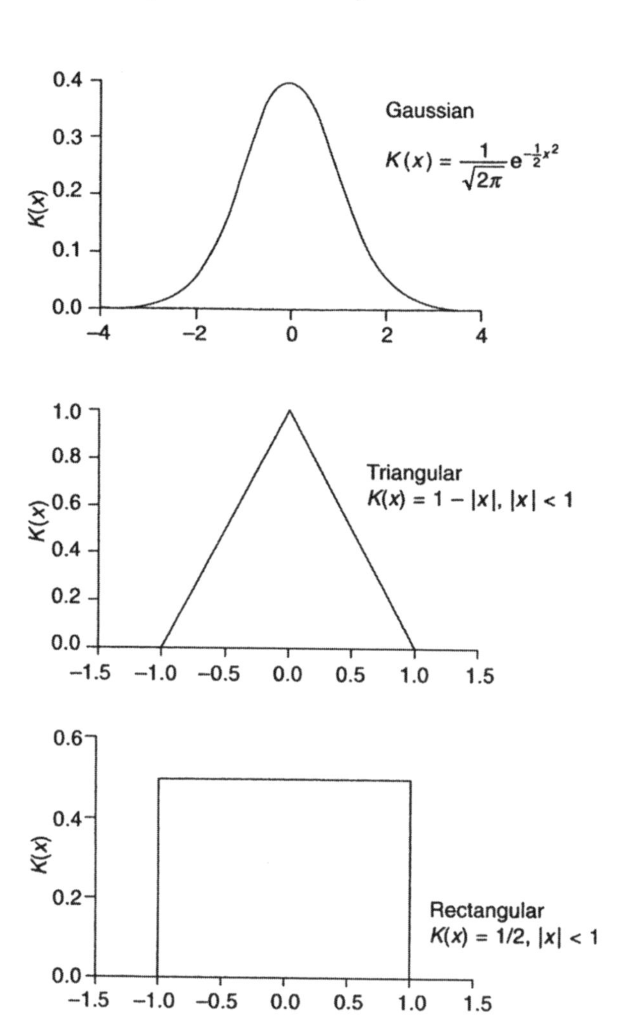

- In general, the choice of the shape of the kernel function is not usually of great importance. In contrast, the choice of bandwidth can be critical.
- There are situations in which it is satisfactory to choose the bandwidth relatively subjectively to achieve a 'smooth' estimate. More formal methods are available, however. For details, see Silverman (1986).

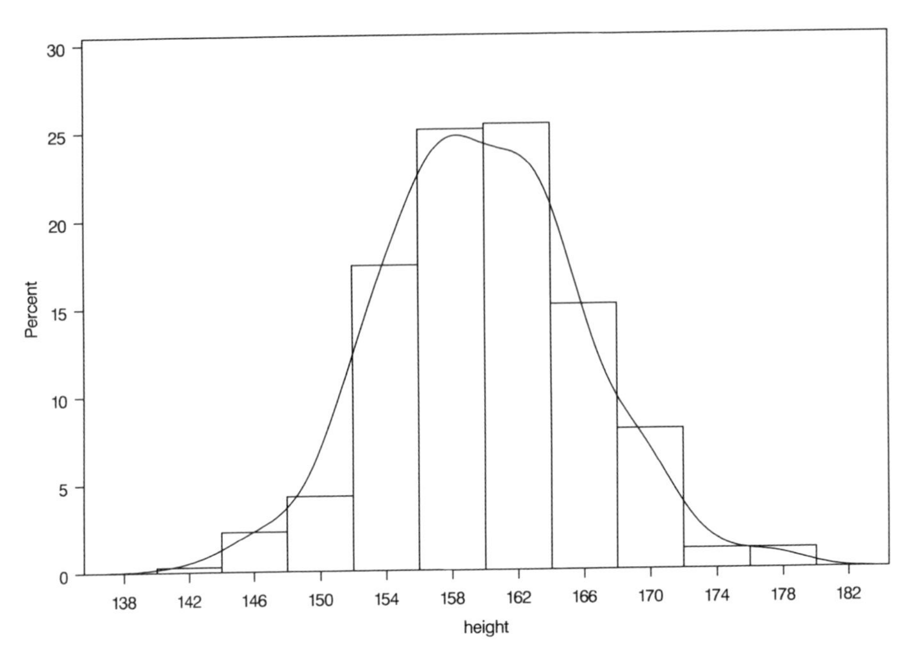

FIGURE 2.6
Histogram of height data with fitted kernel density estimate, using a normal kernel and bandwith of 1.9.

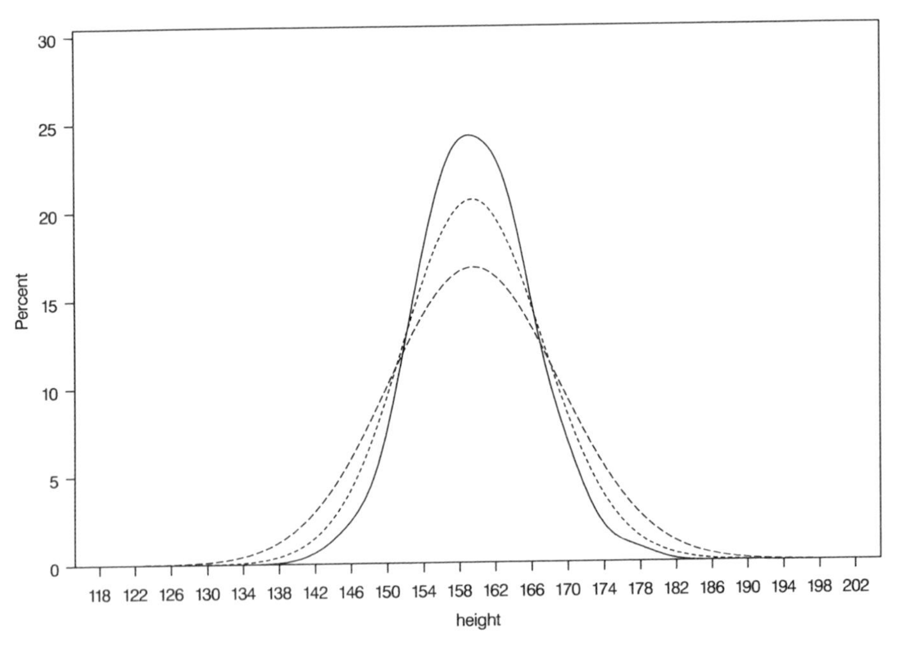

FIGURE 2.7
Histogram of height data with fitted kernel density estimate, using a normal kernel and bandwidths of 2.5, 5, and 7.4.

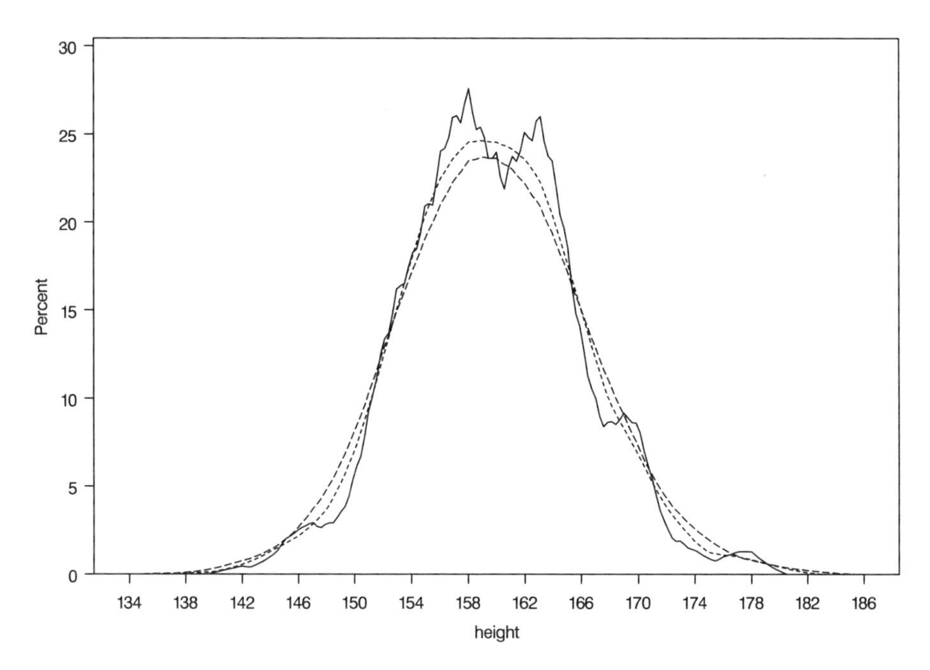

FIGURE 2.8
Histogram of height data with fitted kernel density estimate, using a triangular kernel and bandwidths of 2.5, 5, and 7.4.

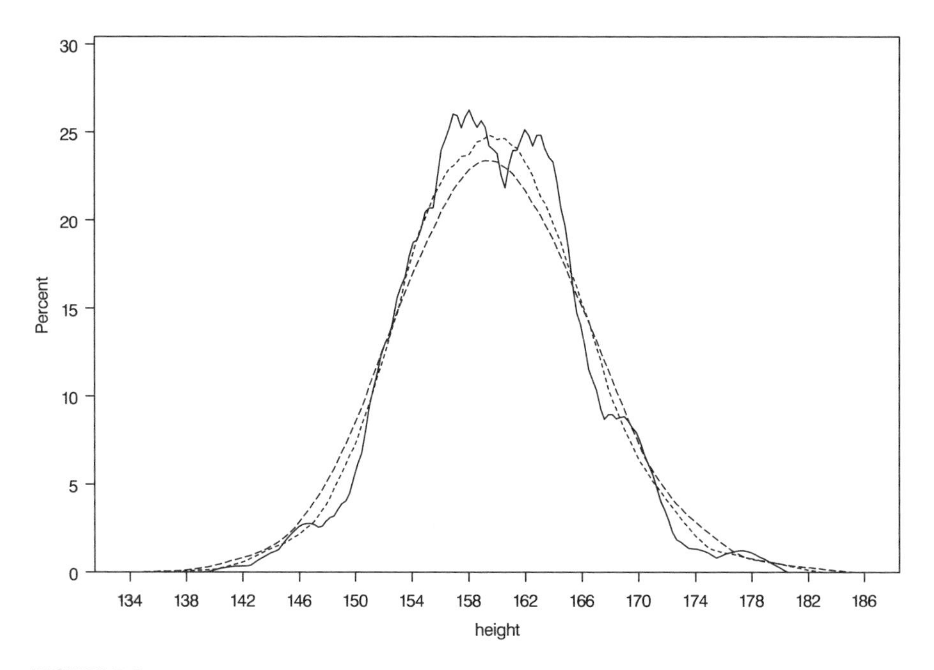

FIGURE 2.9
Histogram of height data with fitted kernel density estimate, using a quadratic kernel and bandwidths of 2.5, 5, and 7.4.

DISPLAY 2.3

Constructing a Boxplot

- The plot is based on a five-number summary of a data set: 1, minimum; 2, lower quartile; 3, median; 4, upper quartile; 5, maximum.
- The distance between the upper and lower quartiles, the *interquartile range*, is a measure of the spread of a distribution that is quick to compute and, unlike the range, is not badly affected by outliers.
- The median and upper and lower quartiles can be used to define rather arbitrary but still useful limits, L and U, to help identify possible outliers in the data:

$$U = UQ + 1.5 \times IQR$$

$$L = LQ - 1.5 \times IQR$$

  where UQ is the upper quartile, LQ is the lower quartile, and IQR the interquartile range, UQ – LQ.
- Observations outside the limits L and U are regarded as potential outliers and identified separately on the box plot (and known as *outside values*), which is constructed as follows:
- To construct a boxplot, a "box" with ends at the lower and upper quartiles is first drawn. A horizontal line (or some other feature) is used to indicate the position of the median in the box. Next, lines are drawn from each end of the box to the most remote observations that, however, are *not* outside observations as defined in the text. The resulting diagram schematically represents the body of the data *minus* the extreme observations. Finally, the outside observations are incorporated into the final diagram by representing them individually in some way (lines, stars, etc.).

```
412   246   180   2970  40
51    166   537   456   727
1112  63    519         3808
46    64    455         791
103   155   406         1804
876   859   365         3460
146   151   942         719
340   166   776
396   37    372
      223   163
```

TABLE 2.5

Survival Times (Days) of Cancer Patients

Stomach	Bronchus	Colon	Ovary	Breast
124	81	248	1234	1235
42	461	377	89	24
25	20	189	201	1581
45	450	1843	356	1166
412	246	180	2970	40
51	166	537	456	727
1112	63	519		3808
46	64	455		791
103	155	406		1804
876	859	365		3460
146	151	942		719
340	166	776		
396	37	372		
	223	163		
	138	101		
	72	20		
	245	283		

```
      138    101
      72     20
      245    283
;
proc format;
  value organ 1='Stomach' 2='Bronchus' 3='Colon'
4='Ovary' 5='Breast';
run;
```

The do loop reads five data values from each line in the file. The trailing single @ holds the line for rereading until the end of the data step. If a nonmissing value has been read, the output statement writes an observation to the data set.

The proc format step defines a format to label the values of the variable organ. The fact that the format and the variable can have the same name can be a useful *aide memoire.*

The required boxplots are obtained using

```
proc sort data=patient;
  by organ;
run;
proc boxplot data=patient;
  plot days*organ / boxstyle=schematic;
  format organ organ.;
run;
```

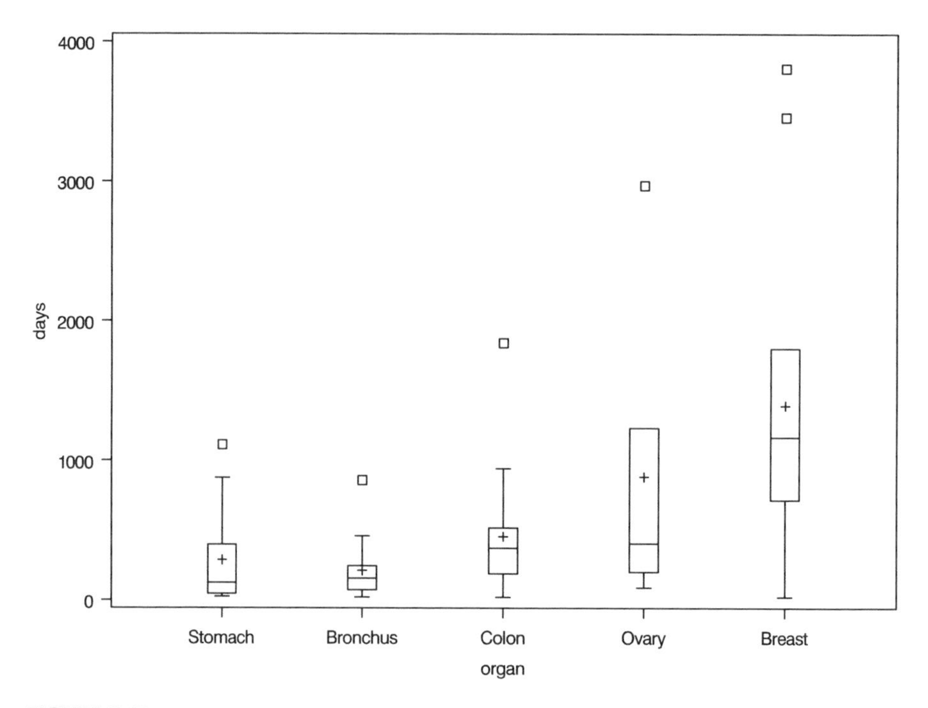

FIGURE 2.10
Boxplots of survival times for patients with different types of cancer.

The boxplot procedure needs the data to be presorted by the grouping variable. The type of boxplot described in Display 2.3 is specified with the `boxstyle=schematic` option. The default type extends the whiskers to the extreme observations. The `format` statement applies the format `organ` to the values of the variable `organ`. The name of the format is distinguished by the dot that follows and in the enhanced editor is given a different colour ('teal' by default). The boxplots are shown in Figure 2.10.

The plot shows that the survival times for stomach and ovary are particularly skew and that the variation of the survival times differs considerably for each organ. We can now examine how the data look after taking a log transformation and creating boxplots of the transformed data.

```
data patient;
  set patient;
  logdays=log(days);
run;
proc boxplot data=patient;
  plot logdays*organ / boxstyle=schematic;
  format organ organ.;
run;
```

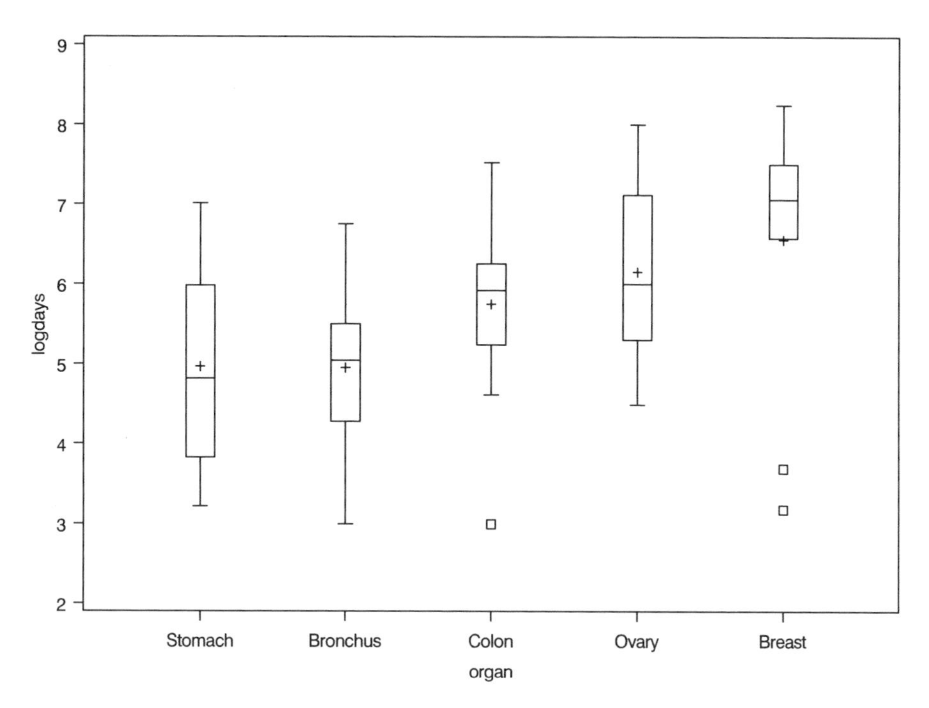

FIGURE 2.11
Boxplots of transformed survival times for different types of cancers.

The resulting set of boxplots is shown in Figure 2.11. The transformed data are now far less skew and might be more suited for techniques such as analysis of variance (see Chapter 5) that assume normality.

2.3 Categorical Data

The data given in Table 2.6 were collected in Bradford, England, between 1968 and 1977, and relate to 13,384 women giving birth to their first child. The women were classified according to social class (five categories on the Registrar General's scale of I to V) and according to the number of cigarettes smoked per day during pregnancy (on a three-level categorization: 1 means no smoking, 2 means 1 to 19 cigarettes per day, and 3 means 20 or more cigarettes per day). The data for each category consists of counts of women showing toxaemic signs (hypertension and/or proteinuria) during pregnancy. The question of interest is how the toxaemic signs vary with social class and pregnancy. For the moment we can address this question with some simple *component bar charts* (see Everitt, 2001). We might, for example, construct such a plot to show the proportion of women having both hypertension and proteinuria by smoking and social class using the following code.

TABLE 2.6

Toxaemia of Pregnancy

		Signs of Toxaemia			
Class	Smoking	Hypertension and Proteinuria	Proteinuria Only	Hypertension Only	Neither Sign Exhibited
1	1	28	82	21	286
1	2	5	24	5	71
1	3	1	3	0	13
2	1	50	266	34	785
2	2	13	92	17	284
2	3	0	15	3	34
3	1	278	1101	164	3160
3	2	120	492	142	2300
3	3	16	92	32	383
4	1	63	213	52	656
4	2	35	129	46	649
4	3	7	40	12	163
5	1	20	78	23	245
5	2	22	74	34	321
5	3	7	14	4	65

```
data toxaemia;
 infile 'N:\sasbook\data\toxaemia.dat' expandtabs;
 input class  smoking group1-group4;
run;
proc gchart data=toxaemia;
 vbar class /subgroup=smoking freq=group1 discrete;
run;
```

The `gchart` procedure can be used to produce a range of chart types, including various types of bar chart. The `vbar` statement specifies a vertical bar chart, and the variable that is to form the horizontal axis is `class`. By default this variable is expected to be continuous, and the procedure will group the values automatically to form the bars. In this case `class` has five discrete values, and we use the `discrete` option so that each value of `class` forms a separate bar. We also want the bars divided into components defined by the level of smoking; this is done with the `subgroup=smoking` option. The data consist of frequency counts, so the `freq=group1` option specifies the variable that contains the counts from which the chart is to be built. The resulting graph is shown in Figure 2.12.

By default, the procedure differentiates the subgroups by different patterns of hatching, although pattern statements can be used to change this.

Similar graphs can be constructed showing the proportions with proteinuria only, hypertension only, and with neither sign; see Figure 2.13, Figure 2.14, and Figure 2.15.

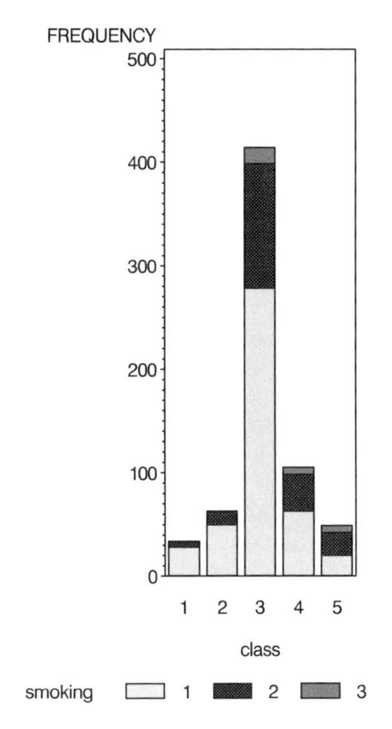

FIGURE 2.12
Component bar chart for smoking data showing proportion of women with both hypertension and proteinuria.

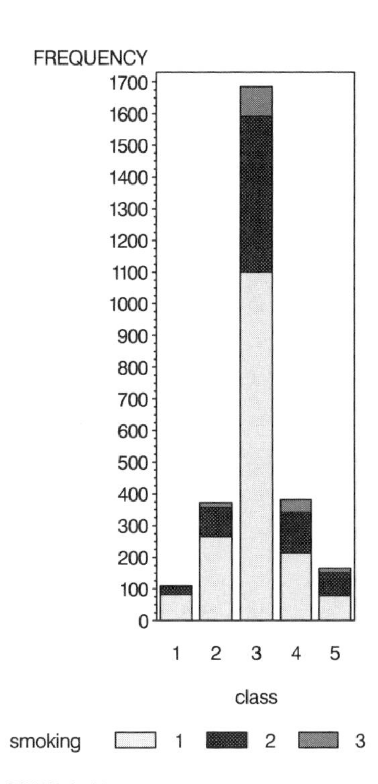

FIGURE 2.13
Component chart for smoking data showing proportion of women with proteinuria only.

An alternative graphical representation of these data is obtained using a horizontal bar chart, a form which is usually preferable when the bars are to be labelled. We can illustrate this plot using the data shown in Table 2.7, which gives the standardized mortality rate for 25 occupation categories. The necessary SAS code to produce the plot (Figure 2.16) is as follows:

```
data cancer;
 infile cards;
 input  smr occupation  :$15.;
cards;
 84   Farmers
116   Miners
. . . .
120   Service
 60   Administrators
 51   Professional
```

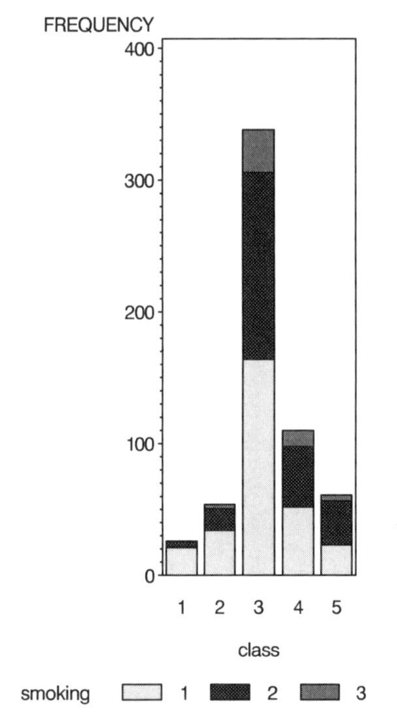

FIGURE 2.14
Component chart for smoking data showing proportion of women with hypertension only.

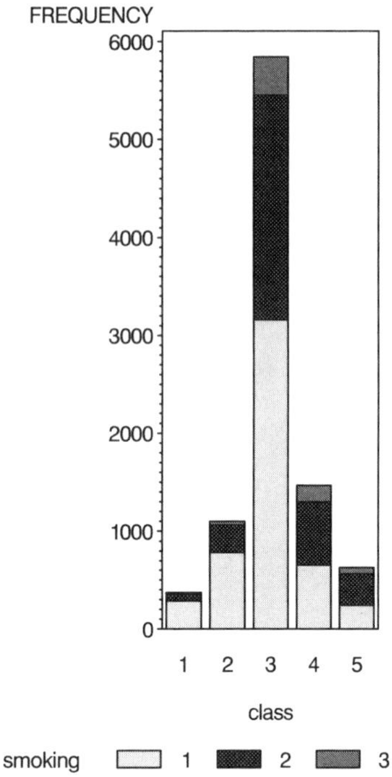

FIGURE 2.15
Component chart for smoking data showing proportion of women with neither proteinuria nor hypertension.

```
;
run;
pattern1 v=s;
proc gchart data=cancer;
  hbar occupation  /discrete descending type=sum
sumvar=smr;
run;
```

The pattern statement `value=` option `v=s` specifies solid bars for this chart. Other possibilities are `v=e` (empty), `l1-l5`, `r1-r5`, and `x1-x5` for left-slanting, right-slanting and cross-hatched lines of varying thickness. When working in colour or grey scales, the `c=` option can be used to control the colour of the bars.

The syntax of the `hbar` statement for a horizontal bar chart is much the same as the `vbar` statement above. The variable `occupation` is again discrete so the `discrete` option is used. The default type of bar chart is one

TABLE 2.7

Standardized Mortality Rate (SMR) for Deaths from Lung Cancer for 25 Occupation Categories

84	Farmers
116	Miners
123	Chemical
128	Glass
155	Furnace
101	Electrical
118	Engineering
113	Woodworkers
104	Leather
88	Textile
104	Clothing
129	Food
86	Paper
96	Other
144	Construction
139	Decorators
113	Crane drivers
146	Labourers
128	Transport
115	Warehousemen
79	Clerical
85	Sales
120	Service
60	Administrators
51	Professional

where the heights of the bars reflect frequency counts. Here the heights of the bars will correspond to the values of a second variable. This variable is specified with the `sumvar=` option, and the `type=sum` option specifies that the heights of the bars should correspond to the sum of the values for that variable. As there is only one observation for each occupation, `type=mean` would have given the same result. The `descending` option orders the bars. The descriptive statistics on the right of the chart can be suppressed with the `nostats` option.

The data could also be displayed as a *dotplot*. To illustrate this, we have provided a SAS macro to produce dotplots, which is invoked as follows:

```
%include 'c:\sasbook\macros\dotplot.sas';
%dotplot(data=cancer,xvar=smr,label=occupation);
```

The three parameters for the macro are the name of the data set, the variable to be plotted along the x axis, and a variable to be used to label the y axis. The resulting plot is shown in Figure 2.17.

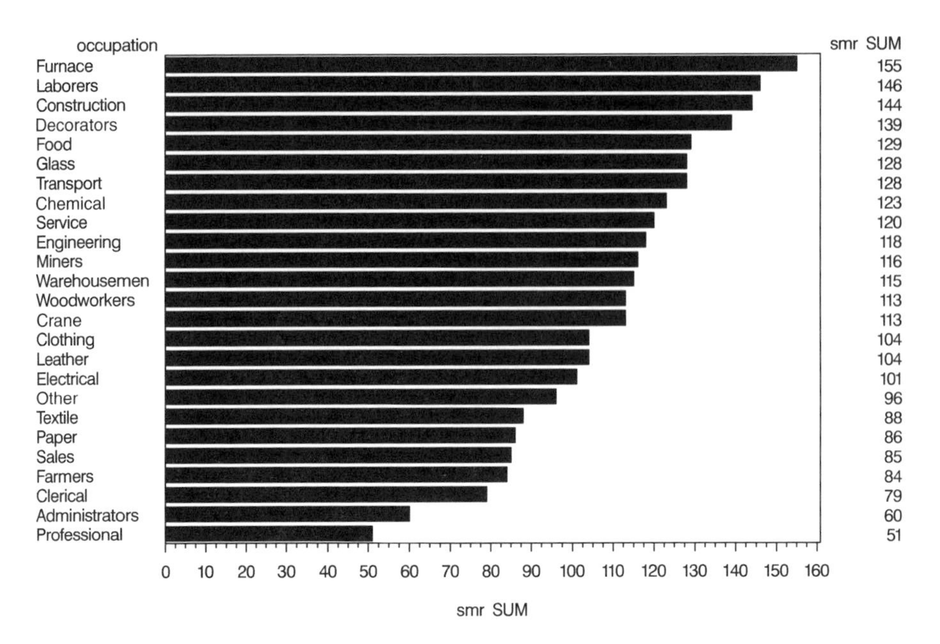

FIGURE 2.16
Plot of standardized mortality rate for a variety of occupations.

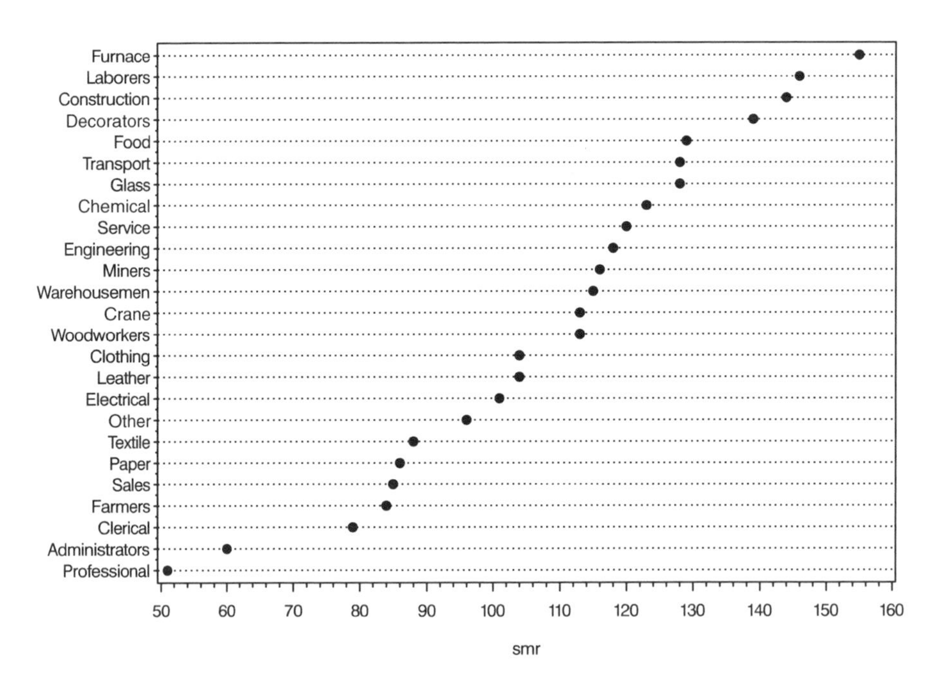

FIGURE 2.17
Dot plot of standardized mortality rate for a variety of occupations.

2.4 Summary

Data analysis usually begins by calculating some appropriate summary statistics and plotting some relatively simple graphs. Using a package such as SAS makes the production of such summaries and graphs very straightforward. In this chapter, only simple data sets have been considered, but as we shall see in later chapters, even when the data and the necessary analyses become more complex, the methods outlined in this chapter remain important in the initial stage of an investigation in which researchers are attempting to understand the main characteristics of their observations.

3

Basic Inference

3.1 Introduction

Inference — the process of drawing conclusions about a population on the basis of measurements or observations made on a sample of individuals from the population — is central to statistics in general and medical statistics in particular. In this chapter we shall look at some basic inferential methods, i.e., *statistical tests,* for both continuous and categorical data.

3.2 Simple Inference for Continuous Variables

3.2.1 Tests for Independent Samples

The data shown in Table 3.1 are taken from a study in which urinary-thromboglobulin excretion in 12 normal and 12 diabetic patients was measured. One of the questions of interest about the data is whether there is a difference in average urinary-thromboglobulin excretion in the normal and diabetic populations from which the samples were taken.

To begin, let us look at the boxplots for both groups produced in SAS as shown in the previous chapter. The two boxplots are shown in Figure 3.1 and provide a relatively clear indication that the diabetics have higher excretion levels than the normals do. The boxplots also suggest that the distribution of urinary excretion in the diabetic group is somewhat skew and that the variance of the excretion level for diabetics is greater than that for normals.

Most medical researchers would be unwilling to accept the informal evidence of a difference in excretion levels between diabetics and normals provided by Figure 3.1 and would therefore turn to a significance test to assess the evidence more formally. The most likely test such researchers would use in this situation is the *two-sample* t-test, hopefully accompanied by the calculation of a confidence interval for the difference in average excretion level in normals and diabetics. Details of the test and the construction of the confidence interval are given in Display 3.1.

TABLE 3.1

Urinary-Thromboglobulin Excretion

Normal	Diabetic
4.1	11.5
6.3	12.1
7.8	16.1
8.5	17.8
8.9	24.0
10.4	28.8
11.5	33.9
12.0	40.7
13.8	51.3
17.6	56.2
24.3	61.7
37.2	69.2

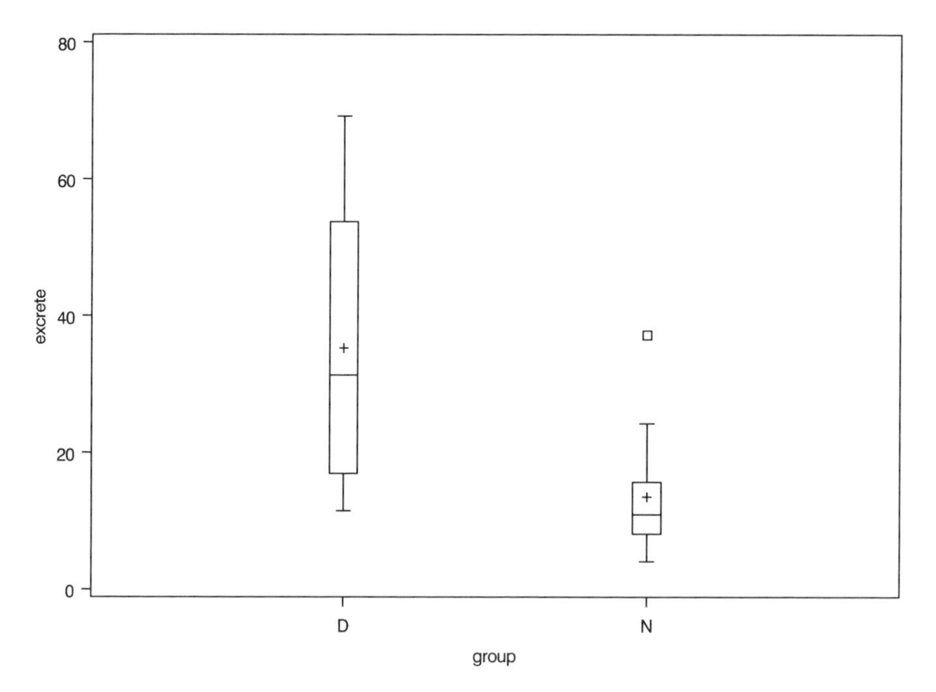

FIGURE 3.1
Boxplots for urinary-thromboglobulin excretion.

DISPLAY 3.1

Independent Samples t-Test

- The independent samples t-test is used to test the null hypothesis that the means of two populations are the same, $H_0 : \mu_1 = \mu_2$, when a sample of observations from each population is available. The subjects of one population must not be individually matched with subjects from the other population, and the subjects within each group should not be related to each other.
- The variable to be compared is assumed to have a normal distribution with the same standard deviation in both populations.
- The test-statistic is

$$t = \frac{\bar{y}_1 - \bar{y}_2}{s\sqrt{\frac{1}{n_1} + \frac{1}{n_2}}}$$

where $\bar{y}_1$ and $\bar{y}_2$ are the means in groups 1 and 2, n_1 and n_2 are the sample sizes, and s is the pooled standard deviation defined by

$$s = \sqrt{\frac{(n_1 - 1)s_1^2 + (n_2 - 1)s_2^2}{n_1 + n_2 - 2}}$$

where s_1 and s_2 are the standard deviation in the two groups.

- Under the null hypothesis, the t-statistic has a Student's t-distribution with $n_1 + n_2 - 2$ degrees of freedom.
- A 100(1 – α)% confidence interval for the difference between two means can be constructed as follows:

$$\bar{y}_1 - \bar{y}_2 \pm t_{\alpha, n_1 + n_2} - 2S\sqrt{\frac{1}{n_1} + \frac{1}{n_2}}$$

where $t_{\alpha, n_1 + n_2 - 2}$ is a percentage point of the t-distribution such that the cumulative distribution function, $P(t < t_{\alpha, n_1 + n_2 - 2})$, equals $1 - \alpha / 2$.

- If the two populations are suspected of having different variances, a modified form of the t-statistic may be used, namely

DISPLAY 3.1 (continued)

Independent Samples *t*-Test

$$t = \frac{\bar{y}_1 - \bar{y}_2}{\sqrt{\frac{s_1^2}{n_1} + \frac{s_2^2}{n_2}}}$$

- In this case, t has a Student's t-distribution with υ degrees of freedom, where

$$\upsilon = \left[\frac{c}{n_1 - 1} + \frac{(1-c)^2}{n_2 - 1} \right]^{-1}$$

with

$$c = \frac{s_1^2 / n_1}{s_1^2 / n_1 + s_2^2 / n_2}$$

- This is called the Satterthwaite method in SAS

The SAS code for applying the t-test and constructing the associated confidence interval is as follows;

```
data diabetes;
 input v1 v2;
 excrete=v1; group='N'; output;
 excrete=v2; group='D'; output;
 drop v1 v2;
cards;
 4.1 11.5
 6.3 12.1
 7.8 16.1
 8.5 17.8
 8.9 24.0
10.4 28.8
11.5 33.9
12.0 40.7
13.8 51.3
17.6 56.2
24.3 61.7
```

```
37.2 69.2
;
proc ttest data=diabetes;
  var excrete;
  class group;
run;
```

We first read in the data into two variables, v1 and v2, but these values belong to different individuals so we need to create two separate observations in the data set for each line of data read in. The output statement writes an observation to the data set, so the two output statements write out two observations with appropriate values of excrete and group. The variables v1 and v2 are no longer needed in the data set and so are excluded by the drop statement. The drop statement is effective even though it follows the output statements.

For the ttest procedure the var statement specifies the variable to be analysed and the class statement specifies the variable that divides the sample into two groups.

The results are shown in Table 3.2. Here the test for the equality of variances indicates that there is a significant difference ($p = 0.0144$) suggesting that it is more appropriate to use the version of the t-test that does not make the equal variance assumption. The p-value associated with this test is 0.004, and we can conclude that there is strong evidence of a difference in the average urinary-thromboglobulin levels between diabetics and normals. The confidence interval shown in Table 3.2 indicates that, on average, normals have an excretion level between about 8 and 35 units lower than that of diabetics.

TABLE 3.2

Results of Applying the t-test to the Data in Table 3.1

Statistics

Variable	group	N	Mean	Lower CL Mean	Upper CL Mean	Std Dev	Lower CL Std Dev	Upper CL Std Dev	Std Err
excrete	D	12	22.396	35.275	48.154	14.359	20.27	34.416	5.8514
excrete	N	12	7.6914	13.533	19.375	6.5133	9.1945	15.611	2.6542
excrete	Diff (1-2)		8.4164	21.742	35.067	12.172	15.739	22.276	6.4253

T-Tests

Variable	Method	Variances	DF	t Value	Pr > |t|
excrete	Pooled	Equal	22	3.38	0.0027
excrete	Satterthwaite	Unequal	15.3	3.38	0.0040

Equality of Variances

Variable	Method	Num DF	Den DF	F Value	Pr > F
excrete	Folded F	11	11	4.86	0.0144

We should now perhaps consider whether simply assuming that the normality assumption is valid for these data is justified. The boxplots in Figure 3.1, for example, suggest a fair degree of skewness in the data implying that the normality assumption may be suspect. This may not be of too much concern here since

1. The *t*-test is known to be relatively robust against departures from normality.
2. The evidence in favour of a difference in excretion rates in the two populations is so strong.

But in cases where the latter is not the case and the data show a marked departure from normality, we might consider two other approaches;

- Apply the *t*-test after a transformation of the data aimed at achieving a more normally distributed data set (see Chapter 2).
- Use a nonparametric, distribution-free test that does not assume normality.

Such tests have properties that hold under relatively minor assumptions regarding the underlying populations from which the data are obtained. In particular, distribution-free methods forgo the traditional assumption that the underlying populations are normal. A vast range of distribution-free methods are now available (see Hollander and Wolf, 1999).

Here we shall illustrate the second of these options and use the *Wilcoxon Mann–Whitney rank sum test* (see Display 3.2) on the excretion data. To do this we use the npar1way procedure with the wilcoxon option.

```
proc npar1way data=diabetes wilcoxon;
  var excrete;
  class group;
run;
```

The relevant results from SAS are that the normal approximation described in Display 3.2 takes the value 3.06 with associated two-sided *p*-value of 0.0022. The conclusion again is that normals and diabetics differ in their urinary-thromboglobulin excretion rates.

3.2.2 Tests for Dependent Samples

Consider the data in Table 3.3. These data arise from eight people who each had one eye affected with glaucoma and one not, and the corneal thickness (in microns) of both eyes has been measured. In many respects these data look of a similar form to those in Table 3.1, so it might be thought that their

DISPLAY 3.2

Wilcoxon Mann–Whitney Rank Sum Test

- The null hypothesis to be tested is that the two populations being compared have identical distributions. (For two normally distributed population with common variance, this would be equivalent to the hypothesis that the means of the two populations are the same.)
- The alternative hypothesis is that the population distributions differ in location (the median).
- Samples of observations are available from each of the two populations being compared.
- The test is based on the joint ranking of the observations from the two samples (as if they were from a single sample). If there are ties, the tied observations are given the average of the ranks for which the observations are competing.
- The test-statistic is the sum of the ranks of one sample (the lower of the two rank sums is generally used).
- For small samples, *p*-values for the test-statistic can be assigned relatively simply.
- A large sample approximation is available that is suitable when the two sample sizes n_1 and n_2 are both greater than 15, and there are no ties. The test-statistic Z is given by

$$Z = \frac{S - n_1(n_1 + n_2 + 1)/2}{\sqrt{n_1 n_2 (n_1 + n_2 + 1)/12}}$$

  where S is the test-statistic based on the sample with n_1 observations. Under the null hypothesis, Z has approximately a standard normal distribution.
- A modified Z-statistic is available when there are ties; see Hollander and Wolfe (1999).

analysis should again involve the independent samples *t*-test or the Wilcoxon Mann–Whitney test as described above for the urinary-thromboglobulin excretion data. But use of the *t*-test described in Display 3.1 would be an error here since in this case the pairs of observations on a subject are unlikely to be independent. The observations are essentially paired, producing dependent samples, and we need to therefore use a test in which this aspect of the data is accounted for. The relevant parametric test is the *paired t*-test described in Display 3.3 and the analogous distribution-free test is the *Wilcoxon signed*

DISPLAY 3.3

Paired t-Test

- A paired t-test is used to compare the means of two populations when samples from the populations are available, in which each individual in one sample is paired with an individual in the other sample. Examples are anorexic girls and their healthy sisters or the same patients before and after treatment.
- If the values of the variable of interest y for the members of the ith pair in groups 1 and 2 are denoted as y_{1i} and y_{2i}, then the differences $d_i = y_{1i} - y_{2i}$ are assumed to have a normal distribution.
- The null hypothesis here is that the mean difference is zero, i.e., $H_0 : \mu_d = 0$.
- The paired t-statistic is

$$t = \frac{\bar{d}_i}{s_d / \sqrt{n}}$$

where $\bar{d}_i$ is the mean difference between the paired groups and s_d is the standard deviation of the differences d_i. Under the null hypothesis, the test-statistic has a t-distribution with $n - 1$ degrees of freedom.

- A 100(1 – α)% confidence interval can be constructed as follows:

$$\bar{d}_i \pm t_{\alpha,n-1} \frac{sd}{\sqrt{n}}$$

where $P\left(t < t_{\alpha,n-1}\right) = 1 - \alpha / 2$.

TABLE 3.3

Corneal Thickness of Eyes

Affected with Glaucoma	Not Affected with Glaucoma
488	484
478	478
480	492
426	444
440	436
410	398
458	464
460	476

DISPLAY 3.4

Wilcoxon Signed Rank Test

- Assume, we have two observations, x_i and y_i, on each of n subjects in our sample, e.g., before and after treatment. We first calculate the differences, $z_i = x_i - y_i$, between each pair of observations.
- To compute the Wilcoxon signed-rank statistic T^+, form the absolute values of the differences, z_i, and then order them from least to greatest.
- If there are ties among the calculated differences, assign each of the observations in a tied group the average of the integer ranks that are associated with the tied group.
- Now assign a positive or negative sign to the ranks of the differences according to whether the corresponding difference was positive or negative. (Zero values are discarded, and the sample size n altered accordingly.)
- The statistic T^+ is the sum of the positive ranks. Tables are available for assigning p-values. See Table A.4 in Hollander and Wolfe (1999).
- A large sample approximation involves testing the statistic Z as a standard normal:

$$Z = \frac{T^+ - n(n+1)/4}{\sqrt{n(n+1)(2n+1)/24}}$$

rank test (see Display 3.4). Both tests can be applied to the glaucoma data using the following SAS instructions;

```
data glaucoma;
 input affected unaffected;
 difference=affected-unaffected;
cards;
488 484
478 478
480 492
426 444
440 436
410 398
458 464
```

```
460 476
;
proc ttest data=glaucoma;
  paired affected*unaffected;
run;
proc univariate data=glaucoma;
  var difference;
run;
```

In this data set, unlike the previous example, both measurements are made on the same individual, so it is appropriate that they should be read into two variables within the same observation. The syntax for a paired t-test is largely self explanatory, but note that the paired variables need to be joined with an asterisk. The same result, plus the Wilcoxon signed rank test, is obtained using `proc univariate` on the difference between the paired variables.

Extracting the results for the paired t-test from the SAS output shows that the t-statistic takes the value –1.05 with an associated p-value of 0.33. There is no evidence of a difference in average corneal thickness in the affected and unaffected eyes. The test-statistic for the signed rank test takes the value –6.5 with p-value 0.34, leading to the same conclusion.

3.3 Simple Inference for Categorical Data

3.3.1 Testing for Independence in Contingency Tables

The data in Table 3.4 come from a clinical trial and show the effect of the drug sulphinpyrazone on deaths after myocardial infarction; this is an example of a 2 × 2 contingency table. The question of interest is whether the drug reduces mortality. The appropriate test is a chi-squared test for a difference in the proportion of deaths in the populations of patients treated with the drug and the placebo — see Display 3.5. The test can be applied using the following SAS code:

TABLE 3.4

Sulphinpyrazone and Heart Attacks

	Deaths	Survivors
Sulphinpyrazone	41	692
Placebo	60	682

DISPLAY 3.5

Chi-Squared Test for a 2 × 2 Contingency Table

- The general 2 × 2 contingency table can be written as

		Variable 2		
		1	2	
Variable1	1	a	b	a + b
	2	c	d	c + d
		a + c	b + d	a + b + c + d = N

- The null hypothesis is that the two variables are independent.
- The test statistic is

$$X^2 = \frac{N(ad - bc)^2}{(a+b)(c+d)(a+c)(b+d)}$$

- Under the null hypothesis of independence, the statistic has a chi-squared distribution with a single degree of freedom.

```
data MIdeaths;
  input group$ outcome$ n;
cards;
Sulp Dead 41
Sulp Alive 692
Placebo Dead 60
Placebo Alive 682
;
proc freq data=MIdeaths order=data;
  tables group*outcome / chisq;
  weight n;
run;
```

`Proc freq` is used both to produce contingency tables and to analyse them. The `tables` statement defines the table to be produced and specifies the analysis of it. The variables that form the rows and columns are joined with an asterisk. These may be numeric or character variables. One-way frequency distributions are produced, where variables are not joined by asterisks. Several tables may be specified on a single `tables` statement.

TABLE 3.5

Part of SAS Output for the Analysis of the Data in Table 3.4

```
                  Table of group by outcome

            group     outcome

            Frequency,
            Percent  ,
            Row Pct  ,
            Col Pct  ,Dead     ,Alive   ,  Total
            --------- -------- --------
            Sulp     ,      41 ,     692 ,     733
                     ,    2.78 ,   46.92 ,   49.69
                     ,    5.59 ,   94.41 ,
                     ,   40.59 ,   50.36 ,
            --------- -------- --------
            Placebo  ,      60 ,     682 ,     742
                     ,    4.07 ,   46.24 ,   50.31
                     ,    8.09 ,   91.91 ,
                     ,   59.41 ,   49.64 ,
            --------- -------- --------
            Total          101      1374      1475
                          6.85     93.15    100.00


          Statistics for Table of group by outcome

   Statistic                     DF       Value      Prob
   ------------------------------------------------------
   Chi-Square                     1      3.5923    0.0580
             Table Probability (P)       0.0137
             Two-sided Pr <= P           0.0636

                    Sample Size = 1475
```

The options after the '/' specify the type of analysis. The `chisq` option requests chi-square tests of independence and measures of association based on chi-square.

The `weight` statement specifies a variable that contains weights for each observation. The default weight is 1, so the `weight` statement is not usually needed when the data set consists of observations on individuals. In this example the data are in the form of a contingency table, and the `weight` statement is used to specify the cell counts.

The `order=data` option on the `proc` statement specifies that the rows and columns are to be laid out in the order that they occur in the data. The default would be alphabetical order. This is for purely cosmetic purposes so that the table in the output matches Table 3.4.

Part of the SAS output is shown in Table 3.5. The results of the test are $X^2 = 3.59$ $df = 1$, $p = 0.058$. The test fails to reach significance at the 5% level, and the conclusion is that there is no convincing evidence that treatment of this type of patient with sulphinpyrazole reduces mortality.

DISPLAY 3.6

Testing for Independence in an $r \times c$ Contingency Table

- The general $r \times c$ contingency table can be written as

		Column variable			
		1	...	c	
Row variable	1	n_{11}	...	n_{1c}	$n_{1.}$
	2	n_{21}	...	n_{2c}	$n_{2.}$
	⋮	⋮	⋮	⋮	
	r	n_{r1}	...	n_{rc}	$n_{2.}$
		$n_{.1}$	...	$n_{.2}$	N

where n_{ij} is the count in the ijth cell, n_i is the row total for category i of the row variable and n_j is the corresponding term for the jth category of the column variable.

- Under the null hypothesis that the row and column classifications are independent, estimated expected values, E_{ij}, for the ith cell can be found as

$$E_{ij} = \frac{n_{i.}n_{.j}}{N}$$

- The test statistic for assessing independence is

$$X^2 = \sum_{i=1}^{r}\sum_{j=1}^{c}\frac{\left(n_{ij} - E_{ij}\right)^2}{E_{ij}}$$

- Under the null hypothesis of independence, X^2 has a chi-square distribution with $(r - 1)(c - 1)$ degrees of freedom.

The test for a difference in two proportions in a 2×2 contingency table is also a test that the row and column classifications are *independent*. The test of independence is also important in contingency tables with more than two rows and two columns, and details of the relevant chi-squared test are given in Display 3.6. The test can be illustrated on data recorded during a study of Hodgkin's disease and shown in Table 3.6. (The study is described in detail in Hancock et al., 1979.) Each of 538 patients with the disease was classified by histological type, and their response to treatment 3 months after it had begun was recorded. The histological types are:

- LP: lymphocyte predominance
- NS: nodular sclerosis
- MC: mixed cellularity
- LD: lymphocyte depletion

TABLE 3.6

Hodgkin's Disease

Histological Type	Response			
	Positive	Partial	None	Total
LP	74	18	12	104
NS	68	16	12	96
MC	154	54	58	266
LD	18	10	44	72
Total	314	98	126	538

The question of interest is whether or not the response is related to histological type. To apply the test to the data in Table 3.6 using SAS requires the following instructions:

```
data Hodgkins;
 input type$ v1-v3;
 response='Positive'; n=v1; output;
 response='Partial';  n=v2; output;
 response='None';     n=v3; output;
 drop v1-v3;
cards;
LP  74  18  12
NS  68  16  12
MC 154  54  58
LD  18  10  44
;
proc freq data=Hodgkins order=data;
  tables type*response /chisq;
  weight n;
run;
```

The only difference from the previous example is in the way that the data are read in. Here we read in a row of the table, which contains three cells, and use three `output` statements to write out three observations with appropriate values to the data set.

Extracting just the results of the chi-square test from the SAS output gives a value of 75.89 for the test statistic, which with 6 degrees of freedom has an associated p-value less than 0.0001. Clearly, response and histological type are not independent. But to discover more about the reasons for the clear departure from independence of response and histological type, we need to examine the pattern of differences of the observed and expected values in each cell of the table. It is also often useful to look at these differences after they have been "standardized" by dividing them by the square root of the corresponding expected value. The following SAS code provides the required expected values, differences, and standardized differences:

```
proc freq data=Hodgkins order=data;
  tables type*response /expected deviation cellchi2
                        norow nocol nopercent
                        out=tabout outexpect;
  weight n;
run;
data resids;
  set tabout;
  residual=(count-expected)/sqrt(expected);
run;
proc tabulate data=resids order=data;
  class type response;
  var residual;
  table type,
        response*residual*mean='';
run;
```

The `norow`, `nocol` and `nopercent` options suppress the printing of the percentages, and the `expected deviation` and `cellchi2` options print the expected value, the deviation (i.e., observed – expected) and the cell contribution to the chi-square statistic. There is no option to print the required cell "residual" (i.e., deviation/sqrt[expected]), but a table of residuals can be produced by writing out the observed and expected values to a data set using the `out=` and `outexpect` options, then calculating them in a data step and tabulating them with `proc tabulate`.

The results are shown in Table 3.7. It is clear from examination of the residuals that the lymphocyte depletion condition, in particular, has a considerable excess of patients who show no response than would be expected if condition and response were independent.

3.3.2 Fisher's Exact Test

One of the requirements of the chi-squared test used in the examples above is that the expected values are not too small. Historically, this has been interpreted as requiring values greater than 5 for the test to be valid. Although there is some evidence that this recommendation is rather too conservative, very sparse contingency tables can be a problem for the usual chi-squared test. For a 2×2 table, the usual alternative suggested is Fisher's exact test. A brief account of this test is given in Display 3.7. The test can be illustrated on the data shown in Table 3.8, which came from a study comparing the health of juvenile delinquent boys with that of a nondelinquent

TABLE 3.7

Expected Values, Observed–Expected Value Differences, and Standardized Residuals for the Histological Type Data in Table 3.6

```
                                        The FREQ Procedure

                              Table of type by response

                    type            response

                    Frequency       ,
                    Expected        ,
                    Deviation       ,
                    Cell Chi-Square,Positive,Partial ,None     ,  Total
                    --------------- -------- -------- --------
                    LP              ,     74 ,     18 ,     12 ,    104
                                    , 60.699 , 18.944 , 24.357 ,
                                    , 13.301 , -0.944 , -12.36 ,
                                    , 2.9147 , 0.0471 ,  6.269 ,
                    --------------- -------- -------- --------
                    NS              ,     68 ,     16 ,     12 ,     96
                                    ,  56.03 , 17.487 , 22.483 ,
                                    ,  11.97 , -1.487 , -10.48 ,
                                    , 2.5573 , 0.1264 ,  4.888 ,
                    --------------- -------- -------- --------
                    MC              ,    154 ,     54 ,     58 ,    266
                                    , 155.25 , 48.454 , 62.297 ,
                                    , -1.249 , 5.5465 , -4.297 ,
                                    ,   0.01 , 0.6349 , 0.2964 ,
                    --------------- -------- -------- --------
                    LD              ,     18 ,     10 ,     44 ,     72
                                    , 42.022 , 13.115 , 16.862 ,
                                    , -24.02 , -3.115 , 27.138 ,
                                    , 13.732 ,   0.74 , 43.674 ,
                    --------------- -------- -------- --------
                    Total                314       98      126      538

----------------------------------------------------------
                               response
                    ------------ ------------ ------------
                      Positive  ,  Partial   ,    None
                    ------------ ------------ ------------
                      residual  ,  residual  ,  residual
------------------- ------------ ------------ ------------
type               ,            ,            ,
-------------------             ,            ,
LP                 ,        1.71,       -0.22,       -2.50,
------------------- ------------ ------------ ------------
NS                 ,        1.60,       -0.36,       -2.21,
------------------- ------------ ------------ ------------
MC                 ,       -0.10,        0.80,       -0.54,
------------------- ------------ ------------ ------------
LD                 ,       -3.71,       -0.86,        6.61,
------------------- ------------ ------------ ------------
```

control group. They relate to the subset of the boys who failed a vision test and show the numbers who did and did not wear glasses. The question of interest is whether delinquents with poor eyesight are more or less likely to wear glasses than are nondelinquents with poor eyesight. Fisher's test is computed by default when the `chisq` option is used with a 2×2 table.

DISPLAY 3.7

Fisher's Exact Test for a 2×2 Table

- The probability of any particular arrangement of the frequencies $a, b, c,$ and d in a 2×2 contingency table, when the marginal totals are fixed and the two variables are independent, is

$$P = \frac{(a+b)!(a+c)!(c+d)!(b+d)!}{a!b!c!d!N!}$$

where ! denotes the factorial of a number, i.e., $x! = x(x-1)(x-2) \ldots 3 \cdot 2 \cdot 1$

- This is known as a hypergeometric distribution.
- Fisher's exact test employs this distribution to find the probability of the observed arrangement of frequencies and of every arrangement giving as much or more evidence of a departure from independence, when the marginal totals are fixed.

TABLE 3.8

Spectacle Wearing and Delinquency

Spectacle Wearers	Juvenile Delinquents	Nondelinquents	Total
Yes	1	5	6
No	8	2	10
Total	9	7	16

```
data delinquency;
  input specs$ delinquent$ n;
cards;
Y Y 1
Y N 5
N Y 8
N N 2
;
proc freq data=delinquency;
  tables specs*delinquent / chisq;
  weight n;
run;
```

The two-sided p-value obtained by applying Fisher's exact test can be found in the SAS output to be 0.035.There is some evidence of a difference

TABLE 3.9

Oral Lesions Data Set

Site of Lesion	Kerala	Gujarat	Andhra
Buccal mucosa	8	1	8
Commisure	0	1	0
Gingiva	0	1	0
Hard palate	0	1	0
Soft palate	0	1	0
Tongue	0	1	0
Floor of mouth	1	0	1
Alveolar ridge	1	0	1

Source: Cytel Software STATXACT Manual. With permission.

in spectacle wearing between juvenile delinquents and nondelinquents with poor eyesight. A lower proportion of the delinquents wear spectacles. (For interest, the chi-squared test in this case gives a *p*-value of 0.051.)

Although in the past Fisher's test has been largely applied to sparse 2×2 tables, it can also be applied to larger tables when there is concern about small values in some cells. The last decade has seen a large amount of work on exact tests for contingency tables in which the counts are small (see, for example, Mehta and Patel, 1986). To illustrate this use of Fisher's exact test, we shall use the data shown in Table 3.9 showing the distribution of the oral lesion site found in house-to-house surveys in three geographic regions of rural India. Application of Fisher's test to the data requires the following SAS code:

```
data lesions;
  length region $8.;
  input site $ 1-16 n1 n2 n3;
  region='Keral';   n=n1;  output;
  region='Gujarat'; n=n2;  output;
  region='Anhara';  n=n3;  output;
  drop n1-n3;
cards;
Buccal Mucosa    8  1  8
Labial Mucosa    0  1  0
Commissure       0  1  0
Gingiva          0  1  0
Hard palate      0  1  0
Soft palate      0  1  0
Tongue           0  1  0
Floor of mouth   1  0  1
```

```
Alveolar ridge   1  0  1
;
run;
proc freq data=lesions order=data;
  tables site*region /exact;
  weight n;
run;
```

For tables larger than 2×2, exact tests are requested by using the `exact` option on the `tables` statement.

The resulting p-value of 0.01 taken from the SAS output indicates a strong association between site of lesion and geographic region. For comparison, the chi-square statistic for these data takes the value 22.01, which with 14 degrees of freedom has an associated p-value of 0.14, suggesting no association. Here, the contingency table is so sparse that the usual chi-squared asymptotic distribution with 14 *df* is unlikely to yield accurate p-values.

3.3.3 The Mantel–Haenszel Test

A commonly occurring form of data in medical studies is a set of 2×2 contingency tables. Table 3.10 gives an example from a study involving cases of bronchitis by level of organic particles in the air and by age (Somes and O'Brien, 1985). Three 2×2 tables are available, one from each of three age groups. The data could be collapsed over age and the aggregate 2×2 table analysed as described previously. But the dangers of this are well documented (see, for example, Everitt, 1992). In particular, such pooling of tables can generate an association when in the separate tables there is none. A more appropriate test of association in this situation is the *Mantel–Haenszel* test described in Display 3.8.

TABLE 3.10

Number of Cases of Bronchitis by Level of Organic Particulates in the Air and by Age

Age (years)	Organic Particulates Level	Bronchitis		Total
		Yes	No	
15 to 24	High	20	382	402
	Low	9	214	223
23 to 30	High	10	172	182
	Low	7	120	127
40+	High	12	237	339
	Low	6	183	189

Source: *Encyclopedia of Statistical Science,* Wiley. With permission.

DISPLAY 3.8

Mantel–Haenszel Test

- For a series of k 2 × 2 contingency tables, the Mantel–Haenszel statistic for testing the hypothesis of no association is

$$X^2 = \frac{\left[\sum_{i=1}^{k} a_i - \sum_{i=1}^{k} \frac{(a_i + b_i)(a_i + c_i)}{N_i}\right]^2}{\sum_{i=1}^{k} \frac{(a_i + b_i)(c_i + d_i)(a_i + c_i)(b_i + d_i)}{N_i^2 (N_i - 1)}}$$

  where a_i, b_i, c_i, d_i represent the counts in the four cells of the ith table and N_i is the total number of observations in the ith table.
- Under the null hypothesis, this statistic has a chi-squared distribution with a single degree of freedom.
- The test is only appropriate if the degree and direction of the association between the two variables is the same in each stratum. A possible test of this assumption is that due to Breslow and Day (see Agresti, 1996).

```
data bronchitis;
  input agegrp level $ bronch $ n;
cards;
1 H Y 20
1 H N 382
1 L Y 9
1 L N 214
2 H Y 10
2 H N 172
2 L Y 7
2 L N 120
3 H Y 12
3 H N 327
3 L Y 6
3 L N 183
;
```

```
proc freq data=bronchitis order=data;
  Tables agegrp*level*bronch / cmh noprint;
  weight n;
run;
```

The `tables` statement specifies a three-way tabulation, with `agegrp` defining the strata. The `cmh` option requests the Cochran–Mantel–Haenszel statistics, and the `noprint` option suppresses the tables.

The SAS output gives the value of the Breslow–Day test statistic for homogeneity of odds ratios as 0.117, with an associated p-value of 0.94. There is no evidence against the homogeneity assumption. The value of the Mantel–Haenszel test statistic (called the Cochran–Mantel–Haenszel statistic in the SAS output) is 0.22 with p-value 0.64, indicating a lack of association between bronchitis and level of organic particulates in the air.

3.3.4 McNemar's Test for Correlated Proportions

The tests on categorical data described previously have assumed that the observations are independent. Often, however, categorical data arise from *paired observations*, for example, cases matched with controls on variables such as sex, age, and so on, or observations made on the same subjects on two occasions (cf., paired t-test). Such a set of data is shown in Table 3.11. Here, the cases were 175 women of reproductive age (15 to 44 years) discharged alive from 43 hospitals in five cities after initial attacks of idiopathic thrombophlebitis, pulmonary embolism, or cerebral thrombosis or embolism. The controls were matched with their cases for hospital, residence, time of hospitalisation, race, age, marital status and a number of other variables. The history of oral contraceptive use by the women was then determined.

For this type of paired data, the required procedure is McNemar's test — see Display 3.9 — and this is applied using the SAS code

```
data pill_use;
  input caseused $ controlused $ n;
cards;
Y Y 10
```

TABLE 3.11

Post Oral Contraceptive Use in 175 Pairs of Married Women

Oral Contraceptive Use	Number of Pairs
Used by both members of the pair	10
Used by the case only	57
Used by the control only	13
Used by neither the case or the control	95

DISPLAY 3.9

McNemar's Test for Grouped Data

- The frequencies in a matched samples data set can be written as

		Sample 1	
		Present	Absent
Sample 2	Present	*a*	*b*
	Absent	*c*	*d*

- Under the hypothesis that the two populations do not differ in their probability of having the characteristic present, the test-statistic

$$X^2 = \frac{(a-d)^2}{a+d}$$

has a chi-squared distribution with a single degree of freedom.

```
Y N 57
N Y 13
N N 95
;
run;
proc freq data=pill_use order=data;
 tables caseused*controlused / agree;
 weight n;
run;
```

The `agree` option is used for the McNemar test, as well as measures of agreement.

Here, the value of the test-statistic is 27.66 and the associated *p*-value is very small. There is a statistically significant association between thromboembolism and oral contraceptive use. The proportion of pairs in which only the case has used oral contraceptives is greater than the proportion in which only the control has used them.

3.4 Summary

Basic significance tests such as the *t*-test and the chi-squared test are the most frequently used of all statistical techniques. They can be applied extremely simply using any statistical package, including SAS. But users need to remember that the tests are based on underlying assumptions that need to be considered before they are used. When such assumptions are violated, alternative procedures such as transformations or nonparametric tests can be applied.

4

Scatterplots, Correlation, Simple Regression, and Smoothing

4.1 Introduction

Often, the data collected in medical investigations consist of observations on a pair of variables (*bivariate data*), and several issues may be of interest. For example, how are the variables correlated? Can one variable be predicted from another? What form of equation links the two variables? Such questions will be addressed in this chapter. In addition, we will also consider some aspects of the analysis of data sets containing several variables (*multivariate data*), although descriptions of methods needed for a detailed examination of such data will be left until Chapter 15.

4.2 The Scatterplot

The simple xy scatterplot has been in use since at least the eighteenth century and has many virtues — indeed, according to Tufte (1983):

> The relational graphic — in its barest form the scatterplot and its variants — is the greatest of all graphical designs. It links at least two variables encouraging and even imploring the viewer to assess the possible causal relationship between the plotted variables. It confronts causal theories that x causes y with empirical evidence as to the actual relationship between x and y.

The use of the scatterplot can be illustrated on the data given in Table 4.1, which were collected in a study investigating the possible link between alcohol consumption and the death rate per 100,000 of the population from cirrhosis and alcoholism. A scatterplot of the data that includes appropriate labels for each bivariate observation can be constructed using the following SAS code, which also produces the value of the Pearson's correlation coefficient for the two variables.

TABLE 4.1

Average Alcohol Consumption and Death Rate

Country	Alcohol Consumption (litres/person/year)	Cirrhosis and Alcoholism (Death Rate/100,000)
France	24.7	46.1
Italy	15.2	23.6
W. Germany	12.3	23.7
Austria	10.9	7.0
Belgium	10.8	12.3
U.S.	9.9	14.2
Canada	8.3	7.4
England and Wales	7.2	3.0
Sweden	6.6	7.2
Japan	5.8	10.6
Netherlands	5.7	3.7
Ireland	5.6	3.4
Norway	4.2	4.3
Finland	3.9	3.6
Israel	3.1	5.4

Source: Osborn, J.F. (1979) *Statistical Exercises in Medical Research,* Blackwell.

```
data drinking;
 input country $ 1-12 alcohol cirrhosis;
cards;
France        24.7  46.1
Italy         15.2  23.6
W.Germany     12.3  23.7
Austria       10.9   7.0
Belgium       10.8  12.3
USA            9.9  14.2
Canada         8.3   7.4
E&W            7.2   3.0
Sweden         6.6   7.2
Japan          5.8  10.6
Netherlands    5.7   3.7
Ireland        5.6   3.4
Norway         4.2   4.3
Finland        3.9   3.6
Israel         3.1   5.4
;
run;
proc corr; run;
```

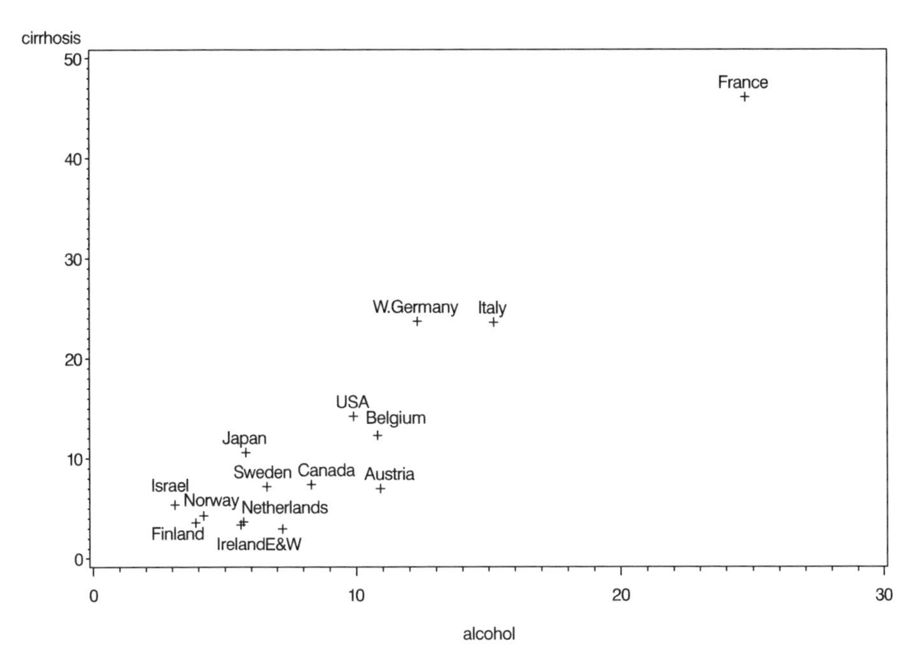

FIGURE 4.1
Scatterplot of death rate from cirrhosis vs. alcohol consumption.

```
symbol1 pointlabel=('#country');
proc gplot data=drinking;
  plot cirrhosis*alcohol;
run;
```

Some of the country names are longer than the default of eight for character variables, so column input is used to read them in. The values of the two numeric variables can then be read in with list input. This is an example of mixing different forms of input on one `input` statement. `Proc corr` produces Pearson correlations by default. A `var` statement would normally be used as the default is to include all numeric variables. The `pointlabel` option on the `symbol` statement specifies a variable whose values are to be used as labels on the plot. Note that the variable name must be enclosed in quotes and preceded by a hash (#) sign.

The scatterplot produced by SAS is shown in Figure 4.1, and the numerical output is shown in Table 4.2.

The scatterplot indicates a that there is a very strong relationship between death rate from cirrhosis and alcohol consumption, and this is underlined by the value of Pearson's correlation coefficient, 0.939, given in Table 4.2; the associated *p*-value is <0.0001. Figure 4.1 also demonstrates that France lies some way from the other countries in terms of the two variables of interest,

TABLE 4.2

Output from `proc corr` Applied to the Data in Table 4.1

```
                    2  Variables:     alcohol    cirrhosis


                                 Simple Statistics

Variable          N          Mean       Std Dev           Sum       Minimum       Maximum

alcohol          15       8.94667       5.53868     134.20000       3.10000      24.70000
cirrhosis        15      11.70000      11.66882     175.50000       3.00000      46.10000


                      Pearson Correlation Coefficients, N = 15
                             Prob > |r| under H0: Rho=0

                                     alcohol      cirrhosis

                     alcohol         1.00000        0.93883
                                                     <.0001

                     cirrhosis       0.93883        1.00000
                                      <.0001
```

so that it might be sensible to recalculate the correlation after excluding France. The necessary SAS code is

```
data drinking2;
 set drinking;
 if country~='France';
run;
proc corr; run;
```

The new value of the correlation coefficient found from the resulting output is 0.832 which, although lower than the previous value, is again highly significant.

This example demonstrates that outliers can often distort the value of a correlation coefficient. A procedure that can sometimes be usefully applied to a set of bivariate data to allow robust estimation of the correlation is *convex hull trimming*. In this approach, the points defining the convex hull of the observations are deleted before the correlation coefficient is calculated. (The convex hull of a set of bivariate data consists of the vertices of the smallest convex polyhedron in variable space within which all data points lie.) The major advantage of this approach is that it eliminates isolated outliers without disturbing the general shape of the bivariate distribution.

We shall apply convex hull trimming to the data in Table 4.1, although it is generally more useful with larger data sets. (An IML function is used to compute the convex hull. SAS/IML is licensed separately from SAS/STAT and so may not be available to all users of SAS.) The code for the function is as follows:

```
proc iml;
  use drinking;
  read all var {alcohol cirrhosis} into xy;
  ptr = cvexhull(xy);
  create hullptr var {ind};
  append from ptr;
quit;
data hull inner;
  set hullptr;
  hull=ind>0;
  pointer=abs(ind);
  set drinking point=pointer;
  if hull then output hull;
     else output inner;
run;
data anno;
  retain xsys ysys '2';
  set hull;
  y=cirrhosis;
  x=alcohol;
  function='polycont';
  if _n_=1 then function='poly';
run;
symbol1 v=circle i=none pointlabel=none;
proc gplot data=drinking;
 plot cirrhosis*alcohol / annotate=anno;
run;
```

`Proc IML` uses a different syntax from SAS. The `use` and `read` statements specify that the variables `alcohol` and `cirrhosis` from the `drinking` data set are to be read into the 2 x N matrix `xy`. The `cvexhull` function returns a vector of length N, whose entries indicate which rows of the `xy` matrix are on the hull and which are internal. The initial entries in the vector list the rows corresponding to points on the hull, and the remaining entries are the internal points. The latter are negative to distinguish them. The `create` and `append` statements create an SAS data set, `hullptr`, from the vector and name the single variable in it `ind`. The following data step uses this data set to create two new data sets, `hull` and `inner`, from the original

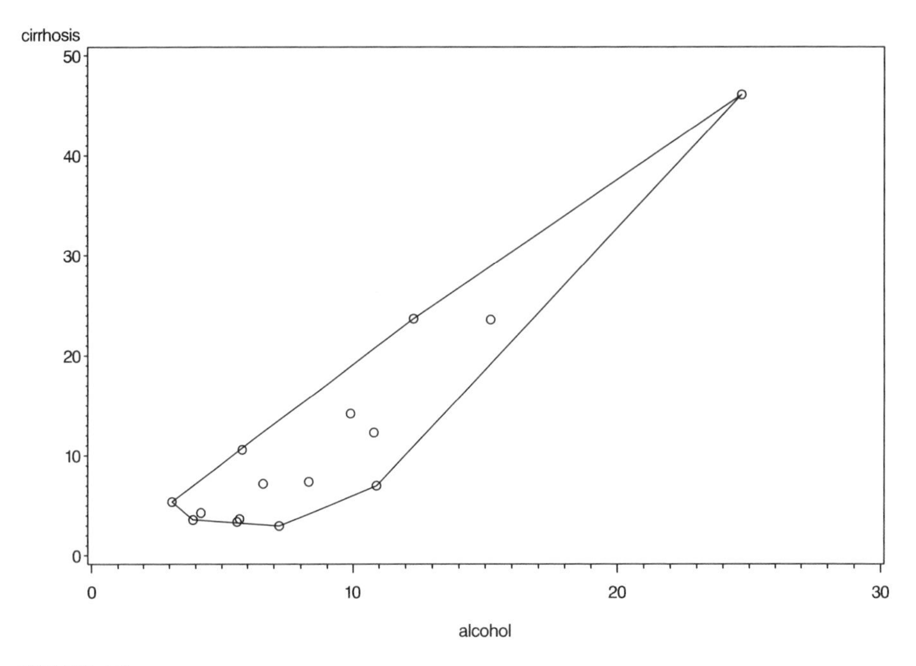

FIGURE 4.2
Convex hull of data in Table 4.1.

`drinking` data set. The `point=` option on the `set drinking` statement allows observations to be retrieved in the order specified by the `pointer` variable. There are some restrictions to the use of the `point=` option; in particular, the data set being accessed must not be compressed.

The following data step uses the `hull` data set to create an annotated data set which will draw a polygon through the points of the hull, as illustrated in Figure 4.2.

Recalculating the correlation coefficient for only the points within the convex hull requires the following code:

```
proc corr data=inner;
  var cirrhosis alcohol;
run;
```

The value of the resulting correlation coefficient is 0.925, which is very similar to the value calculated using all the observations.

4.2.1 The Aspect Ratio of a Scatterplot

An important parameter of a scatterplot that can greatly influence our ability to recognize patterns is the *aspect ratio*, the physical length of the vertical axis divided by that of the horizontal axis. By default SAS scales plots, and

TABLE 4.3

U.S. Monthly Birthrates between 1940 and 1943[a]

1890	1957	1925	1885	1896	1934	2036	2069	2060
1922	1854	1852	1952	2011	2015	1971	1883	2070
2221	2173	2105	1962	1951	1975	2092	2148	2114
2013	1986	2088	2218	2312	2462	2455	2357	2309
2398	2400	2331	2222	2156	2256	2352	2371	2356
2211	2108	2069	2123	2147	2050	1977	1993	2134
2275	2262	2194	2109	2114	2086	2089	2097	2036
1957	1953	2039	2116	2134	2142	2023	1972	1942
1931	1980	1977	1972	2017	2161	2468	2691	2890
2913	2940	2870	2911	2832	2774	2568	2574	2641
2691	2698	2701	2596	2503	2424			

[a] Read along rows for temporal sequence.
Source: Cook and Weisberg, 1994, Wiley.

other graphics, to fill the available graphics area. This will, typically, result in an aspect ratio of 3:4, which may not be the most useful.To illustrate how changing this characteristic of a scatterplot can help understand what the data are trying to tell us, we shall use the example given by Cook and Weisberg (1994) involving the monthly U.S. births per thousand population for the years 1940 to 1948. The data are given in Table 4.3. A scatterplot of the birthrates against month with the default aspect ratio can be obtained using the following SAS instructions:

```
data USbirth;
  retain obs 0;
  do year=1940 to 1947;
   do month=1 to 12;
   input rate @@;
   obs=obs+1;
   datestr=('15'||put(month,z2.)||put(year,4.));
   obsdate=input(datestr,ddmmyy8.);
   output;
   end;
  end;
cards;
1890   1957   1925   1885   1896   1934   2036   2069   2060
1922   1854   1852   1952   2011   2015   1971   1883   2070
2221   2173   2105   1962   1951   1975   2092   2148   2114
2013   1986   2088   2218   2312   2462   2455   2357   2309
2398   2400   2331   2222   2156   2256   2352   2371   2356
2211   2108   2069   2123   2147   2050   1977   1993   2134
2275   2262   2194   2109   2114   2086   2089   2097   2036
1957   1953   2039   2116   2134   2142   2023   1972   1942
1931   1980   1977   1972   2017   2161   2468   2691   2890
2913   2940   2870   2911   2832   2774   2568   2574   2641
2691   2698   2701   2596   2503   2424
;
proc gplot data=usbirth;
```

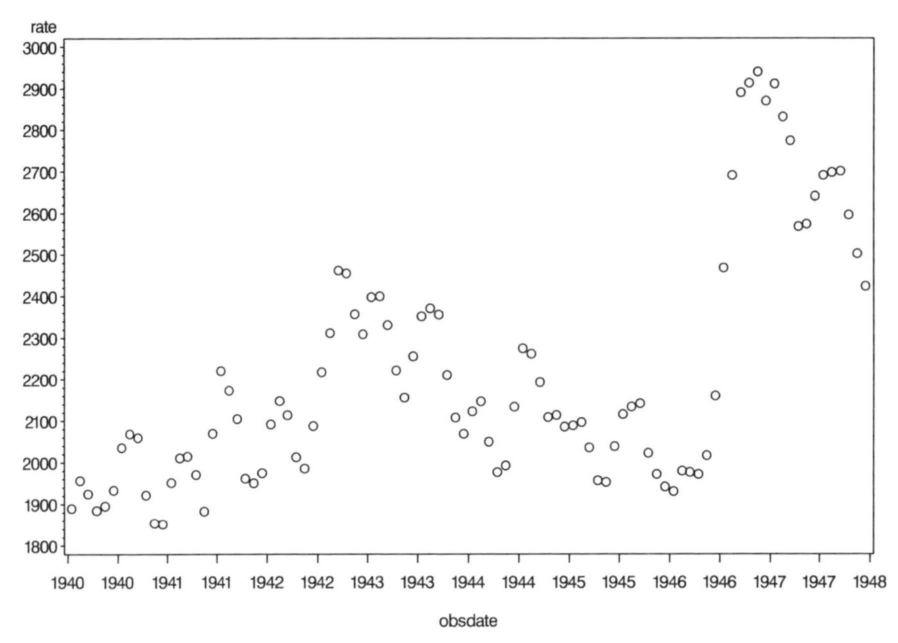

FIGURE 4.3
U.S. birthrate against year with default aspect ratio.

```
  plot rate*obsdate;
  format obsdate year.;
run;
```

The data are read in using two `do` loops to set values of `year` and `month` and each observation is, somewhat arbitrarily, given a date of the 15th of the month. Formatted values of this date variable can then be used to label the x axis of the plots. (Note that the `symbol` statement used for the drinking data has not been reset, so the plotting symbol is a circle as opposed to the default plus sign.)

The resulting plot is shown in Figure 4.3. The plot shows that the U.S. birthrate was increasing between 1940 and 1943, decreasing between 1943 and 1946, rapidly increasing during 1946, and then decreasing again during 1947 to 1948. As Cook and Weisberg comment:

> These trends seem to deliver an interesting history lesson, since the U.S. involvement in World War II started in 1942 and troops began returning home during the part of 1945 about nine months before the rapid increase in the birth rate.

Now let us see what happens when we alter the aspect ratio of the plot. One simple way to do this is to fix the length of the x and y axes with the `length=` option on the `axis` statement. In the following example we use inches (in) to produce a plot with an aspect ratio of .3. Centimeters, abbreviated cm, could also be used.

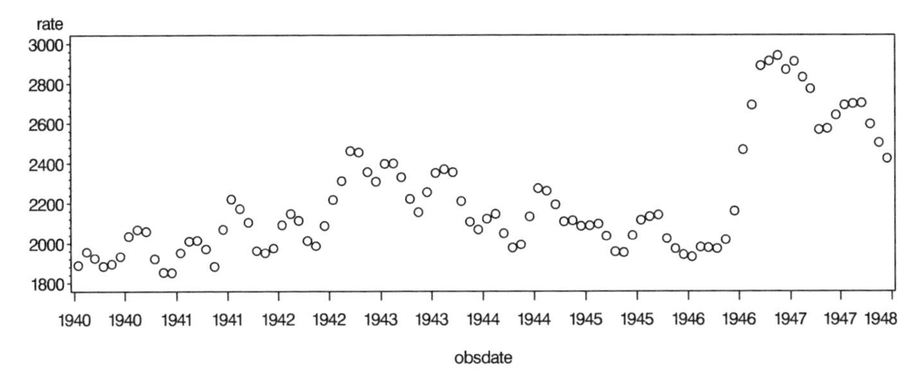

FIGURE 4.4
U.S. birthrate against year with aspect ratio 0.3.

```
axis1 length=10in;
axis2 length=3in;
proc gplot data=usbirth;
 plot rate*obsdate / haxis=axis1 vaxis=axis2;
 format obsdate year.;
run;
```

The resulting graph appears in Figure 4.4. The new plot displays many peaks and troughs and suggests perhaps some minor within-year trends in addition to the global trends apparent in Figure 4.3. A clearer picture is obtained by plotting only a part of the data; here we will plot the observations for the years 1940 to 1943 using the SAS code:

```
proc gplot data=usbirth;
 plot rate*obsdate / haxis=axis1 vaxis=axis2;
 format obsdate monyy7.;
 where year<1943;
run;
```

This plot is shown in Figure 4.5. Now, a within-year cycle is clearly apparent with the lowest within-year birthrate at the beginning of the summer and the highest occurring in the autumn. This pattern can be made clearer by connecting adjacent points in the plot with a line; the necessary SAS instructions are

```
symbol1 i=join v=none;
proc gplot data=usbirth;
 plot rate*obsdate / haxis=axis1 vaxis=axis2;
```

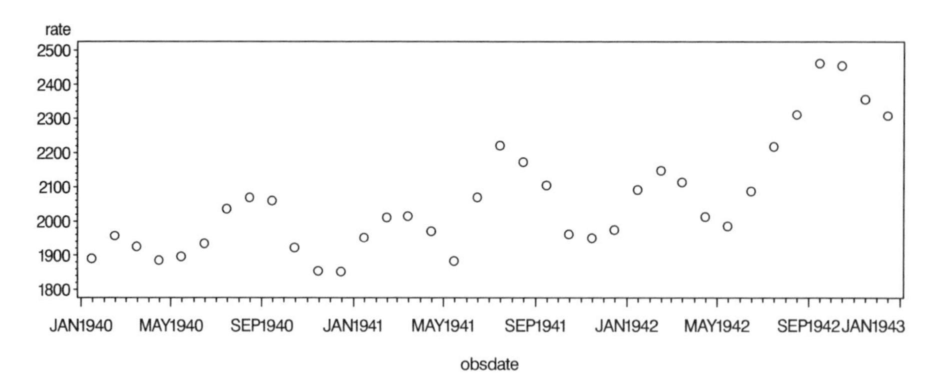

FIGURE 4.5
U.S. birthrate against year (1940 to 1943) with aspect ratio 0.3.

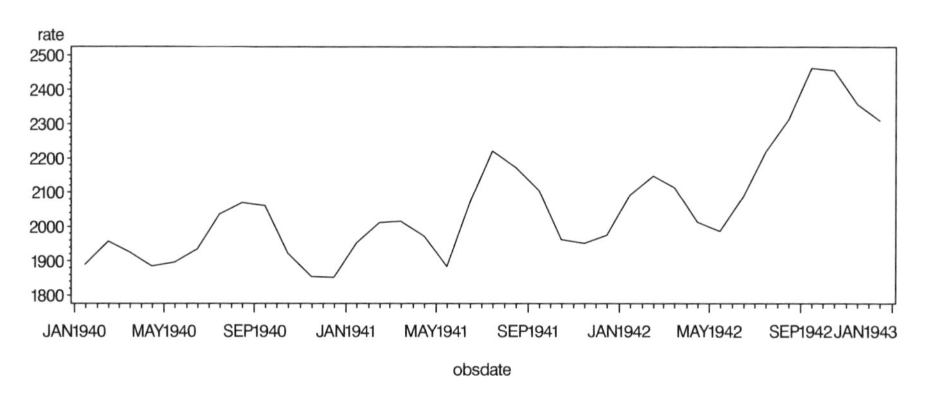

FIGURE 4.6
U.S. birthrate against year (1940 to 1943) with observations joined and aspect ratio 0.3.

```
  format obsdate monyy7.;
  where year<1943;
run;
```

The new plot appears in Figure 4.6. Reducing the aspect ratio to 0.2, replotting all 96 observations, and again joining adjacent points with a line, has made both the within-year and global trends clearly visible. The relevant SAS code is

```
axis3 length=2in;
symbol1 i=join v=none;
proc gplot data=usbirth;
  plot rate*obsdate / haxis=axis1 vaxis=axis3;
  format obsdate yyq7.;
run;
```

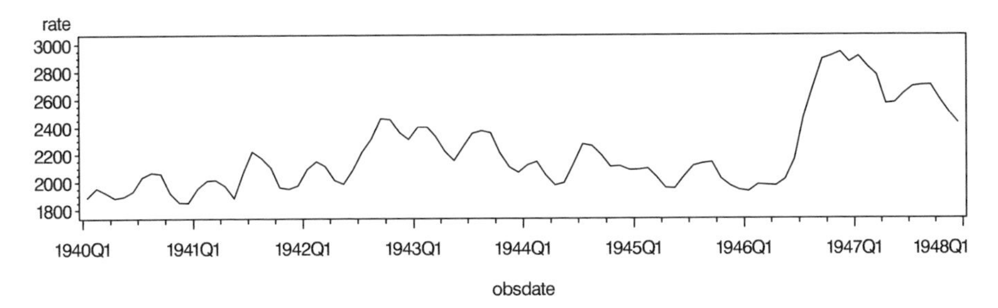

FIGURE 4.7
U.S. birthrate against year with observations joined and aspect ratio 0.2.

The plot appears in Figure 4.7. (In these plots a variety of date formats have been used to label the x axis.)

4.2.2 Estimating Bivariate Densities

Examination of scatterplots often centers on assessing density patterns such as clusters, gaps, or outliers. But humans are not particularly good at visually examining point density, and some type of density estimate added to the scatterplot will frequently be very helpful. There is now a vast literature on density estimation (see, for example, Silverman, 1986); its use in association with univariate data has already been described in Chapter 2. The estimation of bivariate densities is briefly described in Display 4.1.

To illustrate how bivariate density estimation can be used to enhance a scatterplot, we shall use the data on birth rates and death rates for 69 countries given in Table 4.4. The SAS code for reading in the data and calculating the required bivariate density estimate is:

```
data fertility;
  input country$ birth death;
cards;
alg   36.4   14.6
con   37.3   8.0
...
ast   21.6   8.7
nzl   25.5   8.8
;
data anno;
  set fertility;
  retain xsys ysys '2' function 'SYMBOL' text 'CIRCLE';
  y=death;
  x=birth;
```

DISPLAY 4.1

Estimating Bivariate Densities

- The data set whose underlying density is to be estimated is $\mathbf{X}_1, \mathbf{X}_2, \cdots, \mathbf{X}_n$.
- The bivariate kernel density estimator with kernel K and window width h is defined by

$$\hat{f}(\mathbf{x}) = \frac{1}{nh^2} \sum_{i=1}^{n} K\left\{\frac{1}{h}(\mathbf{x} - \mathbf{X}_i)\right\}$$

- The kernel function $K(\mathbf{x})$ is a function, defined for bivariate $\mathbf{x}$, satisfying

$$\int K(\mathbf{x}) d\mathbf{x} = 1$$

- Usually $K(\mathbf{x})$ will be a radially symmetric unimodal probability density function, for example, the standard bivariate normal density function:

$$K(\mathbf{x}) = \frac{1}{2\pi} \exp\left(-\frac{1}{2}\mathbf{x}'\mathbf{x}\right)$$

```
run;
proc kde data=fertility out=kdeout;
  var birth death;
run;
proc gcontour data=kdeout;
  plot death*birth=density /
 nlevels=25 nolegend annotate=anno;
run;
```

`Proc kde` produces univariate and bivariate density estimates using normal kernels. The output data set contains the density estimates, which can then be plotted as a contour plot with `proc gcontour` or as a perspective plot with `proc g3d`. To produce a plot that combines a contour plot of the density estimates with a scatterplot of the data, we use the annotate facility to overlay the scatterplot on the contour plot. The resulting plot is shown in Figure 4.8.

TABLE 4.4

Birthrates and Death Rates for 69 Countries

Country	Birth	Death	Country	Birth	Death
Alg	36.4	14.6	Arg	21.8	8.1
Con	37.3	8.0	Bol	17.4	5.8
Egy	42.1	15.3	Bra	45.0	13.5
Gha	55.8	25.6	Chl	33.6	11.8
Ict	56.1	33.1	Clo	44.0	11.7
Mag	41.8	15.8	Ecu	44.2	13.5
Mor	46.1	18.7	Per	27.7	8.2
Tun	41.7	10.1	Urg	22.5	7.8
Cam	41.4	19.7	Ven	42.8	6.7
Cey	35.8	8.5	Aus	18.8	12.8
Chi	34.0	11.0	Bel	17.1	12.7
Tai	36.3	6.1	Brt	18.2	12.2
Hkg	32.1	5.5	Bul	16.4	8.2
Ind	20.9	8.8	Cze	16.9	9.5
Ids	27.7	10.2	Dem	17.6	19.8
Irq	20.5	3.9	Fin	18.1	9.2
Isr	25.0	6.2	Fra	18.2	11.7
Jap	17.3	7.0	Gmy	18.0	12.5
Jor	46.3	6.4	Gre	17.4	7.8
Kor	14.8	5.7	Hun	13.1	9.9
Mal	33.5	6.4	Irl	22.3	11.9
Mog	39.2	11.2	Ity	19.0	10.2
Phl	28.4	7.1	Net	20.9	8.0
Syr	26.2	4.3	Now	17.5	10.0
Tha	34.8	7.9	Pol	19.0	7.5
Vit	23.4	5.1	Pog	23.5	10.8
Can	24.8	7.8	Rom	15.7	8.3
Cra	49.9	8.5	Spa	21.5	9.1
Dmr	33.0	8.4	Swe	14.8	10.1
Gut	47.7	17.3	Swz	18.9	9.6
Hon	46.6	9.7	Rus	21.2	7.2
Mex	46.1	10.5	Yug	21.4	8.9
Nic	42.9	7.1	Ast	21.6	8.7
Pan	40.1	8.0	Nzl	25.5	8.8
Usa	21.7	9.6			

Source: Hartigan, J.A., 1975, *Clustering Algorithms*. With permission.

As the default bandwidths tend to oversmooth the data, the `bwm=` option can be used to control the bandwidth separately for each variable. Values less than one produce a rougher estimate than the default and those greater than one a smoother estimate. To change the bandwidths and replot requires the SAS code that follows:

```
proc kde data=fertility out=kdeout2 bwm=.5,.5;
  var birth death;
run;
```

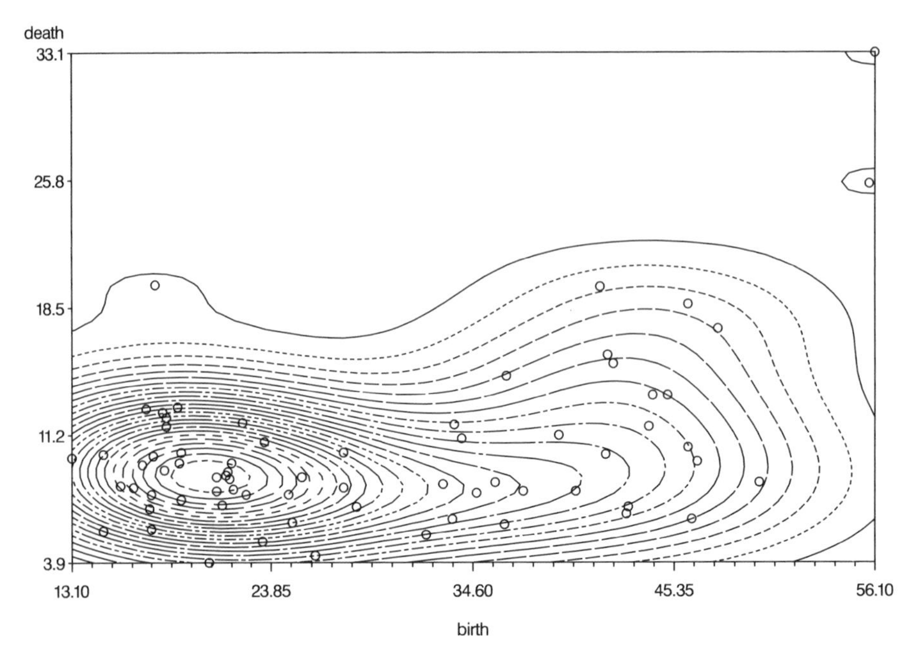

FIGURE 4.8
Estimated bivariate density for birth and death rate data in Table 4.4.

```
proc gcontour data=kdeout2;
  plot death*birth=density /
 nlevels=25 nolegend  annotate=anno;
run;
```

Figure 4.9 in particular gives some evidence that there are two modes in the data, perhaps indicating the presence of "clusters" of countries.

The density estimates can also be presented in the form of perspective plots as shown in Figure 4.10 and Figure 4.11, obtained using

```
proc g3d data=kdeout;
 plot death*birth=density /rotate=30 tilt=45;
run;
proc g3d data=kdeout2;
 plot death*birth=density /rotate=30 tilt=45;
run;
```

We have used the `rotate` and `tilt` options to give a better view of the plots. With the default values, too much detail was hidden behind the main peak. The `rotate` option turns the y axis the specified number of degrees anticlockwise from the vertical. The `tilt` option tilts the graph away from you, starting from the viewpoint directly above.

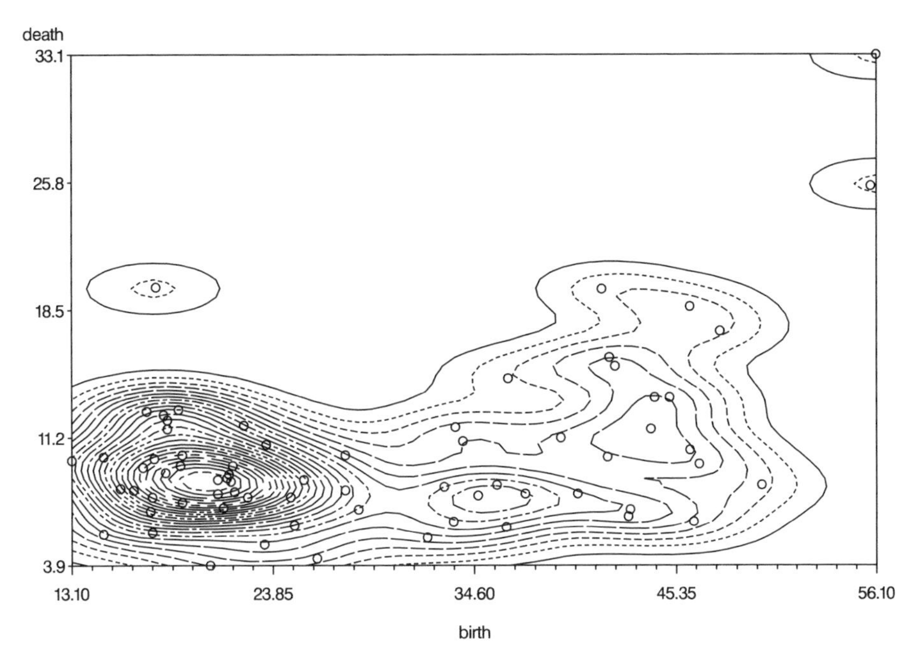

FIGURE 4.9
Estimated bivariate density for the birth and death rate data.

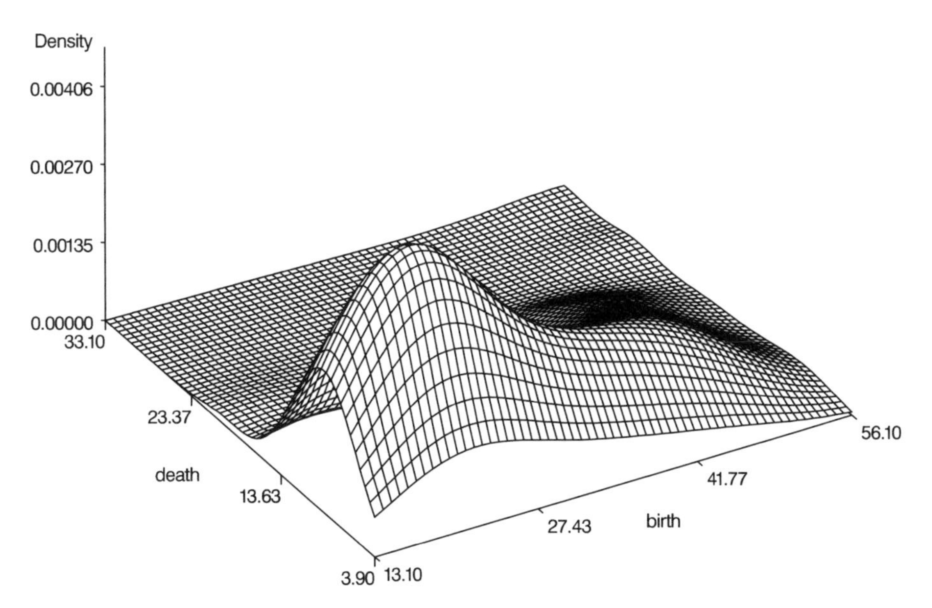

FIGURE 4.10
Perspective plot of estimated bivariate density for birth and death rate data.

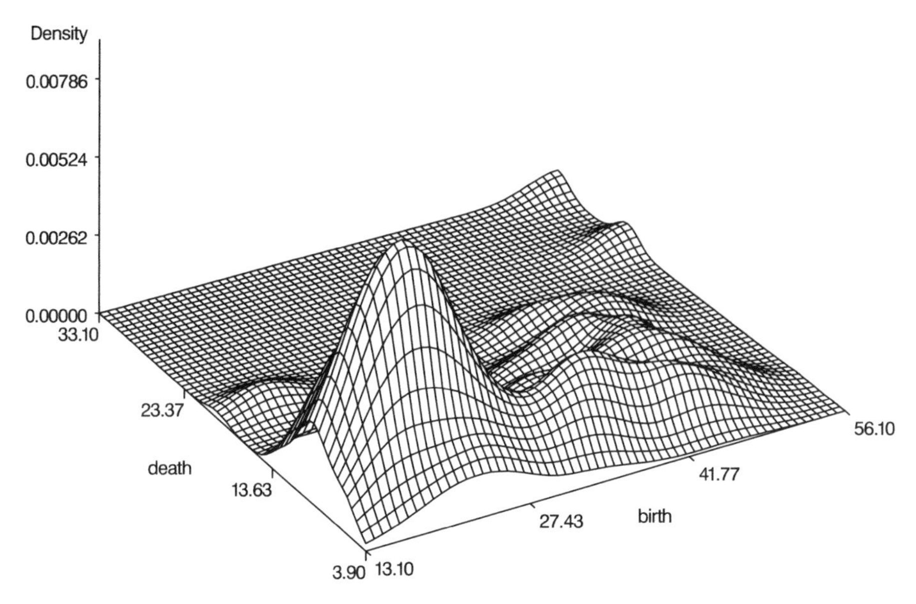

FIGURE 4.11
Perspective plot of estimated bivariate density for birth and death rate data.

4.3 Scatterplot Matrices

The data in Table 4.4 are reported in Begg and Hearns (1966) and were collected in an investigation of the relative contributions of haematocrit (packed cell volume, PCV) and fibrinogen and other proteins (albutin and globulin) to the viscosity of blood. The four observed variables generate between them six possible scatterplots, and it is very important that the separate bivariate displays be presented in a way that aids in overall comprehension and understanding of the data. The scatterplot matrix is intended to accomplish exactly this objective.

A scatterplot matrix is defined as a square, symmetric grid of bivariate scatterplots. This grid has p rows and columns, each one corresponding to a different variable. Each of the grid's cells shows a scatterplot of two variables. Variable j is plotted against variable i in the ijth cell, and the same variables appear in cell ji with the x- and y-axes of the scatterplots interchanged. The reason for including both the upper and lower triangles of the grid, despite the seeming redundancy, is that it enables a row and column to be visually scanned to see one variable against all others, with the scales of the one variable lined up along the horizontal or the vertical.

A scatterplot matrix of the data can be generated in SAS using a macro:

```
data blood;
  input patid viscosity PCV fibrinogen protein;
```

```
cards;
1   3.71   40   344   6.27
2   3.78   40   330   4.86
. . . .
30   5.77   57   1070   4.82
31   5.90   54   488   5.70
32   5.90   54   488   5.70
;
%inc 'c:\sasbook\macros\plotmat.sas';
%inc 'c:\sasbook\macros\template.sas';
%plotmat(blood,viscosity--protein);
```

The `plotmat` macro itself uses the `template` macro, so both have to be included before it is used. The macro has two parameters: the first is the name of the SAS data set and the second a list of variables to be used for the scatterplot matrix. The result is shown in Figure 4.12.

The scatterplot matrix is a useful graphic when interpreting the correlation matrix of a set of variables. Such a matrix can be found for the data in Table 4.4 using the SAS constructions:

```
proc corr data=blood;
 var viscosity--protein;
run;
```

The resulting output is shown in Table 4.5 and indicates that substantial correlations exist between several pairs of variables, for example, fibrinogen and viscosity.

When three or more variables are measured as in Table 4.4, it is often of interest to calculate *partial correlation coefficients* (see Display 4.2). Here of most interest is to see whether the association of blood viscosity and fibrinogen remains after allowing for the association with PCV. The SAS code needed to get the relevant coefficients is

```
proc corr data=blood;
 var viscosity fibrinogen protein;
 partial pcv;
run;
```

The output is shown in Table 4.6. Note that the partial correlation between viscosity and fibrinogen is now reduced to 0.222, which is not significantly different from zero.This suggests that the association between blood viscosity and fibrinogen can be largely explained by variation in PCV.

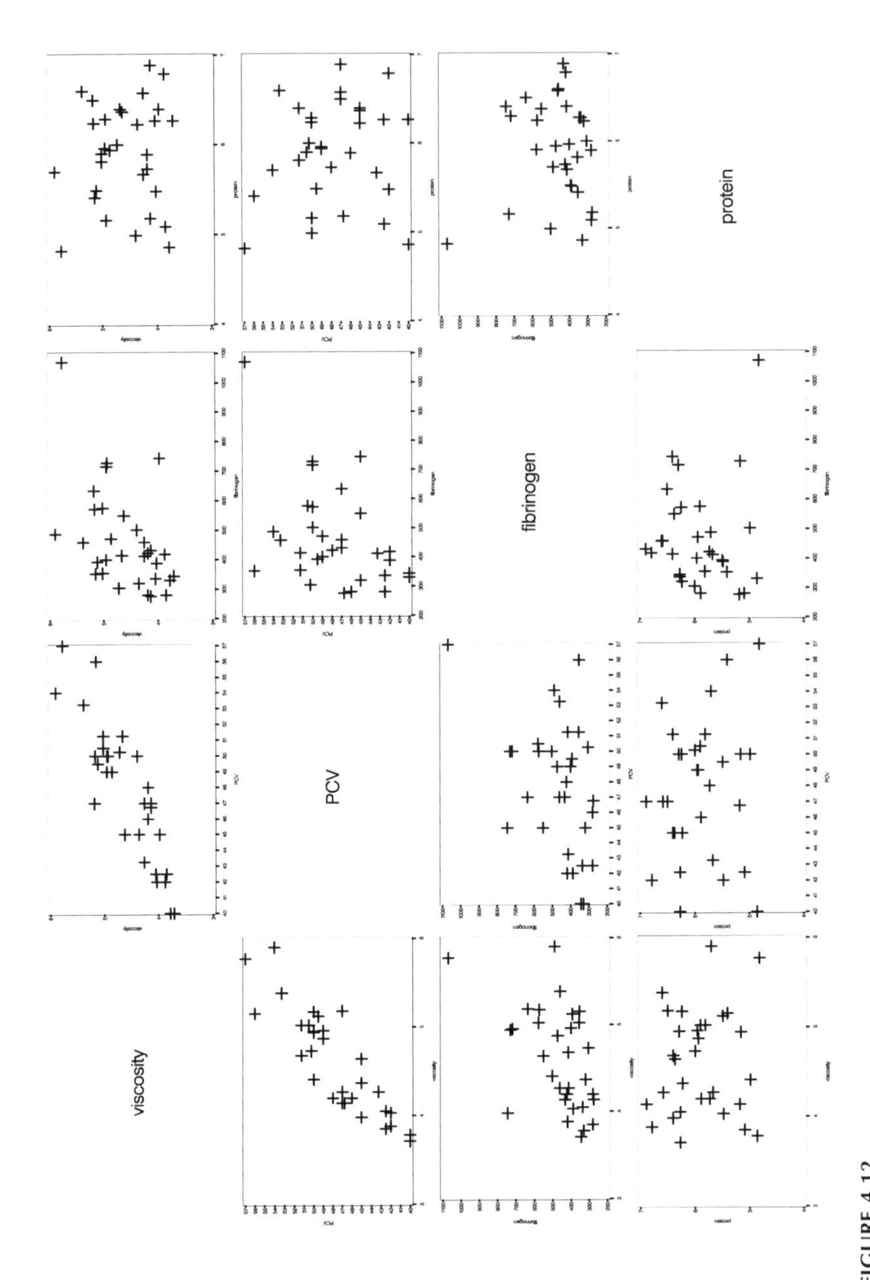

FIGURE 4.12
Scatterplot matrix of blood viscosity data.

TABLE 4.5

Data on Blood Viscosity, Packed Cell Volume (PCV), Plasma Fibrinogen, and Other Proteins from 32 Hospital Patients

Patient	Blood Viscosity (cP)	PCV (100%)	Plasma Fibrinogen (mg/100 ml)	Plasma Protein (g/100 ml)
1	3.71	40	344	6.27
2	3.78	40	330	4.86
3	3.85	42.5	280	5.09
4	3.88	42	418	6.79
5	3.98	45	744	6.40
6	4.03	42	388	5.48
7	4.05	42.5	336	6.27
8	4.14	47	431	6.89
9	4.14	46.75	276	5.18
10	4.20	48	422	5.73
11	4.20	46	280	5.89
12	4.27	47	460	6.58
13	4.27	43.25	412	5.67
14	4.37	45	320	6.23
15	4.41	50	502	4.99
16	4.64	45	550	6.37
17	4.68	51.25	414	6.40
18	4.73	50.25	304	6.00
19	4.87	49	472	5.94
20	4.94	50	728	5.16
21	4.95	50	716	6.29
22	4.96	49	400	5.96
23	5.02	50.5	576	5.90
24	5.02	51.25	354	5.81
25	5.12	49.5	392	5.49
26	5.15	56	352	5.41
27	5.17	50	572	6.24
28	5.18	47	634	6.50
29	5.38	53.25	458	6.60
30	5.77	57	1070	4.82
31	5.90	54	488	5.70
32	5.90	54	488	5.70

Source: Begg and Hearns, 1966. *Clinical Science.* With permission.

4.4 Simple Linear Regression and Locally Weighted Regression

The correlation coefficients calculated for data sets in previous sections indicate the strength of the relationship between a pair of variables. But other questions may also be of interest about such data; for example, how can one of the variables best be predicted from the other? To answer this question requires the use of some form of regression; here we shall concentrate on

DISPLAY 4.2

Partial Correlation Coefficients

- For three variables x, y, and z, with correlation coefficients for a sample of n observations of r_{xy}, r_{xz} and r_{yz}, the partial correlations are calculated as follows:

$$r_{xy|z} = \frac{r_{xy} - r_{xz}r_{yz}}{\sqrt{\left(1-r_{xz}^2\right)\left(1-r_{yz}\right)^2}}$$

$$r_{xz|y} = \frac{r_{xz} - r_{xy}r_{yz}}{\sqrt{\left(1-r_{xy}^2\right)\left(1-r_{yz}^2\right)}}$$

$$r_{yz|x} = \frac{r_{yz} - r_{xy}r_{xz}}{\sqrt{\left(1-r_{xy}^2\right)\left(1-r_{xz}^2\right)}}$$

- Hypotheses tests on the partial correlation are performed in the same way as for the usual correlation coefficient except that there are $n - 3$ degrees of freedom.
- So, for example, to test the hypothesis $\rho_{xy|z} = 0$, the test statistic is

  $r_{xy|z}\sqrt{\frac{n-3}{1-r_{xy|z}^2}}$ tested against a t distribution with $n - 3$ degrees of freedom.

the use of the technique for two variables and leave until later chapters accounts of using regression techniques in more complex situations.

Simple linear regression is described in Display 4.3. We can fit such a model to the data in Table 4.1 (leaving out France), using `proc reg` as follows.

```
goptions reset=symbol;
proc reg data=drinking2;
  model cirrhosis=alcohol;
  output out=regout p=pr uclm=upper lclm=lower;
  plot cirrhosis*alcohol / conf;
run;
```

Basic use of `proc reg` need only involve the `model` statement. In this example we also illustrate the use of the `plot` statement, which can be used

TABLE 4.6

Correlation Matrix, Etc., for Data in Table 4.5

```
4 Variables:    viscosity PCV    fibrinogen protein
```

Simple Statistics

Variable	N	Mean	Std Dev	Sum	Minimum	Maximum
viscosity	32	4.64563	0.62088	148.66000	3.71000	5.90000
PCV	32	47.93750	4.45678	1534	40.00000	57.00000
fibrinogen	32	465.96875	169.43292	14911	276.00000	1070
protein	32	5.89406	0.56861	188.61000	4.82000	6.89000

Pearson Correlation Coefficients, N = 32
Prob > |r| under H0: Rho=0

	viscosity	PCV	fibrinogen	protein
viscosity	1.00000	0.87882 <.0001	0.46791 0.0069	-0.10107 0.5820
PCV	0.87882 <.0001	1.00000	0.42332 0.0158	-0.15749 0.3893
fibrinogen	0.46791 0.0069	0.42332 0.0158	1.00000	-0.05680 0.7575
protein	-0.10107 0.5820	-0.15749 0.3893	-0.05680 0.7575	1.00000

DISPLAY 4.3

Simple Linear Regression

- Assume y_i represents the value of the response variable on the ith individual (plotted on the vertical axis), and that x_i represents the individual's values on an explanatory variable (plotted on the horizontal axis).
- The simple regression model is

$$y_i = \beta_0 + \beta_i x_i + \varepsilon_i$$

where β_0 is the intercept, β_1 is the slope of the linear relationship, and ε_i is an error term or residual.

- The residuals are assumed to be independent random variables having a normal distribution with mean zero and constant variance σ^2.

DISPLAY 4.3 (continued)

Simple Linear Regression

- The *regression coefficients*, β_0 and β_1, may be estimated as $\hat{\beta}_0$ and $\hat{\beta}_1$ using *least squares*. Here, the sum of squared differences between the observed values of the response variable y_i and the values 'predicted' by the regression equation $\hat{y}_i = \hat{\beta}_0 + \hat{\beta}_1 x_i$ is minimized, leading to the estimates

$$\hat{\beta}_0 = \bar{y} - \hat{\beta}_1 \bar{x}$$

$$\hat{\beta}_1 = \frac{\sum (y_i - \bar{y})(x_i - \bar{x})}{\sum (x_i - \bar{x})^2}$$

- The predicted values of y from the model are

$$\hat{y}_i = \hat{\beta}_0 + \hat{\beta}_1 x_i$$

- The variance σ^2 is estimated as s^2 given by

$$s^2 = \sum_{i=1}^{n} (y_i - \hat{y}_i)^2 / (n-2)$$

- The estimated variance of the estimate of the slope parameter is

$$\text{Var}(\hat{\beta}_1) = \frac{s^2}{\sum_{i=1}^{n} (x_i - \bar{x})^2}$$

- The estimated variance of a predicted value y_{pred} at a given value of x, say x_0 is

$$\text{Var}(y_{\text{pred}}) = s^2 \sqrt{\frac{1}{n} + \frac{(x_0 - \bar{x})^2}{\sum_{i=1}^{n} (x_i - \bar{x})^2}}$$

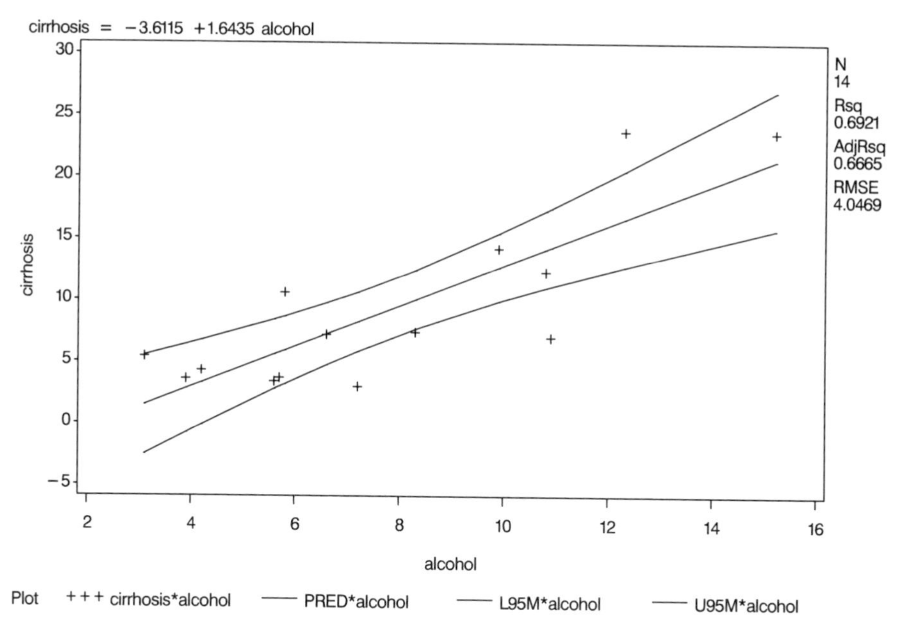

FIGURE 4.13
Scatterplot of death rate from cirrhosis against alcohol consumption showing fitted linear regression and confidence interval.

to produce a wide range of diagnostic plots. Here we reproduce the scatter plot of the original data supplemented, via the `conf` option, with the addition of the fitted regression line and 95% confidence intervals — see Figure 4.13. (The `goptions` statement resets any symbol definitions that remain active from previous analyses in this chapter.)

The SAS output is shown in Table 4.7. The regression coefficient of death rate on alcohol consumption is highly significant. The value of R-squared (where R is the multiple correlation coefficient — see Chapter 6) indicates that 69% of the variation in death rates among the countries is due to variation in alcohol consumption.

Another way to plot the results of the regression is to save the predicted values and confidence limits in an output data set, as the `output` statement does, and then use `proc gplot` as follows:

```
symbol1 v=circle i=none;
symbol2 v=none i=join;
symbol3 v=none i=join l=3 r=2;
proc gplot data=regout;
  plot (cirrhosis pr upper lower)*alcohol / overlay;
run;
```

The resulting plot is shown in Figure 4.14.

TABLE 4.7

Partial Correlation Coefficients

```
1 Partial Variables:    PCV
3         Variables:    viscosity  fibrinogen protein
```

Simple Statistics

Variable	N	Mean	Std Dev	Sum	Minimum	Maximum
PCV	32	47.93750	4.45678	1534	40.00000	57.00000
viscosity	32	4.64563	0.62088	148.66000	3.71000	5.90000
fibrinogen	32	465.96875	169.43292	14911	276.00000	1070
protein	32	5.89406	0.56861	188.61000	4.82000	6.89000

Simple Statistics

Variable	Partial Variance	Partial Std Dev
PCV		
viscosity	0.09070	0.30116
fibrinogen	24349	156.04034
protein	0.32581	0.57079

Pearson Partial Correlation Coefficients, N = 32
Prob > |r| under H0: Partial Rho=0

	viscosity	fibrinogen	protein
viscosity	1.00000	0.22180 0.2304	0.07922 0.6718
fibrinogen	0.22180 0.2304	1.00000	0.01103 0.9530
protein	0.07922 0.6718	0.01103 0.9530	1.00000

TABLE 4.8

Linear Regression Results for Cirrhosis and Alcohol Consumption Data

Model: MODEL1
Dependent Variable: cirrhosis

Analysis of Variance

Source	DF	Sum of Squares	Mean Square	F Value	Pr > F
Model	1	441.84624	441.84624	26.98	0.0002
Error	12	196.52804	16.37734		
Corrected Total	13	638.37429			

Root MSE	4.04689	R-Square	0.6921
Dependent Mean	9.24286	Adj R-Sq	0.6665
Coeff Var	43.78400		

Parameter Estimates

Variable	DF	Parameter Estimate	Standard Error	t Value	Pr > |t|
Intercept	1	-3.61154	2.70081	-1.34	0.2060
alcohol	1	1.64348	0.31641	5.19	0.0002

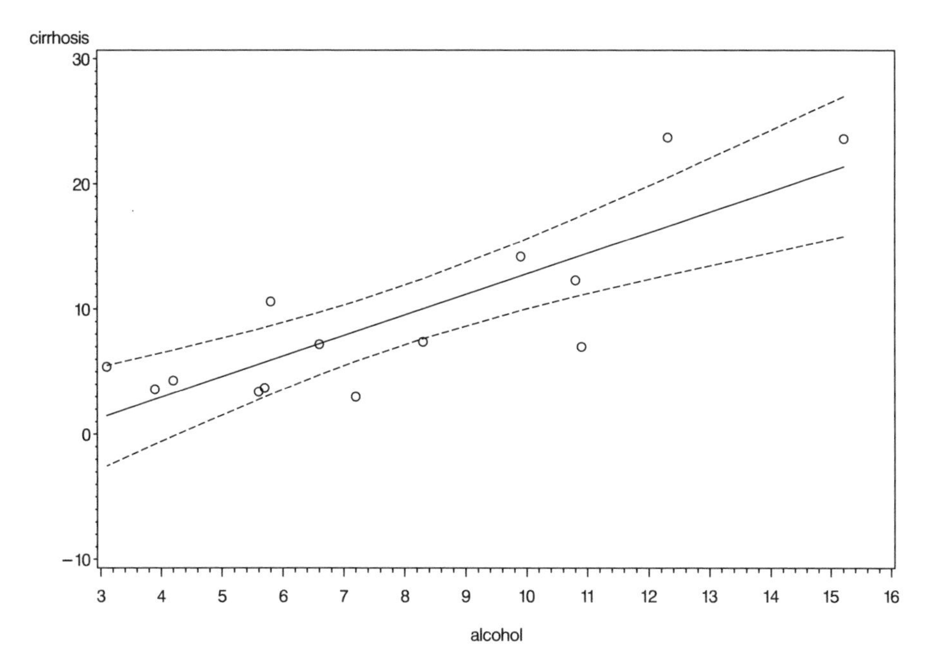

FIGURE 4.14
Scatterplot of death rate from cirrhosis against alcohol consumption showing fitted linear regression and confidence interval.

Parametric regression models are very useful but are not adequate for all data sets. The patterns in many bivariate relationships are too complex to be described by a simple parametric family. An alternative approach to dealing with such data is to fit a curve to the observations *locally,* so that at any point the curve at that point depends only on the observations at that point and some specified neighboring points. Because such a fit produces an estimate of the response that is less variable than the original observed response, the result is often called a *smooth,* and procedures for producing such fits are called *scatterplot smoothers.* A brief description of one such technique, the Lowess fit, is given in Display 4.4.

A lowess curve can be fitted to the alcohol consumption and cirrhosis data in Table 4.1 and then plotted along with the simple refitted regression line on a scatterplot of the data as follows.

```
proc loess data=drinking2;
  model cirrhosis=alcohol /  smooth=.5;
ods output Outputstatistics=lofit;
run;
data both;
```

DISPLAY 4.4

Local Regression Models (Lowess)

- We assume we have observations on a response variable y and an explanatory variable x.
- We assume that y and x are related by

$$y_i = g(x_i) + \varepsilon_i$$

where g is a 'smooth' function and the ε_i are random variables with mean zero and constant scale.
- Fixed values $\hat{y}_i$ are used to estimate the y_i at each x_i by fitting polynomials using weighted least squares with large weights for points near to x_i and small otherwise.
- Two parameters need to be chosen to fit a lowess curve; the first is a smoothing parameter with larger values leading to smoother curves, and the second is the degree of certain polynomials that are fitted by the method.

```
  set regout;
  set lofit;
run;
proc gplot data=both;
  plot (cirrhosis pr pred)*alcohol / overlay;
run;
```

`Proc loess` is used to fit the locally weighted curve. Unlike `proc reg`, `proc loess` does not have an `output` statement, so the fitted values are saved with an `ods output` statement. The two output data sets are combined with a short data step. With more complex data it would be safer to use a `merge` statement, but in this simple example two `set` statements will do. Both fitted lines are then overlaid on the scatter plot. Note that circles are used as the plotting symbols, rather than the default plus, because the symbol definition from the previous example is still active.

The resulting plot is shown in Figure 4.15. There is some deviation of the locally weighted regression line from the simple linear regression fit, but with such a small number of observations this is not convincing evidence that the relationship between death rate and alcohol consumption is not linear.

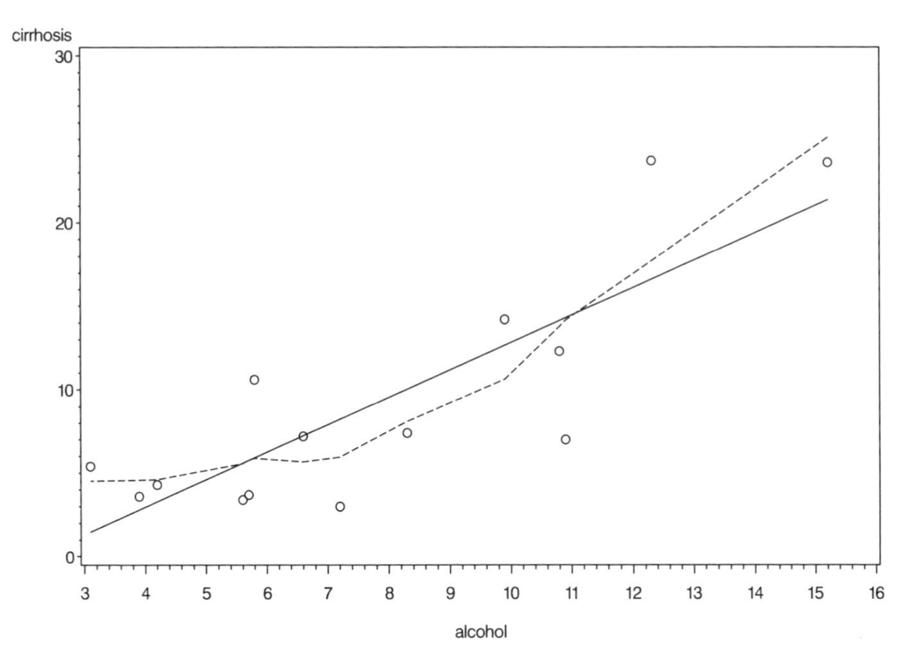

FIGURE 4.15
Scatterplot of death rate against alcohol consumptions showing both the fitted linear regression and the locally weighted regression fit.

4.5 Summary

The scatterplot is the basic tool for exploring bivariate data. From it the form of the relationship between the two variables is often apparent, and this will often indicate what is, and what is not, a sensible model to fit to the data. Other information such as an estimate of the bivariate density or a fitted regression line can often be added to the scatterplot to increase its usefulness. As we shall see in Chapter 7, the scatterplot also forms the basis of other more ambitious graphic procedures for exploring complex data sets.

5

Analysis of Variance and Covariance

5.1 Introduction

This chapter is concerned with the analysis of studies in medicine in which a continuous response variable is observed under the levels of one or more categorical variables (factors). The appropriate statistical procedure for such data is *analysis of variance*. In addition, it is often the case that other continuous variables thought to be associated with the response variable need to be accounted for in any analysis, in which case the relevant methodology is *analysis of covariance.*

5.2 A Simple One-Way Example

The data shown in Table 5.1 are steady-state haemoglobin levels for patients with different types of sickle cell disease: HB SS, HB S/– thalassaemia, and HB SC. One question of interest about these data is whether the steady state haemoglobin levels differ significantly between patients with different types of disease.

The formal procedure for analyzing the data in Table 5.1 is a one-way analysis of variance, described briefly in Display 5.1. Before applying this procedure, however, it will be useful to look at boxplots of the observations available for the three types of sickle cell disease. The necessary SAS code to read in the data and construct the boxplots is

```
data sickle;
  do type=1 to 3;
  input hglevel 5. @;
  if hglevel~=. then output;
  end;
cards;
  7.2  8.1 10.7
```

TABLE 5.1

Sickle Cell Disease

HB SS	HB S/-Thalassaemia	HB SC
7.2	8.1	10.7
7.7	9.2	11.3
8.0	10.0	11.5
8.1	10.4	11.6
8.3	10.6	11.7
8.4	10.9	11.8
8.1	11.1	12.0
8.5	11.9	12.1
8.6	12.0	12.3
8.7	12.1	12.6
9.1		12.6
9.1		13.3
9.1		13.3
9.8		13.8
10.1		13.9
10.3		

Source: Taken with permission from Small Datasets.

```
  7.7  9.2 11.3
  8.0 10.0 11.5
  8.1 10.4 11.6
  8.3 10.6 11.7
  8.4 10.9 11.8
  8.4 11.1 12.0
  8.5 11.9 12.1
  8.6 12.0 12.3
  8.7 12.1 12.6
  9.1      12.6
  9.1      13.3
  9.1      13.3
  9.8      13.8
 10.1      13.9
 10.3
;
proc sort data=sickle;
  by type;
run;
proc boxplot data=sickle;
  plot hglevel*type / boxstyle=schematic;
run;
```

DISPLAY 5.1

One-Way Analysis of Variance

- Let y_{ij} be the jth observation in the ith group. The model assumed is

$$y_{ij} = \mu + \alpha_i + \varepsilon_{ij}$$

where is the overall mean, α_i is the group effect, and ε_{ij} is a random error term, assumed to be normally distributed with mean zero and variance σ^2.
- Because the model is overparameterized, the group effects need to be constrained in some way, most usually by requiring that $\sum_{i=1}^{k} \alpha_i = 0$, where k is the number of groups.
- The hypothesis of the equality of group means can be written in terms of the group effects as

$$H_0 : \alpha_1 = \alpha_2 = \cdots = \alpha_k = 0$$

- The total variation in the observations is partitioned into that due to differences in the group means and that due to differences among observations within groups. Under the hypothesis of the equality of group means, both the between-group variance and the within-group variance are estimates of σ^2. Thus, an F-test of the equality of the two variances provides a test of H_0.
- The necessary terms for the F-test are usually arranged in an analysis of variance table as follows (N is the total number of observations):

Source	**DF**	**SS**	**MS**	**MSR**
Between groups	$k - 1$	$\sum_{i=1}^{k} n_i (\bar{y}_i - \bar{y})^2$	SS/DF(1)	(1)/(2)
Within groups	$N - k$	$\sum_{i=1}^{k} \sum_{j=1}^{n_i} (y_{ij} - \bar{y}_i)^2$	SS/DF(2)	
Total	$N - 1$	$\sum_{i=1}^{k} \sum_{j=1}^{n_i} (y_{ij} - \bar{y}_i)^2$		

where ni is the number of observations in the ith group
- If H_0 is true and the assumptions below are valid, then MSR has an F-distribution with $k - 1$ and $N - k$ degrees of freedom.

DISPLAY 5.1 (continued)

One-Way Analysis of Variance

- The assumptions made in a one-way analysis of variance are as follows:
  - The observations in each group come from a normal distribution.
  - The population variances of each group are the same.
  - The observations are independent of one another.
- In some studies, the interest is not in testing the equality of means but in testing a more specific hypothesis about these means by way of what is generally known as a planned comparison. Such a test can be formulated in terms of testing for the statistical significance of one or more linear combinations of the means, i.e.,

$$H_0 : c_1\mu_1 + c_2\mu_2 + \cdots + c_k\mu_k = 0$$

- When the constants $c_1,\ldots,c_k$ sum to zero this linear combination of the means is known as a *contrast*. An estimate of the contrast is obtained by replacing the population means, $\mu_1,\ldots,\mu_k$, with their sample estimates, $\bar{x}_1,\ldots,\bar{x}_k$.
- Two contrasts with defining coefficients $c_{11},\ldots,c_{1k}$ and $c_{21}, c_{22},\ldots,c_{2k}$ are said to be *orthogonal* if $c_{11}c_{21} + c_{12}c_{22} \cdots + c_{1k}c_{2k} = 0$. Such contrasts can be tested independently of each other.
- The sum of squares for a contrast is given by

$$SS_c = \sum_{i=1}^{k} \left(c_i \bar{y}_i\right)^2 / \left(N \sum_{i=1}^{k} c_i^2 \right)$$

with 1 degree of freedom, and the F-statistic is obtained by dividing this by the within-groups sum of squares.

The data are read using formatted input. Each data value occupies five columns, including the spaces and the decimal point. The trailing @ holds the line for further data to be read from it.

For the `proc boxplot` the data must be sorted in order of the x-axis variable. The resulting diagram is shown in Figure 5.1.

The boxplots show clear evidence of increasing haemoglobin levels from Type HB SS to HB SC and also some suggestion of skewness in the distribution of haemoglobin level in disease types 2 and 3.

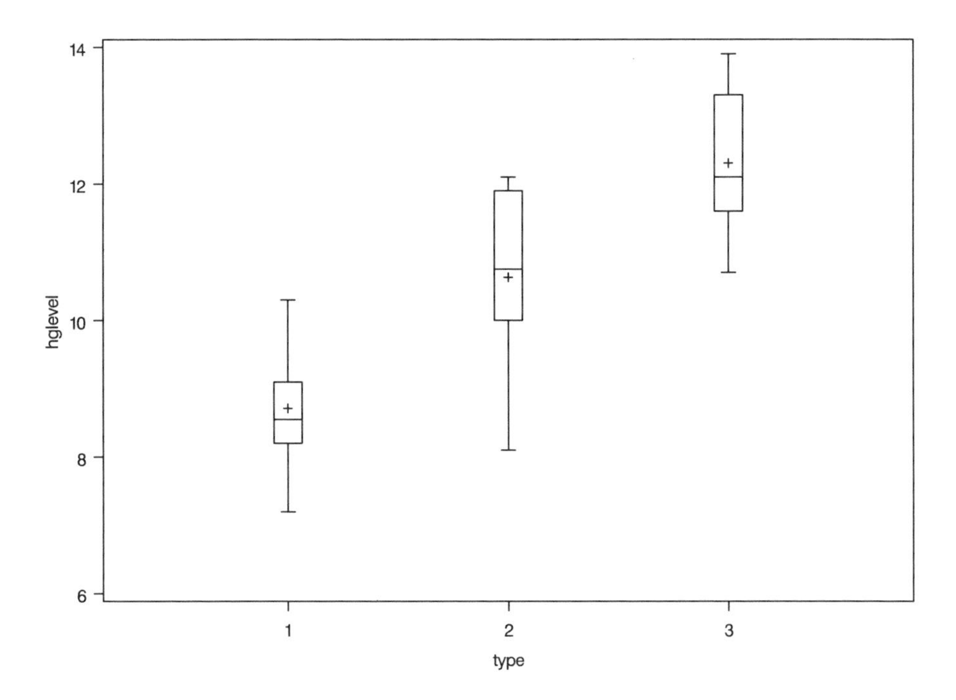

FIGURE 5.1
Boxplots of haemoglobin levels for patients with different types of sickle cell disease: 1 = HB SS, 2 = HB S/-thalassaemia, 3 = HB SC.

A one-way analysis of variance of the data in Table 5.1 can be applied to these data using proc glm with the following SAS code:

```
proc glm data=sickle;
  class type;
  model hglevel=type;
run;
```

`proc glm` can be used to fit the whole class of models that fall within the framework of the *General Linear Model*, including linear regression and analysis of covariance as well as ANOVA. The `class` statement specifies categorical variables, or factors, which may be numeric or character variables. In this example, the `model` statement simply specifies the outcome variable and the single categorical predictor.

The results are given in Table 5.2. The p-value associated with the F statistic for these data is very small and there is clear evidence that there is a difference in the average haemoglobin level in the three disease types. Later in the chapter, we will say more about the Type I and Type III sums of squares that appear in Table 5.2.

TABLE 5.2

One-Way Analysis of Variance of Haemoglobin Levels in Three Types of Sickle Cell Disease

The GLM Procedure

Class Level Information

Class	Levels	Values
type	3	1 2 3

Number of Observations Read	41
Number of Observations Used	41

Dependent Variable: hglevel

Source	DF	Sum of Squares	Mean Square	F Value	Pr > F
Model	2	99.8893049	49.9446524	50.00	<.0001
Error	38	37.9585000	0.9989079		
Corrected Total	40	137.8478049			

R-Square	Coeff Var	Root MSE	hglevel Mean
0.724635	9.525245	0.999454	10.49268

Source	DF	Type I SS	Mean Square	F Value	Pr > F
type	2	99.88930488	49.94465244	50.00	<.0001

Source	DF	Type III SS	Mean Square	F Value	Pr > F
type	2	99.88930488	49.94465244	50.00	<.0001

5.3 Multiple Comparison Procedures

When the F-test in an analysis of variance produces evidence of a difference between the levels of a factor, the investigator usually needs to proceed further to determine both the details of the differences and how large they are. There are two different approaches. One is to carry out a small number of planned comparisons (see Display 5.1) to test a set of specific hypotheses via contrasts. To illustrate this approach we shall assume that in the sickle cell disease example we want to compare the haemoglobin level of the HB SC group with the average haemoglobin level of the other two types and then to compare types I and II with each other. The required contrast coefficients are –1, –1, 2 and 1, –1, 0, respectively. The two contrasts are orthogonal.

`Proc glm` is still running after the previous `proc` step so the sums of squares associated with each contrast can be found simply by submitting the following SAS statements:

```
   contrast '3 vs 1 & 2' type -1 -1 2;
   contrast '1 vs 2'     type  1 -1 0;
run;
```

The `contrast` statement comprises some text in quotes to identify the results in the output, the effect or variable to be used for the contrast, and the values of the contrast coefficients. There is no limit to the number of `contrast` statements that can be used, but they must follow the `model` statement. For some procedures it is possible to submit additional statements in this way, as long as the procedure is still running; this is shown in the title bar of the editor window. A procedure that is still running can be stopped by submitting a `quit` statement.

The results of applying these two contrasts are as follows;

Contrast	DF	Contrast SS	Mean Square	F Value	Pr > F
3 vs 1 & 2	1	64.41	64.41	64.48	<.0001
1 vs 2	1	22.63	22.63	22.65	<.0001

Both are highly significant. The haemoglobin levels of disease types 1 and 2 are different and that of disease type 3 different from the average of types 1 and 2. In this case, of course, the strong evidence of a difference for types 1 and 2 makes the latter test of little real interest.

When the investigator has no *a priori* planned comparisons in mind but would still like to investigate the reasons for a significant overall F statistic, then it is possible to compare *all* pairs of groups, although care is needed because this approach results in a large number of tests if the number of groups is large and the probability of finding at least one pairwise difference when there are no true differences between the groups can become far larger than the nominal significance level being used. Various safeguards against such false-positive findings are needed. The first is to carry out the pairwise tests *only* if the F-test of the ANOVA is significant and to reduce the significance level of the individual pairwise comparisons in an effort to maintain the overall significance level at its intended value. There are many different ways of adjusting the significance levels, resulting in many different *multiple comparison* procedures. All of these procedures produce intervals or bounds for the difference in (usually) one pair of means of the form (estimate) ± (critical point) × (standard error of estimate). The critical point used depends on the specified multiple comparison method. One of the most commonly used is that due to Scheffé (1953); this is described briefly in Display 5.2. To apply this technique we note that `proc glm` is still running so the Scheffé procedure can be applied to the haemoglobin levels in Table 5.1 by submitting a `means` statement with the `scheffe` option as follows;

```
means type / scheffe;
run;
```

DISPLAY 5.2

Scheffé's Multiple Comparison Procedure

- Multiple comparison tests aim to retain the nominal significance level at the required value when undertaking tests of mean differences.
- One such test is due to Scheffé and here the the t-statistic used is

$$t = \frac{\text{mean difference}}{s\left(1/n_1 + 1/n_2\right)^{\frac{1}{2}}}$$

where s^2 is the error mean square and n_1 and n_2 are the number of observations in the two groups being compared.

- Each test-statistic is compared with the critical value

$$\left[\left(k-1\right)F_{k-1,N-k}\left(\alpha\right)\right]^{\frac{1}{2}},$$

where $F_{k-1,N-k}(\alpha)$ is the F-value with $k-1$, $N-k$ degrees of freedom, corresponding to a significance level α. (Details are given by Maxwell and Delaney, 1990.)

- The confidence interval for two means is in this case

$$\text{mean difference} \pm \text{critical value} \times s\left(\frac{1}{n_1} + \frac{1}{n_2}\right)^{\frac{1}{2}}$$

where the critical value is as described above.

The results are shown in Table 5.3 and show that in this case *all* the pairwise comparisons are significant. The haemoglobin levels of each group differ from the other two groups. The confidence intervals quantify the differences.

5.4 A Factorial Experiment

Maxwell and Delaney (1990) report a study designed to investigate the effects of three possible treatments on hypertension. The three treatments were as follows:

TABLE 5.3

Results from Scheffé's Multiple Comparison Test for the Sickle Cell Disease Example

```
                         Scheffé's Test for hglevel

NOTE: This test controls the Type I experimentwise error rate, but it generally has a higher
            Type II error rate than Tukey's for all pairwise comparisons.


                         Alpha                          0.05
                         Error Degrees of Freedom         38
                         Error Mean Square          0.998908
                         Critical Value of F         3.24482

            Comparisons significant at the 0.05 level are indicated by ***.


                               Difference
                    type          Between      Simultaneous 95%
                 Comparison         Means     Confidence Limits

                   3 - 2          1.6700       0.6306    2.7094   ***
                   3 - 1          3.5875       2.6724    4.5026   ***
                   2 - 3         -1.6700      -2.7094   -0.6306   ***
                   2 - 1          1.9175       0.8911    2.9439   ***
                   1 - 3         -3.5875      -4.5026   -2.6724   ***
                   1 - 2         -1.9175      -2.9439   -0.8911   ***
```

1. *Drug medication*: drug X, drug Y, drug Z
2. *Biofeed*: physiological feedback, present or absent
3. *Diet*: present, absent

All 12 combinations of treatments were included in the study. So here we are dealing with a $3 \times 2 \times 2$ design. Six subjects were randomly allocated to each cell of the design, and the response variable measured was blood pressure. The data are given in Table 5.4. The data can be read in as follows;

```
data hyper;
  input n1-n12;
  if _n_<4 then biofeed='P';
           else biofeed='A';
  if _n_ in(1,4) then drug='X';
  if _n_ in(2,5) then drug='Y';
  if _n_ in(3,6) then drug='Z';
  array nall {12} n1-n12;
  do i=1 to 12;
      if i>6 then diet='Y';
         else diet='N';
  bp=nall{i};
  cell=drug||biofeed||diet;
  output;
```

TABLE 5.4

Blood Pressure Data

Biofeedback			No Biofeedback		
Drug X	**Drug Y**	**Drug Z**	**Drug X**	**Drug Y**	**Drug Z**
Diet Absent					
170	186	180	173	189	202
175	194	187	194	194	228
165	201	199	197	217	190
180	215	170	190	206	206
160	219	204	176	199	224
158	209	194	198	195	204
Diet Present					
161	164	162	164	171	205
173	166	184	190	173	199
157	159	183	169	196	170
152	182	156	164	199	160
181	187	180	176	180	179
190	174	173	175	203	179

Source: Maxwell and Delaney, 1990. *Designing Experiments and Analysing Data*. Wadsworth.

```
    end;
    drop i n1-n12;
  cards;
  170 175 165 180 160 158 161 173 157 152 181 190
  186 194 201 215 219 209 164 166 159 182 187 174
  180 187 199 170 204 194 162 184 183 156 180 173
  173 194 197 190 176 198 164 190 169 164 176 175
  189 194 217 206 199 195 171 173 196 199 180 203
  202 228 190 206 224 204 205 199 170 160 179 179
  ;
```

The 12 blood pressure readings per row, or line, of data are read into variables `n1-n12` and used to create 12 separate observations. The row and column positions in the data are used to determine the values of the factors in the design: drug, biofeedback, and diet.

First, the `input` statement reads the 12 blood pressure values into variables `n1` to `n12`. It uses list input, which assumes the data values to be separated by spaces.

The next group of statements use the SAS automatic variable, `_n_`, to determine which row of data is being processed and hence to set the values of `drug` and `biofeed`. Since six lines of data will be read, one line per iteration of the data step, _n_, will increment from 1 to 6 corresponding to the line of data read with the input statement.

The key elements in splitting the one line of data into separate observations are the array, the do loop, and the output statement.

The array statement defines an array by specifying the name of the array, nall here, the number of variables to be included in it in braces, and the list of variables to be included, n1 to n12 in this case.

In SAS an array is a shorthand way of referring to a group of variables. In effect, it provides aliases for them so that each variable can be referred to by using the name of the array and its position within the array in braces. For example, in this data step, n12 could be referred to as nall{12}, or when the variable i has the value 12 as nall{i}. However, the array only lasts for the duration of the data step in which it is defined.

The main purpose of an iterative do loop, like the one used here, is to repeat the statements between the do and the end a fixed number of times, with an index variable changing at each repetition. When used to process each of the variables in an array, the do loop should start with the index variable equal to 1 and end when it equals the number of variables in the array.

Within the do loop, in this example, the index variable, i, is first used to set the appropriate values for diet. Then a variable for the blood pressure reading (bp) is assigned one of the 12 values input. A character variable, cell, is formed by concatenating the values of the drug, biofeed, and diet variables. The double bar operator (||) concatenates character values.

The output statement writes an observation to the output data set with the current value of all variables. An output statement is not normally necessary, since without it an observation is automatically written out at the end of the data step. Putting an output statement within the do loop results in 12 observations being written to the data set.

Finally, the drop statement excludes the index variable i and n1 to n12 from the output data set as they are no longer needed.

As with any relatively complex data manipulation it is wise to check that the results are as they should be, e.g., by using proc print.

As always, before carrying out any formal analysis, it is worth examining the data graphically. One procedure that is often useful in highlighting whether the data should be transformed before analysis is to plot both cell standard deviations against cell means and cell variances against cell means. (The variance should be constant, i.e., independent of the mean.) These plots can be constructed from the following SAS instructions:

```
proc means data=hyper noprint;
  class cell;
  var bp;
  output out=cellmeans mean= std= var= /autoname;
run;
```

```
proc gplot data=cellmeans gout=meangraphs;
  plot (bp_stddev bp_var)*bp_mean;
run;
proc greplay igout=meangraphs nofs;
 tc sashelp.templt;
 template H2;
 treplay 1:1 2:2;
run;
```

`Proc means` is used to calculate the summary statistics and write them out, via the `output` statement, to a new data set, `cellmeans`. The `autoname` option on the `output` statement constructs variable names for the summary statistics and can be useful when summary statistics are being computed for several variables. The `proc gplot` step will produce and display each plot separately, but they are also saved in a graphics catalog, `meangraphs`, with the `gout` option. The saved plots can now be used to produce a graph that contains both plots side by side using `proc greplay` and a graphics template. `Proc greplay` takes as its input the graphics catalog, and the `nofs` option prevents it from entering interactive mode. The `tc` (template catalog) statement specifies the catalog of graphics templates that is supplied with SAS. The names of these templates, which can be viewed with the SAS explorer, indicate the number of panels and their alignment and order. In this example, the `template` statement specifies the `H2` template, which has two horizontally aligned panels. The `treplay` statement then specifies which graph to display in each panel. The panel numbers are the numbers before the colon. The graph identifier follows the colon and can be its name or number. The resulting graph is shown in Figure 5.2.

There appears to be no obvious relationship between the means and the standard deviations or the means and variances that would indicate the need for a transformation. Figure 5.3 shows another example of a multi-panel plot with boxplots of blood pressure for each of the levels of each treatment. The distributions appear to be symmetric, and there is no suggestion of any outliers. The following SAS code was used to produce Figure 5.3.

```
proc sort data=hyper; by drug; run;
proc boxplot data=hyper gout=boxplots;
  plot bp*drug / boxstyle=schematic;
run;
proc sort data=hyper; by diet; run;
proc boxplot data=hyper gout=boxplots;
  plot bp*diet / boxstyle=schematic;
run;
```

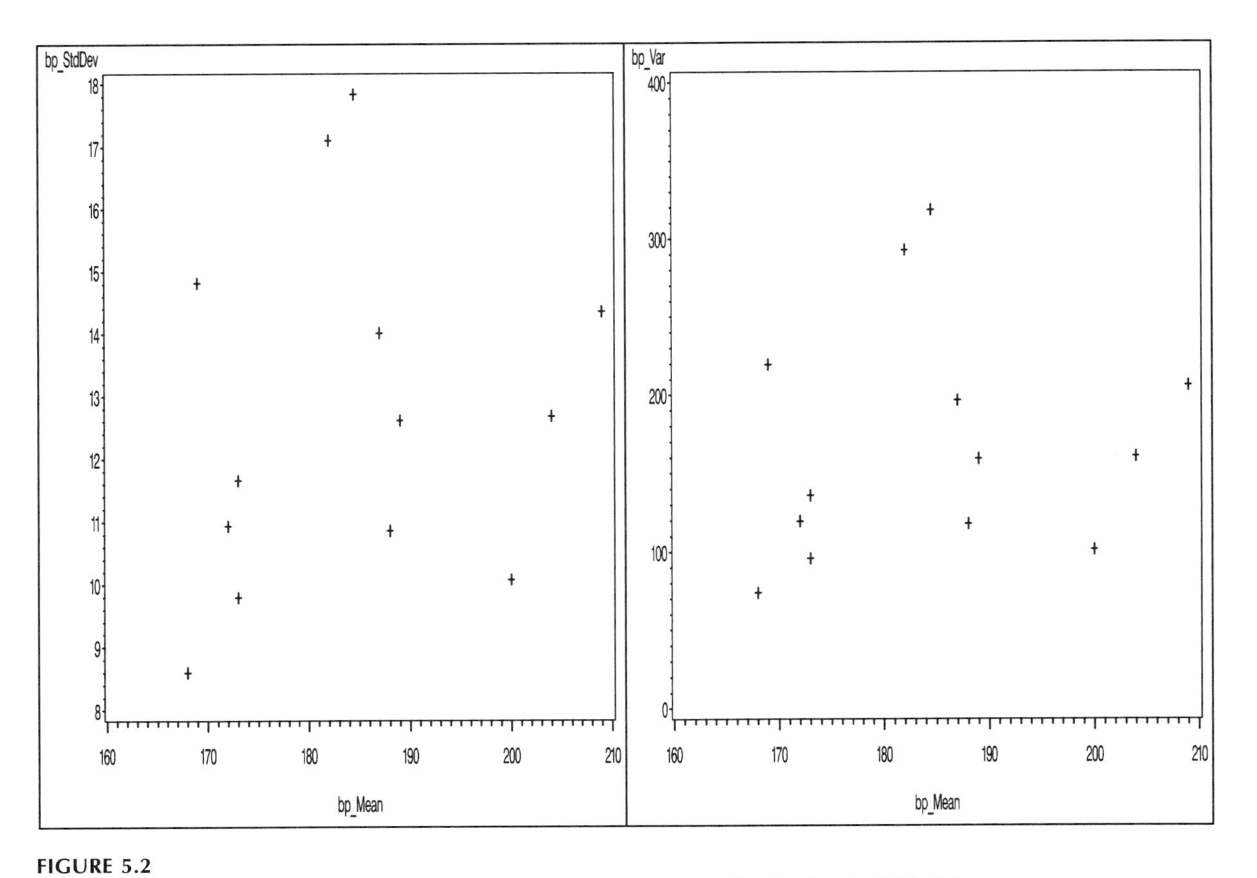

FIGURE 5.2
Plots of means against standard deviations and means against variances for the data in Table 5.4.

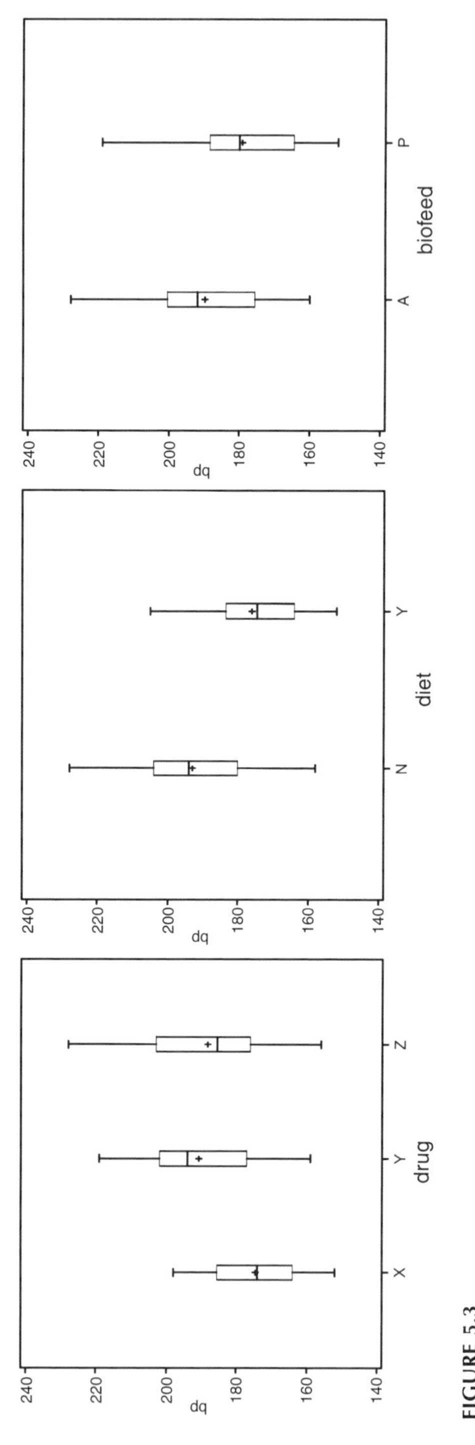

FIGURE 5.3
Boxplots of blood pressure for each treatment level for the data in Table 5.4.

```
proc sort data=hyper; by biofeed; run;
proc boxplot data=hyper gout=boxplots;
  plot bp*biofeed / boxstyle=schematic;
run;
%inc 'c:\sasbook\macros\template.sas';
proc greplay igout=boxplots nofs;
%template(nrows=1,ncols=3);
treplay 1:1 2:2 3:3;
run;
```

The data need to be sorted by the group, or x axis, variable prior to each use of `proc boxplot`. As well as being displayed, the resulting graphs are saved in a graphics catalogue named `boxplots`. These can then be replayed as a single graph, this time using the `template` macro to construct a template with three panels in a row.

A suitable model on which to base the analysis of these data is described in Display 5.3. Here we will use `proc anova`, since the design is balanced although proc glm could be used again.

```
proc anova data=hyper;
  class diet biofeed drug;
  model bp=diet|drug|biofeed;
run;
```

The bar operator used on the model statement is a shorthand way of specifying an interaction and including all the lower order interactions and main effects implied by it. The results are shown in Table 5.5.

Several of the main effects are highly significant, but it is the significant second-order interaction term drug × biofeed × diet that first requires interpretation. Perhaps the simplest approach to trying to understand the meaning of this interaction is to examine the plots of the cell means. Since `proc anova` is still running, the cell means for this interaction can be generated and saved in the `cellmeans2` data set by submitting the following statements:

```
  means diet*drug*biofeed;
ods output means=cellmeans2;
run;
ods output close;
```

The resulting means can be plotted stacked in a multipanel plot as follows.

DISPLAY 5.3

Model for Three-Factor Design

- The model for the observations is

$$y_{ijkl} = \mu + \alpha_i + \beta_j + \gamma_k + \delta_{ij} + \tau_{ik} + \omega_{jk} + \theta_{ijk} + \varepsilon_{ijkl}$$

where α_i, β_j and γ_k represent main effects, δ_{ij}, τ_{ik} and ω_{jk} represent first-order interactions, θ_{ijk} represents the second-order interaction, and ε_{ijkl} are random error terms assumed to be normally distributed with zero mean and variance σ^2. (Once again, the parameters have to be constrained in some way; for details, see Maxwell and Delaney, 1990.)
- The hypothesis of interest can be written in terms of the parameters of the model as

$$H_0^{(1)}: \alpha_1 = \alpha_2 = \cdots = \alpha_a = 0$$

$$H_0^{(2)}: \beta_1 = \beta_2 = \cdots = \beta_b = 0$$

$$H_0^{(3)}: \gamma_1 = \gamma_2 = \cdots = \gamma_c = 0$$

$$H_0^{(4)}: \delta_{11} = \delta_{12} = \cdots = \delta_{ab} = 0$$

$$H_0^{(5)}: \tau_{11} = \tau_{12} = \cdots = \tau_{ac} = 0$$

$$H_0^{(6)}: \omega_{11} = \omega_{12} = \cdots = \omega_{bc} = 0$$

$$H_0^{(6)}: \theta_{111} = \theta_{112} = \cdots = \theta_{abc} = 0$$

where a, b, and c are the numbers of levels of the three factors.
- The analysis of variance table is as follows:

Source	SS	DF	MS
A	ASS	$a-1$	ASS/ $(a-1)$
B	BSS	$b-1$	BSS/ $(b-1)$
C	CSS	$c-1$	CSS/ $(c-1)$
A×B	ABSS	$(a-1)(b-1)$	ABSS/ $(a-1)(b-1)$
A×C	ACSS	$(a-1)(c-1)$	ACSS/ $(a-1)(c-1)$
B×C	BBSS	$(b-1)(c-1)$	ABSS/ $(a-1)(b-1)$
A×B×C	ABCSS	$(a-1)(b-1)(c-1)$	ABSS/ $(a-1)(b-1)(c-1)$
Within cell (error)	WCSS	$abc(n-1)$	WCSS/ $abc(n-1)$

For each term, the *F*-statistic is the ratio of the MS divided by the Error MS.

TABLE 5.5

Analysis of Variance of the Blood Pressure Data in Table 5.4

```
                     The ANOVA Procedure

                   Class Level Information

                 Class         Levels    Values

                 diet               2    N Y

                 biofeed            2    A P

                 drug               3    X Y Z

            Number of Observations Read          72
            Number of Observations Used          72

                     The ANOVA Procedure

Dependent Variable: bp

                                     Sum of
   Source                DF         Squares     Mean Square    F Value    Pr > F

   Model                 11     13194.00000      1199.45455       7.66    <.0001

   Error                 60      9400.00000       156.66667

   Corrected Total       71     22594.00000

             R-Square     Coeff Var      Root MSE      bp Mean

             0.583960      6.784095      12.51666     184.5000

   Source                DF        Anova SS     Mean Square    F Value    Pr > F

   diet                   1     5202.000000     5202.000000      33.20    <.0001
   drug                   2     3675.000000     1837.500000      11.73    <.0001
   diet*drug              2      903.000000      451.500000       2.88    0.0638
   biofeed                1     2048.000000     2048.000000      13.07    0.0006
   diet*biofeed           1       32.000000       32.000000       0.20    0.6529
   biofeed*drug           2      259.000000      129.500000       0.83    0.4425
   diet*biofeed*drug      2     1075.000000      537.500000       3.43    0.0388
```

```
proc sort data=cellmeans2; by drug; run;
symbol1 i=join v=none l=1;
symbol2 i=join v=none l=2;
proc gplot data=cellmeans2 gout=cellmeans2;
  plot mean_bp*biofeed=diet;
  by drug;
run;
goptions rotate=portrait;
proc greplay igout=cellmeans2 nofs;
%template(nrows=3,ncols=1);
treplay 1:1 2:2 3:3;
run;
```

The resulting diagram is shown in Figure 5.4. For drug X, there is a large difference in means between biofeedback being present and absent when

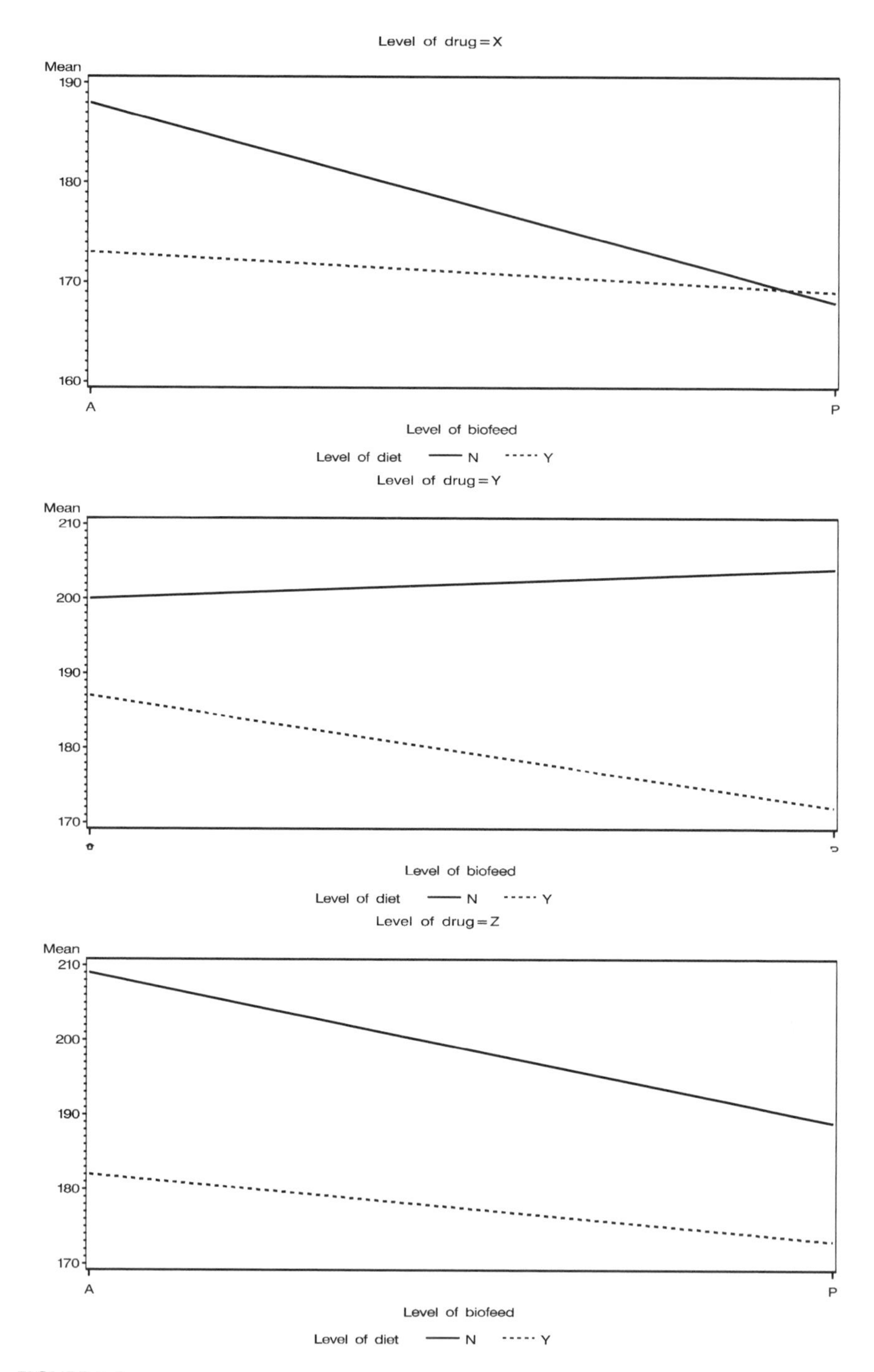

FIGURE 5.4
Diagram of plotted factor level means.

TABLE 5.6

Antipyrine Clearance (Half-Life in Hours)

	1		2		3	
Males	7.4	5.6	3.7	10.9	11.3	13.3
	6.6	6.0		12.2	10.0	
Females	9.1	6.3	7.1	11.0	8.3	
	11.3	9.4	7.9		4.3	

Source: Rifland, A.B. et al., 1976, *Clinical Pharmaceuticals and Therapeutics.*

the diet is not given, but a far smaller difference when the diet is given. For drug Y, the reverse is the case, and for drug Z, the two differences are approximately equal.

5.5 Unbalanced Designs

The data shown in Table 5.6 are from a study reported in Rifland et al. (1976) concerned with antipyrine clearance of people suffering from β– thalassemia, a chronic type of anaemia. In this disease, abnormally thick red blood cells are produced. The treatment of the disease has undesirable side effects, including liver damage. Antipyrine is a drug used to assess liver function, with a high clearance rate indicating satisfactory liver function. The main question of interest is whether there is any difference in clearance rate among the pubertal stages (1 = infant, 2=adolescent, 3 = adult) or between the sexes.

The data in Table 5.6 involve two factors, sex and pubertal stage, but the unbalanced nature of the observations presents considerably more problems for analysis than would a balanced 2 × 3 design. The main difficulty is that when the data are unbalanced, there is no unique way of finding a 'sum of squares' corresponding to each main effect and their interaction, because these effects are no longer independent of one another. (When the data are balanced, the among-cells sums of squares partition orthogonally into the three component sums of squares.) Several methods have been suggested for dealing with this problem, each leading to a different type of sums of squares.

5.5.1 Type I Sums of Squares

These sums of squares represent the effect of adding a term to an existing model, in one particular order. So, for example, a set of Type I sums of squares such as

Source	Type I SS
A	SSA
B	SSB | A
AB	SSAB | A,B

essentially represents a comparison of the following models:

SSAB | A,B	Model including an interaction and main effects with one including only main effects
SSB | A	Model including both main effects, but no interaction, with one including only the main effect of factor A
SSA	Model containing only the A main effect with one containing only the overall mean

The use of these sums of squares in a series of tables in which the effects are considered in different orders (see later) will often provide the most satisfactory way of answering the question as to which model is most appropriate for the observations.

5.5.2 Type II Sums of Squares

These provide sums of squares for a given term given all other terms in the model except terms of higher order involving the term being tested. So, for example, a set of Type II sums of squares for the example in the previous subsection would be

Source	Type II SS
A	SSA | B
B	SSB | A
AB	SSAB | A,B

5.5.3 Type III Sums of Squares

Type III sums of squares represent the contribution of each term to a model including all other possible terms. So, for a two-factor design the sums of squares represent the following:

Source	Type III SS
A	SSA | B,AB
B	SSB | A,AB
AB	SSAB | A,B

(SAS also has a Type IV sum of squares, which is the same as Type III unless the design contains empty cells.)

In a balanced design Type I and Type III sums of squares are equal, but for an unbalanced design they are not, and there have been numerous discussions over which type is most appropriate for the analysis of such designs. Authors such as Maxwell and Delaney (1990) and Howell (1992) strongly recommend the use of Type III sums of squares and these are the default in SAS. Nelder (1977) and Aitkin (1978), however, are strongly critical of 'correcting' main effects sums of squares for an interaction term involving the corresponding main effect; their criticisms are based on both theoretical and pragmatic grounds. The arguments are relatively subtle but in essence go something like this:

- When fitting models to data the principle of *parsimony* is of critical importance. In choosing among possible models we do not adopt complex models for which there is no empirical evidence.
- So if there is no convincing evidence of an AB interaction, we do not retain the term in the model. Thus additivity of A and B is assumed unless there is convincing evidence to the contrary.
- So the argument proceeds that Type III sum of squares for A, in which it is adjusted for AB, makes no sense.
- First, if the interaction term is necessary in the model, then the experimenter will usually wish to consider simple effects of A at each level of B separately. A test of the hypothesis of no A main effect would not usually be carried out if the AB interaction is significant.
- If the AB interaction is not significant then adjusting for it is of no interest and causes a substantial loss of power in testing the A and B main effects.

(The issue does not arise so clearly in the balanced case, for there the sum of squares for A say is independent of whether interaction is assumed or not. Thus in deciding on possible models for the data, the interaction term is not included unless it has been shown to be necessary, in which case tests on main effects involved in the interaction are not carried out, or if carried out not interpreted — see biofeedback example in previous chapter.)

The arguments of Nelder and Aitkin against the use of Type III sums of squares are powerful and persuasive. Their recommendation to use Type I sums of squares (or Type II sums of squares), considering effects in a number of orders, as the most suitable way in which to identify a suitable model for a data set is also convincing and strongly endorsed by the authors of this book.

5.5.4 Analysis of Antipyrine Data

We first read in the data and then apply proc glm using the following SAS code;

```
data antipyrine;
input sex$ stage hours;
cards;
M 1 7.4
M 1 5.6
. . . .
F 2 11.0
```

TABLE 5.7

Analysis of Variance Results for Antipyrine Data

Source	DF	Type I SS	Mean Square	F Value	Pr > F
sex	1	0.75789474	0.75789474	0.13	0.7289
stage	2	9.59433511	4.79716755	0.79	0.4727
sex*stage	2	46.31816489	23.15908245	3.83	0.0491
Source	**DF**	**Type II SS**	**Mean Square**	**F Value**	**Pr > F**
sex	1	0.43508511	0.43508511	0.07	0.7926
stage	2	9.59433511	4.79716755	0.79	0.4727
sex*stage	2	46.31816489	23.15908245	3.83	0.0491
Source	**DF**	**Type III SS**	**Mean Square**	**F Value**	**Pr > F**
sex	1	4.13281250	4.13281250	0.68	0.4231
stage	2	6.00213652	3.00106826	0.50	0.6196
sex*stage	2	46.31816489	23.15908245	3.83	0.0491

```
F 3 8.3
F 3 4.3
;
proc glm data=antipyrine;
  class sex stage;
  model hours=sex|stage / ss1 ss2 ss3;
run;
```

The default for proc glm is to produce both Type I and Type III sums of squares. Here we specify Type II sums of squares as well. The results are given in Table 5.7. Note the different values for the sums of squares attached to each effect, apart from the interaction term. There is some evidence of a sex x stage interaction in the data — the p-value for the associated F test is 0.049. A plot of the six means may be helpful in interpreting this interaction. Such a plot can be obtained using the following SAS code:

```
  means sex*stage;
  ods output means=antmns;
run;
  ods output close;
proc gplot data=antmns;
  plot mean_hours*stage=sex;
  symbol1 i=join l=1;
  symbol2 i=join l=2;
run;
```

The resulting plot is shown in Figure 5.5. Clearly for males the clearance rate increases with age, but for females, it decreases, at first gradually and then between adolescence and adult stages, more dramatically.

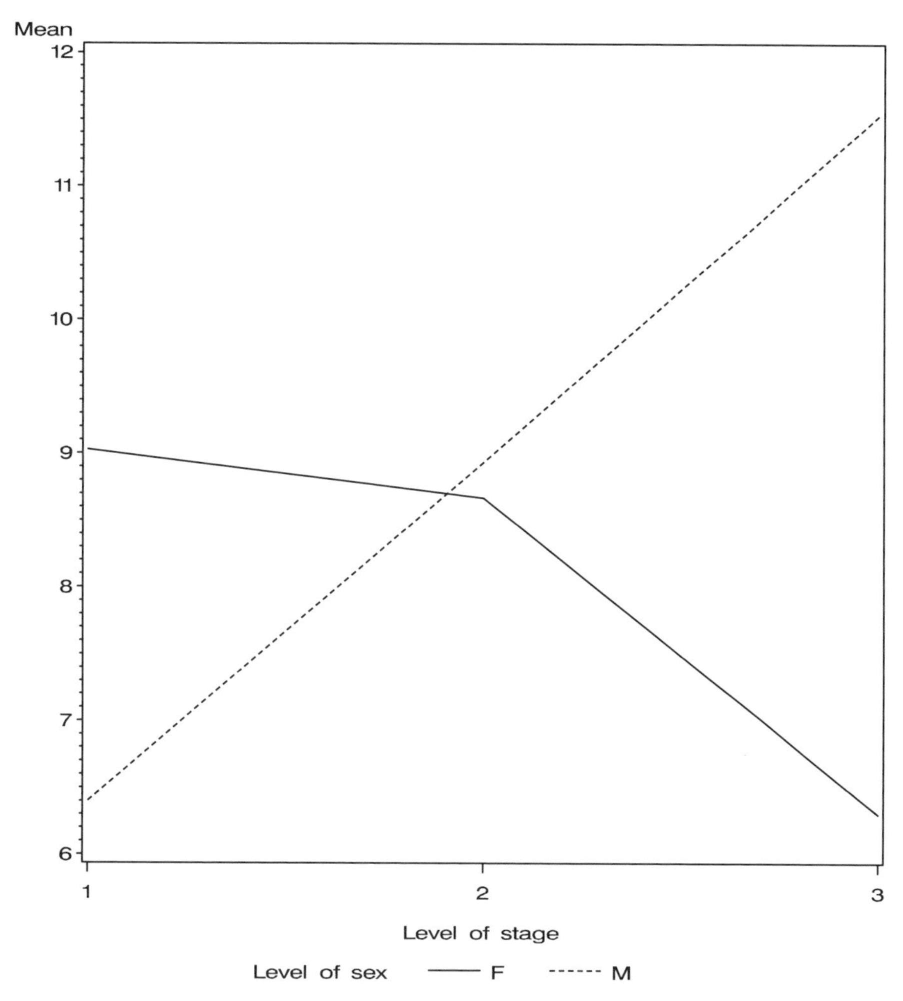

FIGURE 5.5
Plot of mean clearance rate for the three stages and for males and females.

5.6 Nonparametric Analysis of Variance

Although the F-tests used in the analysis of variance are reasonably robust against departures from normality, there may be occasions where the departure is thought to be so extreme that some alternative method of analysis may be required.

To illustrate we shall use the data shown in Table 5.8. These data were collected by Kontula et al. (1980) in a study attempting to develop a more accurate method for determining the number of glucocortical receptor (GR) sites per cell in patients suffering from leukemia. The new methodology was

TABLE 5.8

Number of Glucocorticoid Receptor (GR) Sites per Leukocyte Cell

Normal Subjects	Hairy-Cell Leukemia	Chronic Lymphatic Leukemia	Chronic Myelocytic Leukemia	Acute Leukemia
3500	5,710	2390	6,320	3,230
3500	6,110	3330	6,860	3,880
3500	8,060	3580	11,400	7,640
4000	8,080	3880	14,000	7,890
4000	11,400	4280		8,280
4000		5120		16,200
4300				18,250
4500				29,900
4500				
4900				
5200				
6000				
6750				
8000				

Source: Kontula, K. et al., 1980, *International Journal of Cancer.*

used to count the number of GR sites for samples of leukocyte cells from normal subjects as well as patients with hairy-cell leukemia, chronic lymphatic leukemia, chronic myelocytic leukemia, or acute leukemia.

Rather than use the analysis of variance procedure described in Display 5.1 on these data, we shall use the Kruskal and Wallis distribution-free procedure for one-way designs (see Display 5.4).

The necessary SAS code to read in the data and apply the Kruskal–Wallis procedure is

```
data leukemia;
input group$ ngrs;
cards;
N 3500
N 3500
...
A 16200
A 18250
A 29900
;
proc npar1way data=leukemia wilcoxon;
  class group;
  var ngrs;
run;
```

DISPLAY 5.4

Kruskal–Wallis Distribution-Free Procedure for One-Way Designs

- Assume there are k populations to be compared and that a sample of n_j observations is available from population $j, j = 1,\ldots,k$.
- The hypothesis to be tested is that all the populations have the same probability distribution.
- For the Kruskal–Wallis test to be performed, the observations are first ranked without regard to group membership and then the sums of the ranks of the observations in each group are calculated. These sums will be denoted by $R_1, R_2,\ldots,R_k$.
- If the null hypothesis is true, we would expect the R_js to be more or less equal, apart from differences caused by the different sample sizes.
- A measure of the degree to which the R_js differ from one another is given by

$$H = \frac{12}{N(N+1)} \sum_{j=1}^{k} \frac{R_j^2}{n_j} - 3(N+1)$$

where

- Under the null hypothesis the statistic H has a chi-squared distribution with $k - 1$ degrees of freedom.

By default `proc npar1way` produces analyses based on a number of different rank scoring methods. The `wilcoxon` option restricts it to Wilcoxon scores (i.e., rank sums) and the associated Kruskal–Wallis test. The results are shown in Table 5.9.

The p-value associated with the chi-square test statistic is 0.0022, and so there is strong evidence that the average number of GR sites in the leukocyte cells of the five groups of subjects differ.

5.7 Analysis of Covariance

Analysis of covariance (ANCOVA) is essentially analysis of variance in which differences between levels of a factor are tested, after controlling for other variables, termed covariates. The response variable and the covariate

TABLE 5.9

Results of Kruskal–Wallis Procedure for the Data in Table 5.8

The NPAR1WAY Procedure

Wilcoxon Scores (Rank Sums) for Variable ngrs
Classified by Variable group

Group	N	Sum of Scores	Expected Under H0	Std Dev Under H0	Mean Score
N	14	202.00	266.0	31.911394	14.428571
H	5	133.50	95.0	22.494577	26.700000
C	6	50.50	114.0	24.253494	8.416667
M	4	114.50	76.0	20.431714	28.625000
A	8	202.50	152.0	27.087058	25.312500

Average scores were used for ties.

Kruskal-Wallis Test

Chi-Square	16.6682
DF	4
Pr > Chi-Square	0.0022

are assumed to be related in some way, and from the estimated relationship, the subject's response values are adjusted in an attempt to account for factor level differences in the covariates. Following this adjustment, the usual analysis-of-variance tests are applied to see whether there remains any difference in average response in the different factor levels. For a single factor design and a single covariate, the appropriate model is described in Display 5.5.

DISPLAY 5.5

Analysis of Covariance

- The model assumed is

$$y_{ij} = \mu + \alpha_i + \beta(x_{ij} - \bar{x}) + \varepsilon_{ij}$$

where β is the regression coefficient linking response variable and covariate and $\bar{x}$ is the grand mean of the covariate values.

- NB: The regression coefficient is assumed to be the same in each group.
- The means of the response variable adjusted for the covariate are obtained simply as

$$\text{adjusted group mean} = \text{group mean } + \hat{\beta}(\bar{x}_i - \bar{x})$$

where $\bar{x}_i$ is the mean of the ith group.

TABLE 5.10

Plasma Inorganic Phosphate Levels from 13 Control and 20 Obese Patients

	Hours after Glucose Challenge		
Group	**Patient**	**0**	**3**
Control	1	4.3	2.5
	2	3.7	3.2
	3	4.0	3.1
	4	3.6	3.9
	5	4.1	3.4
	6	3.8	3.6
	7	3.8	3.4
	8	4.4	3.8
	9	5.0	3.6
	10	3.7	2.3
	11	3.7	2.2
	12	4.4	4.3
	13	4.7	4.2
Obese	1	4.3	2.5
	2	5.0	4.1
	3	4.6	4.2
	4	4.3	3.1
	5	3.1	1.9
	6	4.8	3.1
	7	3.7	3.6
	8	5.4	3.7
	9	3.0	26
	10	4.9	4.1
	11	4.8	3.7
	12	4.4	3.4
	13	4.9	4.1
	14	5.1	4.2
	15	4.8	4.0
	16	4.2	3.1
	17	6.6	3.8
	18	3.6	2.4
	19	4.5	2.3
	20	4.6	3.6

Source: Davis, C.S., 2002, *Statistical Methods for the Analysis of Repeated Measurements*, Springer. With permission.

As an illustration of analysis of covariance, the method will be applied to the data shown in Table 5.10. These data show plasma inorganic phosphate measurements obtained from 13 controls and 20 obese patients taken 10 minutes and 3 hours after an oral glucose challenge (data adapted from Zerbe, 1979). Here interest centres on whether there is a difference in average plasma inorganic phosphate level between the control and obese patient populations 3 hours after the challenge after controlling for the difference after 10 minutes.

Before applying analysis of covariance, it will be helpful to examine the data graphically. Here we can plot a scattergram of 10-minute level against 3-hour level, identifying control and obese patients and also showing the simple linear regression line for the two variables, calculated separately in each group. The required SAS code is

```
data pip;
 input pip1 pip2;
 group='C';
 if _n_>13 then group='O';
cards;
4.3     2.5
3.7     3.2
...
3.6     2.4
4.5     2.3
4.6     3.6
;
symbol1 i=rl v=dot;
symbol2 i=rl v=circle L=2;
proc gplot data=pip;
  plot pip2*pip1=group;
run;
```

The data step reads in the two plasma inorganic phosphate measurements. We know that the first 13 observations belong to control subjects and the remainder to obese subjects and so we can use the automatic SAS variable _n_ to assign values to a group variable. The two symbol statements use regression interpolation with a linear fit (quadratic and cubic fits are also possible), and the second uses a different linetype (L=2). The resulting diagram is shown in Figure 5.6.

Figure 5.6 gives little evidence that the regression lines of each group of patients differ in slope, which is reassuring since this is one of the assumptions of the analysis of covariance as outlined in Display 5.5.

Analysis of covariance can be applied to the data using proc glm.

```
proc glm data=pip;
  class group;
  model pip2=pip1 group pip1*group;
```

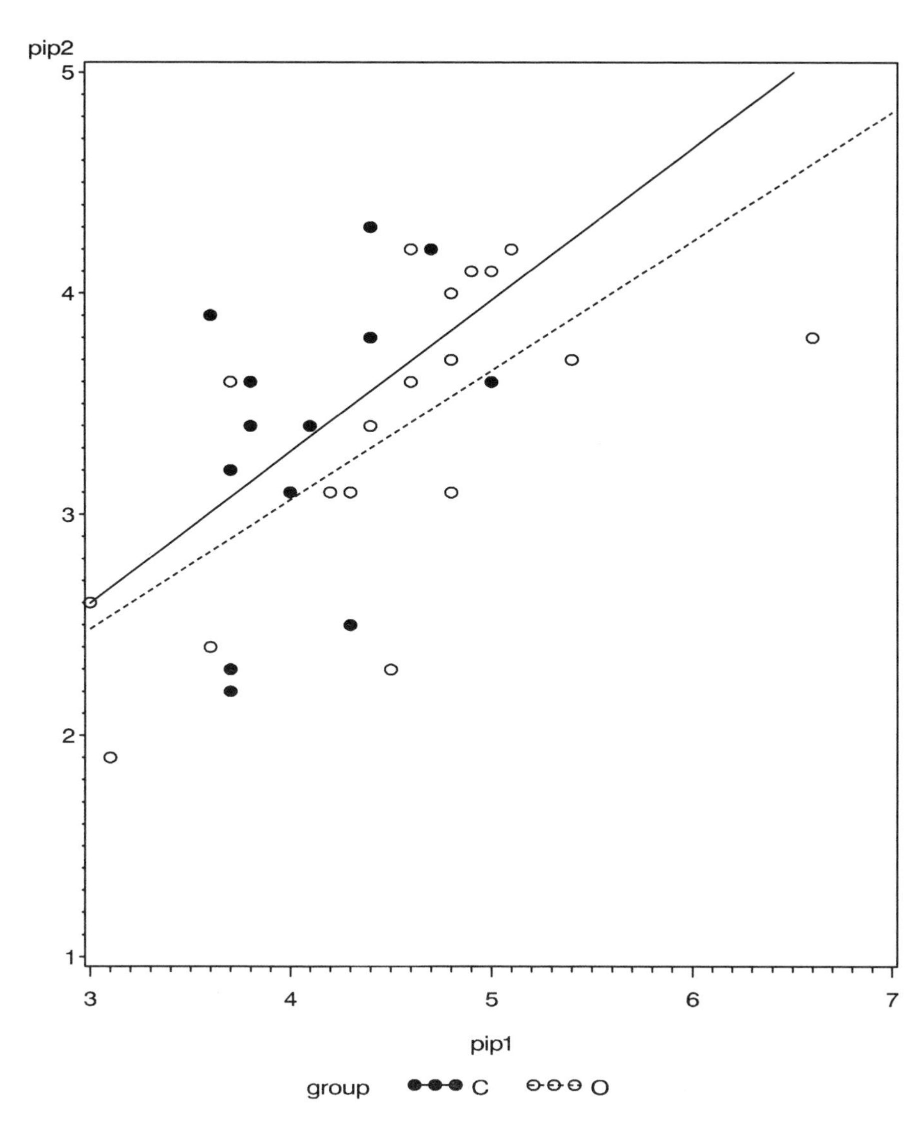

FIGURE 5.6
Plot of the data in Table 5.10.

```
run;
```

As the variable `pip1` is not mentioned on the `class` statement, it is assumed to be continuous. The results are shown in Table 5.11.

Using the Type I sums of squares in Table 5.11, we can conclude that the regression coefficient of the 3-hour phosphate measurement on the 10-minute measurement is significantly different from zero and that after adjusting for the 10-minute level there is no difference between the control and obese patients. The p value of the F statistic for the interaction demonstrates

TABLE 5.11

Analysis of Covariance for the Data in Table 5.10

```
                              The GLM Procedure
                           Class Level Information
                        Class          Levels    Values
                        group               2    C O
                   Number of Observations Read          33
                   Number of Observations Used          33
Dependent Variable: pip2
                                          Sum of
      Source                     DF       Squares     Mean Square    F Value    Pr > F
      Model                       3    5.28062622      1.76020874       5.15    0.0056
      Error                      29    9.91573742      0.34192198
      Corrected Total            32   15.19636364
                    R-Square     Coeff Var      Root MSE     pip2 Mean
                    0.347493      17.38419      0.584741      3.363636
      Source                     DF     Type I SS     Mean Square    F Value    Pr > F
      pip1                        1    4.86961807      4.86961807      14.24    0.0007
      group                       1    0.39083650      0.39083650       1.14    0.2938
      pip1*group                  1    0.02017164      0.02017164       0.06    0.8098
      Source                     DF   Type III SS     Mean Square    F Value    Pr > F
      pip1                        1    3.13693492      3.13693492       9.17    0.0051
      group                       1    0.00398906      0.00398906       0.01    0.9147
      pip1*group                  1    0.02017164      0.02017164       0.06    0.8098
```

that there is no evidence of a difference in the regression slopes of 3-hour value on 10-minute level in the two groups.

5.8 Summary

In this chapter, we have described a number of simple analyses of variance procedures. As we shall see later in Chapter 6, analyses of variance models can be formulated in linear regression terms and are further subsumed under a more general approach, known as *generalized linear models*, to be discussed in Chapter 8.

6

Multiple Regression

6.1 Introduction

Multiple linear regression represents a generalization to more than a single explanatory variable of the simple linear regression model introduced in Chapter 4. The main aim of this type of regression is to model the relationship between a random response variable and a number of explanatory variables. Strictly speaking, the values of the explanatory variable are assumed to be known or under the control of the investigator; in other words, they are not considered to be random variables. In most applications of multiple regression, however, the observed values of the explanatory variables will, like the response variable, be subject to random variation. Parameter estimation and inference are then considered conditional on the observed values of the explanatory variables.

6.2 The Multiple Linear Regression Model

The multiple linear regression model relates a response variable to a set of explanatory variables. The relationship assumed is linear (in terms of the parameters rather than in terms of the explanatory variables), and the parameters in the model (usually known as *regression coefficients*) are generally estimated by least squares. An inferential framework is added by making specific distributional assumptions about the error terms in the model. Details of the structure of the model are given in Display 6.1, and estimation and testing are described in Display 6.2.

DISPLAY 6.1

The Multiple Regression Model

- Assume y_i represents the value of the response variable on the *i*th individual, and that $x_{i1}, x_{i2}, \ldots, x_{ip}$ represent the individual's values on p explanatory variables, with $i = 1, 2 \cdots n$.
- The multiple linear regression model is given by

$$y_i = \beta_0 + \beta_1 x_{i1} + \cdots + \beta_p x_{ip} + \varepsilon_i$$

- The residual or error terms $\varepsilon_i, i = 1, \cdots, n$ are assumed to be independent random variables having a normal distribution with mean zero and constant variance σ^2.
- Consequently, the distribution of the random response variable, y, is also normal with expected value.

$$E(y \mid x_1, x_2, \cdots, x_p) = \beta_0 + \beta_1 x_1 + \cdots + \beta_p x_p$$

and variance σ^2.

- The parameters of the model $\beta_k, k = 1, 2, \cdots, p$ are known as *regression coefficients*. They represent the expected change in the response variable associated with a unit change in the corresponding explanatory variable, when the remaining explanatory variables are held constant.
- The 'linear' in multiple linear regression applies to the regression parameters, not to the response or explanatory variables. Consequently, models in which, for example, the logarithm of a response variable is modeled in terms of quadratic functions of some of the explanatory variables would be included in this class of models. (See also Chapter 10.)
- The multiple regression model can be written most conveniently for all n individuals by using matrices and vectors as

$$\mathbf{y} = \mathbf{X}\beta + \boldsymbol{\varepsilon}$$

where $\mathbf{y}' = [y_1, y_2, \ldots, y_n]$, $\beta' = [\beta_0, \beta_1, \ldots, \beta_p]$, $\boldsymbol{\varepsilon}' = [\varepsilon_1, \varepsilon_2, \ldots, \varepsilon_n]$ and

$$\mathbf{X} = \begin{bmatrix} 1 & x_{11} & x_{12} & \cdots & x_{1p} \\ 1 & x_{21} & x_{22} & \cdots & x_{2p} \\ \vdots & \vdots & \vdots & \vdots & \vdots \\ 1 & x_{n1} & x_{n2} & \cdots & x_{np} \end{bmatrix}$$

DISPLAY 6.1 (continued)

The Multiple Regression Model

- Each row in **X** (sometimes known as the *design matrix*) represents the values of the explanatory variables for one of the individuals in the sample, with the addition of unity to take account of the parameter β_0.

DISPLAY 6.2

Estimation and Testing in Multiple Regression

- Assuming that **X'X** is nonsingular, (i.e., can be inverted), then the least squares estimator of the parameter vector β is

$$\hat{\beta} = \left(\mathbf{X'X}\right)^{-1}\mathbf{X'y}$$

- This estimator $\hat{\beta}$ has the following properties

$$E\left(\hat{\beta}\right) = \beta$$

$$\mathrm{cov}\left(\hat{\beta}\right) = \sigma^2\left(\mathbf{X'X}\right)^{-1}$$

- The diagonal elements of the matrix cov $\left(\hat{\beta}\right)$ give the variances of the $\hat{\beta}_j$, whereas the off-diagonal elements give the covariances between pairs $\hat{\beta}_j, \hat{\beta}_k$. The square roots of the diagonal elements of the matrix are thus the standard errors of the $\hat{\beta}_j$.
- The regression analysis can be assessed using the following analysis of variance table.

Source of Variation	Sum of Squares	Degrees of Freedom	Mean Square
Regression	$\sum_{i=1}^{n}\left(\hat{y}_i - \bar{y}\right)^2$	p	MSR = SS/df
Residual	$\sum_{i=1}^{n}\left(y_i - \hat{y}_i\right)^2$	$n - p - 1$	MSE = SS/df
Total	$\sum_{i=1}^{n}\left(y_i - \bar{y}\right)^2$	$n - 1$	

DISPLAY 6.2 (continued)

Estimation and Testing in Multiple Regression

where $\hat{y}_i$ is the predicted value of the response variable for the ith individual and $\bar{y}$ is the mean value of the response variable.

- The mean square ratio MSR/MSE provides an F-test of the general hypothesis

$$H_0 : \beta_1 = \beta_2 = \cdots = \beta_p = 0$$

- An estimate of σ^2 is provided by s^2 given by

$$s^2 = \frac{1}{n-p-1}\sum_{i=1}^{n}\left(y_i - \hat{y}_1\right)^2$$

- Under H_0, the mean square ratio has an F-distribution with $p, n-p-1$ degrees of freedom.
- The correlation between the observed values y_i and the predicted values $\hat{y}_i, R$ is known as the multiple correlation coefficient. The value of R^2 gives the proportion of variance of the response variable accounted for by the explanatory variables.
- Individual regression coefficients can be assessed by using the ratio $\hat{\beta}_j / SE\left(\hat{\beta}_j\right)$, although these ratios should only be used as rough guides to the 'significance' or otherwise of the coefficients, for reasons discussed in the text.

6.2.1 Anesthesia Example

As a first illustration of the application of the multiple regression model, it will be applied to the data shown in Table 6.1, which arise from a study reported in Cullen and van Belle (1975), dealing with the amount of anesthetic agent administered during an operation. The variables involved are as follows:

- Response variable y: percentage depression of lymphocyte transformation following anesthesia
- Explanatory variable x_1: duration of anesthesia (in hours)
- Explanatory variable x_2: trauma factor rated on a five-point scale

TABLE 6.1
Duration of Anesthetic Data

Duration	Trauma	Depression
4.0	3	36.7
6.0	3	51.3
1.5	2	40.8
4.0	2	58.3
2.5	2	42.2
3.0	2	34.6
3.0	2	77.8
2.5	2	17.2
3.0	3	–38.4
3.0	3	1.0
2.0	3	53.7
8.0	3	14.3
5.0	4	65.0
2.0	2	5.6
2.5	2	4.4
2.0	2	1.6
1.5	2	6.2
1.0	1	12.2
3.0	3	29.9
4.0	3	74.1
3.0	3	11.5
3.0	3	19.8
7.0	4	64.9
6.0	4	47.8
2.0	2	35.0
4.0	2	1.7
2.0	2	51.5
1.0	1	20.2
1.0	1	–9.3
2.0	1	13.9
1.0	1	–19.0
3.0	1	–2.3
4.0	3	41.6
8.0	4	18.4
2.0	2	9.9

Source: Cullen, B.F. and van Belle, G., 1975, *Anesthesiology*.

The multiple regression model can be fitted using the following SAS code:

```
data anasthetic;
  input duration trauma dlt;
cards;
4.0336.7
6.0351.3
...
4.0341.6
```

TABLE 6.2

Results of Applying a Multiple Regression Model to the Anesthesia Data in Table 6.1

The REG Procedure
Model: MODEL1
Dependent Variable: dlt

Analysis of Variance

Source	DF	Sum of Squares	Mean Square	F Value	Pr > F
Model	2	4163.43495	2081.71747	3.19	0.0547
Error	32	20901	653.17162		
Corrected Total	34	25065			

Root MSE	25.55722	R-Square	0.1661
Dependent Mean	25.54571	Adj R-Sq	0.1140
Coeff Var	100.04505		

Parameter Estimates

Variable	DF	Parameter Estimate	Standard Error	t Value	Pr > |t|
Intercept	1	-2.50201	12.34502	-0.20	0.8407
duration	1	1.11313	3.60534	0.31	0.7595
trauma	1	10.31859	7.42995	1.39	0.1745

```
8.0418.4
2.029.9
;
proc reg data=anasthetic;
  model dlt=duration trauma;
run;
```

The output is shown in Table 6.2. Here, the F-test that the regression coefficients β_1 and β_2 are both zero has an associated p-value of 0.055, and the t-statistics given by the ratios of the estimated regression coefficients to their estimated standard errors have associated p-values of 0.76 and 0.17. It appears that neither duration of anesthesia nor degree of trauma are useful for predicting percentage of depression of lymphocyte transformation following anaesthesia although jointly they do approach significance at the 5% level. The R-squared value of just 0.17 underlines that the two explanatory variables have little predictive power for the response variable, accounting as they do for only 17% of the variance in the latter. The number of observations in this example is, however, rather small, and so inferences are not particularly powerful.

6.2.2 Mortality and Water Hardness

The data in Table 6.3 were collected in an investigation of environmental causes of disease. They show the annual mortality rate per 100,000 for males, averaged over the years 1958 to 1964, and the calcium concentration (in parts per million) in the drinking water supply for 61 large towns in England and

TABLE 6.3

Mortality and Water Hardness

Town	Mortality per 100,000	Calcium (ppm)
S	1247	105
N	1668	17
S	1466	5
N	1800	14
N	1609	18
N	1558	10
N	1807	15
S	1299	78
N	1637	10
S	1359	84
S	1392	73
S	1519	21
N	1755	12
S	1307	78
S	1254	96
N	1491	20
N	1555	39
N	1428	39
S	1318	122
S	1260	21
N	1723	44
N	1379	94
N	1742	8
N	1574	9
N	1569	91
S	1096	138
N	1591	16
S	1402	n
N	1702	44
S	1581	14
S	1309	59
S	1259	133
N	1427	27
N	1724	6
S	1175	107
S	1486	5
S	1456	90
N	1696	6
S	1236	101
N	1711	13
N	1444	14
N	1591	49
N	1987	8
N	1495	14
S	1369	68
S	1257	50
N	1587	75
N	1713	71
N	1557	13
N	1640	57

TABLE 6.3 (continued)

Mortality and Water Hardness

Town	Mortality per 100,000	Calcium (ppm)
N	1709	71
S	1625	13
N	1625	20
S	1527	60
S	1627	53
S	1486	122
N	1772	15
N	1828	8
N	1704	26
S	1485	81
N	1378	71

Wales. (The higher the calcium concentration, the harder the water.) Towns at least as far north as Derby are identified in Table 6.3. The questions of interest for these data are whether water hardness is predictive of mortality, and whether there is a geographical factor in the relationship.

In this example one of the explanatory variables is binary (North/South), making the multiple regression model equivalent to the analysis of covariance model encountered in Chapter 5. The presence of the categorical variable raises no real problems in the multiple regression model since no distributional assumptions are made about the explanatory variables (strictly they are not considered to be random variables). However, `proc reg` expects all variables to be numeric, so the character variable `location` is recoded into a 0/1 numeric variable `region` in the data step, as follows.

```
data water;
  input location$ mortality calcium;
  if location='N' then region=1;
     else region=0;
cards;
S 1247  105
N 1668  17
...
N 1486  122
S 1485  81
N 1378  71
;
proc reg data=water;
  model mortality= calcium region;
run;
```

TABLE 6.4

Results from Fitting the Multiple Regression Model to the Water Hardness Data in Table 6.3

```
                           The REG Procedure
                             Model: MODEL1
                    Dependent Variable: mortality

                         Analysis of Variance

                                   Sum of          Mean
Source                   DF       Squares        Square    F Value    Pr > F

Model                     2        914803        457402      22.14    <.0001
Error                    58       1198371         20662
Corrected Total          60       2113174

             Root MSE             143.74130    R-Square     0.4329
             Dependent Mean      1524.14754    Adj R-Sq     0.4133
             Coeff Var              9.43093

                         Parameter Estimates

                            Parameter      Standard
        Variable     DF      Estimate         Error    t Value    Pr > |t|

        Intercept     1    1660.82438      38.01682      43.69      <.0001
        calcium       1      -3.19101       0.49016      -6.51      <.0001
        region        1      24.18383      37.44636       0.65      0.5209
```

The results of this analysis are shown in Table 6.4.

The test for all regression coefficients being zero has an associated *p*-value less than 0.0001. Clearly at least one of the regression coefficients differs from zero. Examination of the *t*-statistics for the individual regression coefficients suggests that it is calcium concentration that is of greatest importance in predicting mortality rate. The R^2 value is 0.43, so that together the two explanatory variables account for over 40% of the variation in mortality rates.

It is of interest here to show the fitted model graphically. This requires the following statements:

```
plot p.*calcium=region;
run;
```

Chapter 4 introduced the `plot` statement within `proc reg`. This example illustrates one of the keywords that can be used. Each ends with a period (here `p.` is an abbreviation for `predicted.` or `pred.`), and there is a wide range of diagnostic and model fit statistics available. The resulting diagram is shown in Figure 6.1 and consists of a scatterplot of mortality and calcium concentration showing the fitted *parallel* regression lines (i.e., with equal slopes) for the two regions assumed in this model.

A more complex model that might be considered for these data is one that allows for a possible interaction between location and hardness. Unlike `proc glm`, `proc reg` does not allow interactions to be specified on the `model` statement in the form `region*calcium`. Instead a separate variable needs to be calculated to represent the interaction, as follows:

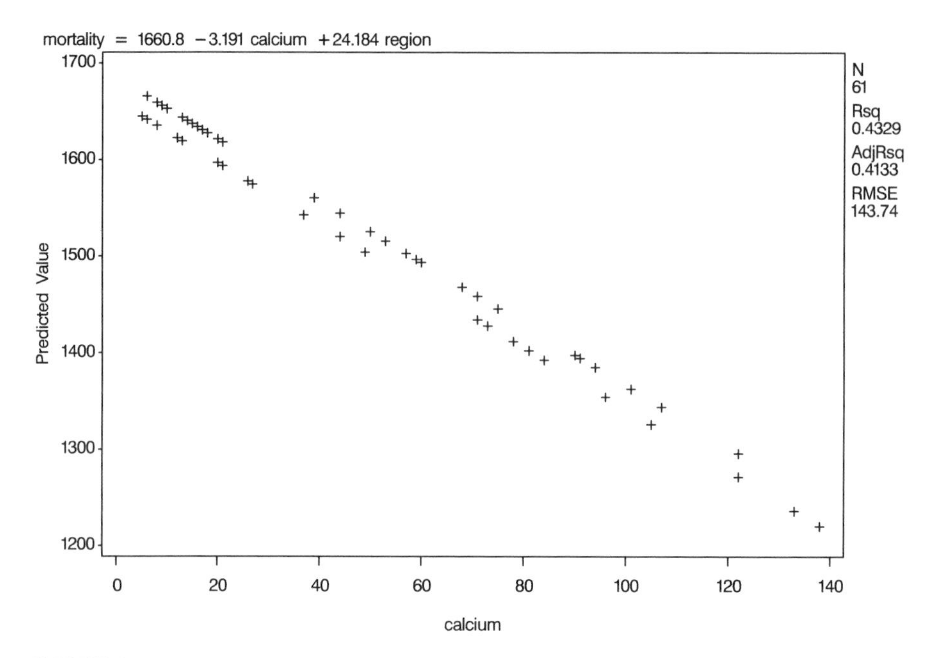

FIGURE 6.1
Multiple regression model for the water hardness data displayed graphically.

```
data water;
  set water;
  reg_calc=region*calcium;
run;
proc reg data=water;
  model mortality= calcium region reg_calc;
  plot p.*calcium=region;
run;
```

The results are given in Table 6.5. Again the overall *F* test provides clear evidence of at least one nonzero regression coefficient. The individual *t*-tests again suggest that only calcium concentration is predictive of mortality. In particular, the interaction term is not needed. This is confirmed by examining the R^2 values for the two models, 0.43 for the first and 0.44 for the second that includes the interaction term. The increase corresponding to the addition of the interaction term to the first model is very small.

The plot illustrating the second model is shown in Figure 6.2. In this case the two regression lines are not assumed to be parallel. But it is clear from our previous discussion that the parallel lines model is adequate for these data; indeed since there is no evidence that region is predictive of mortality, a simple fit of mortality on calcium concentration is all that is required.

TABLE 6.5

Results for Further Multiple Regression Model Fitted to the Water Hardness Data

The REG Procedure
Model: MODEL1
Dependent Variable: mortality

Analysis of Variance

Source	DF	Sum of Squares	Mean Square	F Value	Pr > F
Model	3	931321	310440	14.97	<.0001
Error	57	1181852	20734		
Corrected Total	60	2113174			

Root MSE	143.99392	R-Square	0.4407
Dependent Mean	1524.14754	Adj R-Sq	0.4113
Coeff Var	9.44751		

Parameter Estimates

Variable	DF	Parameter Estimate	Standard Error	t Value	Pr > |t|
Intercept	1	1681.96605	44.84877	37.50	<.0001
calcium	1	-3.59728	0.66954	-5.37	<.0001
region	1	-17.55734	59.95146	-0.29	0.7707
reg_calc	1	0.87905	0.98486	0.89	0.3758

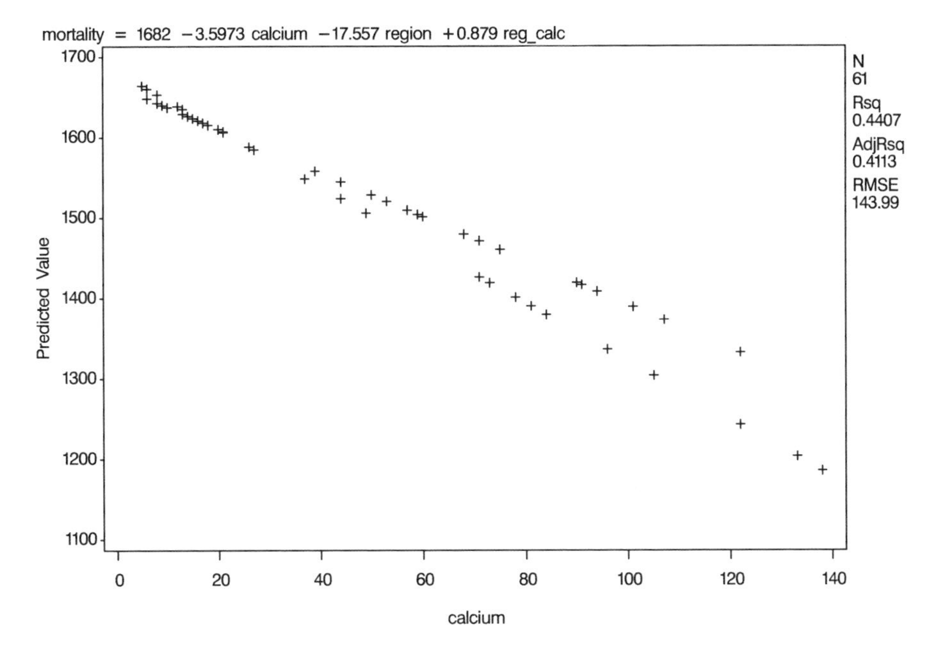

FIGURE 6.2
Graphical illustration of second multiple regression model fitted to water hardness data.

TABLE 6.6

Mass and Physical Measurements in Men

Mass	Fore	Bicep	Chest	Neck	Waist	Height
77	28.5	33.5	100	38.5	178	37.5
85.5	29.5	36.5	107	39	187	40
63	25	31	94	36.5	175	33
80.5	28.5	34	104	39	183	38
79.5	28.5	36.5	107	39	174	40
94	30.5	38	112	39	180	39.5
66	26.5	29	93	35	177.5	38.5
69	27	31	95	37	182.5	36
65	26.5	29	93	35	178.5	34
58	26.5	31	96	35	168.5	35
69.5	28.5	37	109.5	39	170	38
73	27.5	33	102	38.5	180	36
74	29.5	36	101	38.5	186.5	38
68	25	30	98.5	37	188	37
80	29.5	36	103	40	173	37
66	26.5	32.5	89	35	171	38
54.5	24	30	92.5	35.5	169	32
64	25.5	28.5	87.5	35	181	35.5
84	30	34.5	99	40.5	188	39
73	28	34.5	97	37	173	38
89	29	35.5	106	39	179	39.5
94	31	33.5	106	39	184	42

(This is a convenient point to note that categorical explanatory variables with more than two categories can be also be used in multiple linear regression modeling as long as they are representing by a series of dummy variables. To 'dummy-code' a categorical variable with k categories, k – 1 binary dummy variables are created. Each of the dummy variables relates to a single category of the original variable and takes the value '1' when the subject falls into the category and '0' otherwise. The category that is ignored in the dummy coding represents the reference category.)

6.2.3 Weight and Physical Measurement in Men

Larner (1996) measured the weight and various physical measurement for 22 male subjects aged 16 to 30. Subjects were randomly chosen volunteers all in reasonably good health. Subjects were requested to slightly tense each muscle being measured to ensure measurement consistency. The data are shown in Table 6.6.

The question of interest for these data is how weight can best be predicted from the other measurements. To begin it is useful to examine the scatterplot matrix of the data (see Chapter 4). The following SAS code reads in the data and constructs the matrix of scatterplots:

```
data young_man;
  input Mass Forearm Bicep Chest Neck Waist Height;
cards;
7728.533.510038.517837.5
85.529.536.51073918740
...
732834.597  37  173 38
892935.5106 39  179 39.5
943133.5106 39  184 42
;
%inc 'c:\sasbook\macros\plotmat.sas';
%inc 'c:\sasbook\macros\template.sas';
%plotmat(young_man,mass--height);
```

The `plotmat` macro uses the `template` macro, so both must be available or included before `plotmat` can be used. Its two arguments are the name of the data set and the list of variables to be plotted.

The resulting diagram is shown in Figure 6.3. Several pairs of variables are seen to be strongly related. The scatterplot matrix clearly highlights the very strong relationship between most of the variables in Table 6.6. Highly correlated explanatory variables may be an indication of approximate *multicollinearity*, a phenomenon that can cause several problems when applying the multiple regression model, including:

1. It severely limits the size of the multiple correlation coefficient, R, because the explanatory variables are largely attempting to explain much of the same variability in the response variable (see Dizney and Gromen, 1967, for an example).
2. It makes determining the importance of a given explanatory variable (see later) difficult because the effects of explanatory variables are confounded due to their intercorrelations.
3. It increases the variances of the regression coefficients, making using the predicted model for prediction less stable.The parameter estimates become unreliable.

Spotting multicollinearity amongst a set of explanatory variables may not be easy. The obvious course of action is to simply examine the correlations between these variables, but whilst this is often helpful, it is by no means foolproof — more subtle forms of multicollinearity may be missed. An alternative and generally far more useful approach is to examine what are known

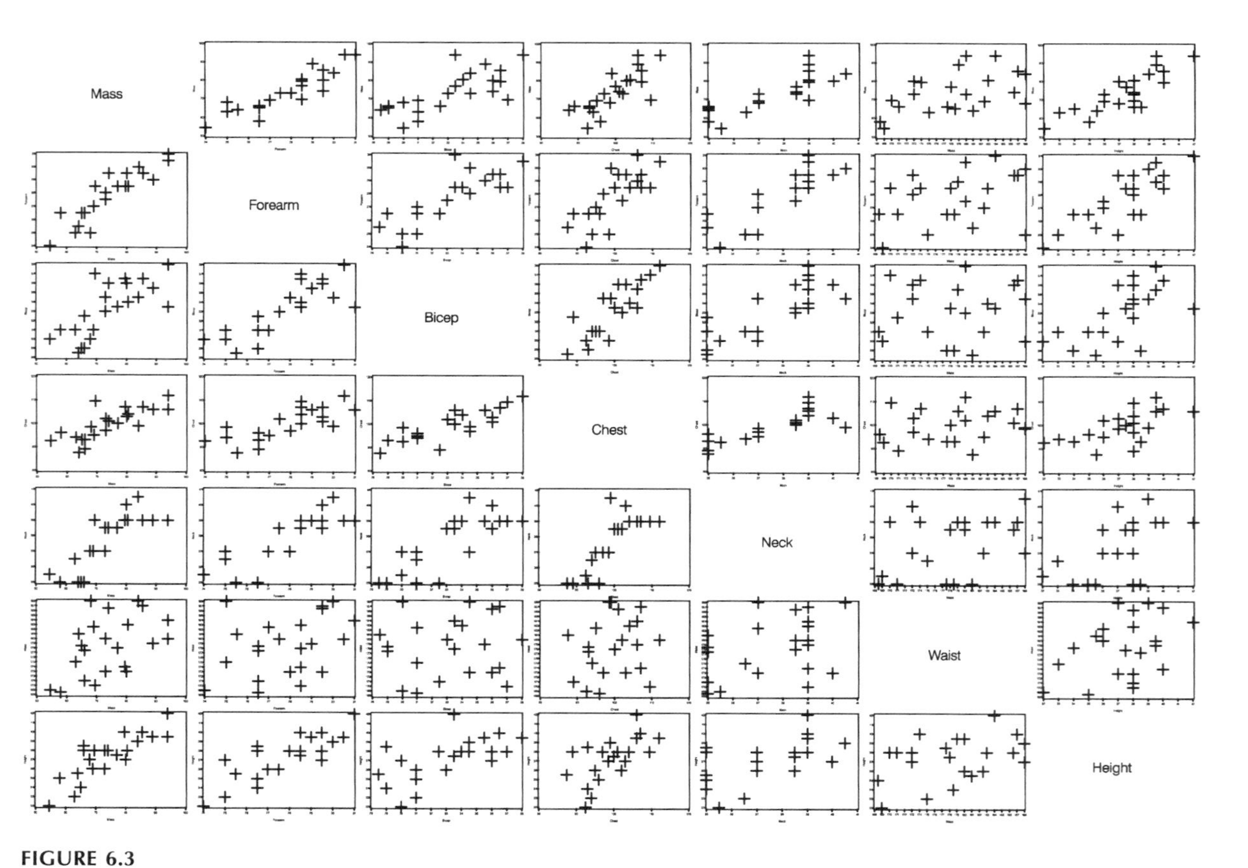

FIGURE 6.3
Scatterplot matrix of physical measurements of young men.

as the *variance inflation factors* of the explanatory variables. The variance inflation factor, VIF_j for the jth variable is given by

$$VIF_j = \frac{1}{1 - R_j^2}$$

where R_j^2, is the square of the multiple correlation coefficient from the regression of the jth explanatory variable on the remaining explanatory variables. The variance inflation factor of an explanatory variable indicates the strength of the linear relationship between the variable and the remaining explanatory variables. A rough rule of thumb is that variance inflation factors greater than 10 give some cause for concern.

How can multicollinearity be combated? One way is to combine in some way explanatory variables that are highly correlated. An alternative is simply to select one of the set of correlated variables. Two more complex possibilities are *regression on principal components* and *ridge regression*, both of which are described in Chatterjee and Price (1998).

We can look at the variance inflation factors for the data in Table 6.6 using the following SAS instructions.

```
proc reg data=young_man;
  model mass=forearm--height /vif;
run;
```

The output is shown in Table 6.7. Concentrating for the moment on the variance inflation factors we see that some are quite large; for example, that for Forearm. But none of the values are greater than 10 and so we can interpret the results of the multiple regression as they are given in Table 6.7. The overall F test indicates that not all the regression coefficients are zero and the R2 value of 0.89 shows that jointly the six explanatory variables account for 89% of the variation in the response, mass. But individually, *none* of the t-statistics is significant at the 5% level. This highlights the problems of using these statistics to decide which of the explanatory variables are most predictive of the response, and to decide on a more parsimonious model for the data (i.e., one with fewer explanantory variables but still adequate to describe the variation on the response). The problem is that the t-statistics are conditional on which explanatory variables are included in the current model. The values of these statistics will change, as will the values of the estimated regression coefficients and their standard errors as other variables are included and excluded from the model. Consequently, other, more involved procedures are needed to focus in on a simpler model that is still able to account adequately for the data.

TABLE 6.7

Results from Multiple Regression Model Fitted to Physical Measurements Data

The REG Procedure
Model: MODEL1
Dependent Variable: Mass

Analysis of Variance

Source	DF	Sum of Squares	Mean Square	F Value	Pr > F
Model	6	2243.01335	373.83556	19.95	<.0001
Error	15	281.13438	18.74229		
Corrected Total	21	2524.14773			

Root MSE	4.32924	R-Square	0.8886
Dependent Mean	73.93182	Adj R-Sq	0.8441
Coeff Var	5.85572		

Parameter Estimates

Variable	DF	Parameter Estimate	Standard Error	t Value	Pr > |t|	Variance Inflation
Intercept	1	-137.49366	29.76445	-4.62	0.0003	0
Forearm	1	2.59669	1.23820	2.10	0.0533	6.32843
Bicep	1	-0.53249	0.86754	-0.61	0.5485	7.12094
Chest	1	0.35216	0.30398	1.16	0.2648	4.69396
Neck	1	0.99038	1.27842	0.77	0.4506	6.17550
Waist	1	0.22585	0.21411	1.05	0.3082	1.97442
Height	1	1.18808	0.72564	1.64	0.1224	3.44696

6.3 Identifying a Parsimonious Model

A multiple regression analysis begins with a set of observations on a response variable and a number of explanatory variables. After an initial analysis has established that some, at least, of the explanatory variables are predictive of the response, the question arises as to whether a subset of the explanatory variables might provide a simpler model that is essentially as useful as the full model in predicting, or explaining, the response. Because as pointed out at the end of the previous section, the *t*-statistics associated with each regression coefficient provide only a partial answer to this question, we need to consider other possible approaches. The best approach is to build a model based on theory, for example, by first considering the most important predictors and confounders and then sequentially considering inclusion of further variables believe to be associated with the response variable. Often, however, this approach is not possible and then the investigator may consider using one of the automatic procedures that are available. These rely on testing many different combinations of variables and therefore suffer from all of the problems of multiple testing; spurious results (false-positives) are likely, and the analysis must be considered exploratory. Nevertheless, we shall briefly examine two automatic selection procedures.

DISPLAY 6.3

Mallows' C_p Statistic

- Mallows' C_p statistic is defined as

$$C_p = \left(\text{RSS}_p / s^2\right) - \left(n - 2p\right)$$

  where RSS_p is the residual sum of squares from a regression model with a particular set of $p - 1$ of the explanatory variables, plus an intercept, and s^2 is the estimate of σ^2 from the model that includes all explanatory variables under consideration.
- C_p is an unbiased estimate of the mean square error, $E\left[\sum \hat{y}_i - E\left(y_i\right)\right]^2 / n$, of the model's fitted values as estimates of the true expectations of the observations.
- 'Low' values of C_p are those that indicate the best models to consider.
- If C_p is plotted against p, the subsets of variables worth considering in searching for a parsimonious model are those lying close to the line $C_p = p$.
- In this plot, the value of p is (roughly) the contribution to C_p from the variance of the estimated parameters, whereas the remaining $C_p - p$ is (roughly) the contribution from the bias of the model.
- This feature makes the plot a useful device for a broad assessment of the C_p values of a range of models.
- The criterion is described in more detail in Mallows (1973, 1995) and Burman (1996).

6.3.1 All Possible Subsets Regression

With p explanatory variables, there are a total of $2^p - 1$ possible regression models — each variable can be in or out of the model, and the model containing no explanatory variables is excluded. In all possible subsets regression *all* of these models are estimated and then compared using some numerical criterion designed to indicate which models are the 'best'. The most commonly used of the criteria that have been proposed is *Mallows' C_p statistic*, which is described fully in Display 6.3.

All possible subsets regression using the C_p criterion can be performed using the `selection=cp` option as follows;

```
proc reg data=young_man;
  model mass=forearm--height / selection=cp;
run;
```

TABLE 6.8

Mallows' C_p Statistics for a Subset of the Models Considered in All Subsets Regression

```
                          The REG Procedure
                            Model: MODEL1
                      Dependent Variable: Mass

                          C(p) Selection Method

Number in
  Model        C(p)     R-Square     Variables in Model

       4      3.7035      0.8834     Forearm Chest Waist Height
       3      3.8823      0.8672     Forearm Chest Waist
       3      4.3273      0.8639     Forearm Neck Height
       4      4.3720      0.8784     Forearm Neck Waist Height
       3      4.6150      0.8618     Forearm Waist Height
       2      5.2274      0.8424     Forearm Waist
       4      5.3677      0.8710     Forearm Bicep Neck Height
       5      5.3767      0.8858     Forearm Chest Neck Waist Height
       5      5.6001      0.8842     Forearm Bicep Chest Waist Height
       3      5.6802      0.8539     Forearm Chest Height
       4      5.7518      0.8682     Forearm Bicep Chest Waist
       2      5.8118      0.8380     Forearm Height
       4      5.8726      0.8673     Forearm Chest Neck Waist
       3      5.9130      0.8521     Forearm Neck Waist
       4      5.9306      0.8669     Forearm Bicep Waist Height
       2      6.0470      0.8363     Neck Height

 ...

       1     28.7418      0.6529     Neck
       2     29.1783      0.6645     Bicep Neck
       2     35.5739      0.6171     Bicep Chest
       1     35.5810      0.6022     Chest
       1     45.5197      0.5284     Bicep
       1     84.0842      0.2420     Waist
```

The output lists the resulting models in ascending order of C_p; part of this output is shown in Table 6.8.

A plot of C_p against p can be generated as follows;

```
plot cp.*np. / cmallows=black;
run;
```

The result is shown in Figure 6.4. Although the model that includes Forearm, Chest, Waist, and Height has the lowest value of C_p, the model including Forearm, Chest, and Waist has a value only slightly larger and lies closer to the line. Both of these models are worth considering as parsimonious descriptions of the data.

6.3.2 Stepwise Methods

Perhaps the most common approach to selecting informative subsets of explanatory variables in a multiple regression is to use a method that relies on a significance test to select a particular explanatory variable for inclusion in, or deletion from, the current regression model. There are three main possibilities:

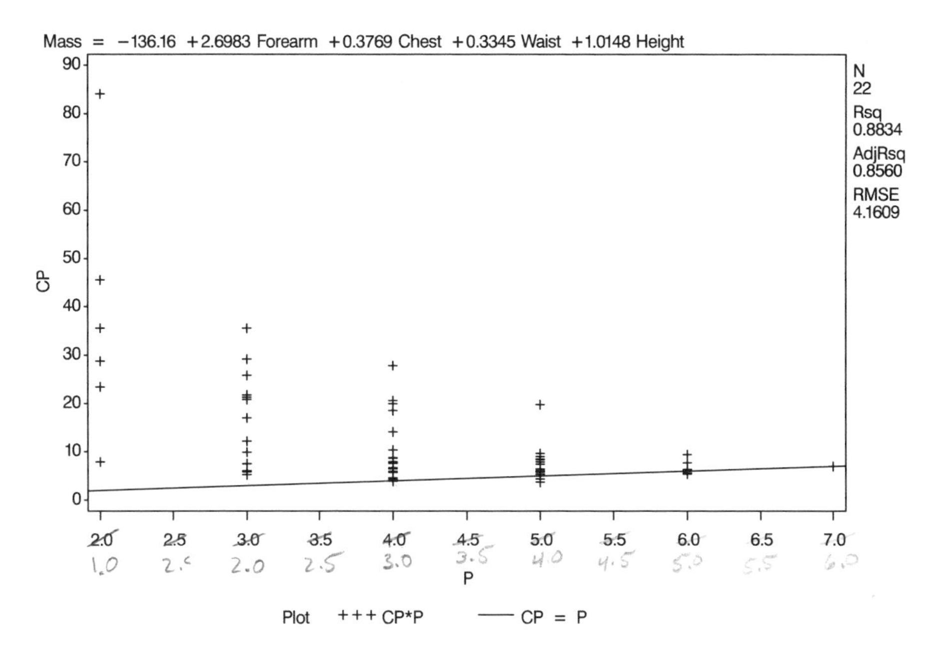

FIGURE 6.4
Plot of number of variables in a model against the value of Mallows' C_p criterion.

- Forward selection
- Backward elimination
- Stepwise regression

The forward selection approach begins with an initial model that contains only a constant term and successively adds explanatory variables to the model from the pool of candidate variables until a stage is reached where none of the candidate variables, if added to the current model, would contribute information that is statistically important concerning the expected value of the response. This is generally decided by comparing a function of the decrease in the residual sum of squares with a threshold value set by the investigator; see Draper and Smith (1998) for details.

The backward elimination method begins with an initial model that contains all explanatory variables and then identifies the single variable that contributes the least information concerning the expected value of the response — again, this is decided by looking at changes in the residual sum of squares, in this case, of course, increases. (Again, details are given in Draper and Smith, 1998.) If the increase in the residual sum of squares is deemed not to be significant, then the variable is eliminated from the current model. Successive iterations of the method result in a 'final' model from which no variables can be eliminated without adversely affecting, in a statistical sense, the predicted value of the expected response.

The stepwise regression method combines elements of both forward selection and backward elimination. The initial model for stepwise regression is one that contains only a constant term. Variables are then considered for inclusion as for forward selection, but in each step, variables included previously are also considered for possible elimination as in the backward method; this will occur if they no longer make any contribution to predicting the expected response.

The three procedures described depend crucially on the thresholds set by the investigator, an obvious danger when seeking a convincing simplified model. A separate factor that influences the results of all such automatic methods in an unpredictable fashion is the underlying correlation of the data. It is highly unlikely, for example, that any of the procedures would produce a final model that included both of two highly correlated explanatory variables. This is, of course, appropriate because including both variables might lead to *collinearity* problems. It does, however, mask the fact that the variable not selected might, if selected, lead to a somewhat different, but equally acceptable, final model. Caution is needed in using any automatic technique for variable selection and users might take heed of the following warning from Agresti (1996):

> Computerized variable selection procedures should be used with caution. When one considers a large number of terms for potential inclusion in a model, one or two that are not of real importance may look impressive simply due to chance. For instance, when all true effects are weak, the largest sample effect may substantially overestimate its true effect. In addition it often makes sense to include certain variables of special interest in a model and report their estimated effects even if they are not statistically significant at some level.

Bearing such warnings in mind we will now investigate the use of all three selection procedures on the physical measurements data. The three methods can all be specified as values for the `selection=` option on the `model` statement, as follows;

```
proc reg data=young_man;
forward:  model mass=forearm--height / selection=f;
backward:  model mass=forearm--height / selection=b;
stepwise:  model mass=forearm--height /
 selection=stepwise;
run;
```

This example also illustrates the fact that several models can be fitted within a single `proc reg` step. To distinguish the output from each of them, it is useful to give each model a label. Note that the label must be the first word on the `model` statement and must end in a colon. The output from forward selection is shown in Table 6.9, that for backward elimination in Table 6.10, and for stepwise regression in Table 6.11.

TABLE 6.9

Results of Forward Selection Applied to the Physical Measurements Data

The REG Procedure
Model: forward
Dependent Variable: Mass

Forward Selection: Step 1

Variable Forearm Entered: R-Square = 0.8078 and C(p) = 7.8915

Analysis of Variance

Source	DF	Sum of Squares	Mean Square	F Value	Pr > F
Model	1	2038.88223	2038.88223	84.03	<.0001
Error	20	485.26550	24.26327		
Corrected Total	21	2524.14773			

Variable	Parameter Estimate	Standard Error	Type II SS	F Value	Pr > F
Intercept	-68.64410	15.58879	470.46866	19.39	0.0003
Forearm	5.13367	0.56002	2038.88223	84.03	<.0001

Bounds on condition number: 1, 1

Forward Selection: Step 2

Variable Waist Entered: R-Square = 0.8424 and C(p) = 5.2274

Analysis of Variance

Source	DF	Sum of Squares	Mean Square	F Value	Pr > F
Model	2	2126.29669	1063.14834	50.77	<.0001
Error	19	397.85104	20.93953		
Corrected Total	21	2524.14773			

Variable	Parameter Estimate	Standard Error	Type II SS	F Value	Pr > F
Intercept	-120.27151	29.12382	357.10480	17.05	0.0006
Forearm	4.73173	0.55620	1515.43992	72.37	<.0001
Waist	0.35181	0.17219	87.41446	4.17	0.0552

Bounds on condition number: 1.143, 4.5719

Forward Selection: Step 3

The REG Procedure
Model: forward
Dependent Variable: Mass

Forward Selection: Step 3
Variable Chest Entered: R-Square = 0.8672 and C(p) = 3.8823

Analysis of Variance

Source	DF	Sum of Squares	Mean Square	F Value	Pr > F
Model	3	2188.99214	729.66405	39.19	<.0001
Error	18	335.15559	18.61975		
Corrected Total	21	2524.14773			

TABLE 6.9 (continued)

Results of Forward Selection Applied to the Physical Measurements Data

Variable	Parameter Estimate	Standard Error	Type II SS	F Value	Pr > F
Intercept	-135.40544	28.67491	415.18526	22.30	0.0002
Forearm	3.60833	0.80616	373.02958	20.03	0.0003
Chest	0.40270	0.21946	62.69545	3.37	0.0831
Waist	0.38661	0.16347	104.14060	5.59	0.0295

Bounds on condition number: 2.7003, 18.964

Forward Selection: Step 4

Variable Height Entered: R-Square = 0.8834 and C(p) = 3.7035

Analysis of Variance

Source	DF	Sum of Squares	Mean Square	F Value	Pr > F
Model	4	2229.82762	557.45690	32.20	<.0001
Error	17	294.32011	17.31295		
Corrected Total	21	2524.14773			

Variable	Parameter Estimate	Standard Error	Type II SS	F Value	Pr > F
Intercept	-136.16141	27.65473	419.70115	24.24	0.0001
Forearm	2.69833	0.97743	131.94313	7.62	0.0134
Chest	0.37687	0.21228	54.56746	3.15	0.0937
Waist	0.33454	0.16124	74.53255	4.31	0.0535
Height	1.01483	0.66079	40.83548	2.36	0.1430

Bounds on condition number: 4.2691, 44.215

No other variable met the 0.5000 significance level for entry into the model.

TABLE 6.10

Results of Backward Elimination for Physical Measurements Data

The REG Procedure
Model: forward
Dependent Variable: Mass

Summary of Forward Selection

Step	Variable Entered	Number Vars In	Partial R-Square	Model R-Square	C(p)	F Value	Pr > F
1	Forearm	1	0.8078	0.8078	7.8915	84.03	<.0001
2	Waist	2	0.0346	0.8424	5.2274	4.17	0.0552
3	Chest	3	0.0248	0.8672	3.8823	3.37	0.0831
4	Height	4	0.0162	0.8834	3.7035	2.36	0.1430

The REG Procedure
Model: backward
Dependent Variable: Mass

Backward Elimination: Step 0

All Variables Entered: R-Square = 0.8886 and C(p) = 7.0000

TABLE 6.10 (continued)

Results of Backward Elimination for Physical Measurements Data

```
                             Analysis of Variance

                                     Sum of           Mean
Source                   DF         Squares         Square    F Value    Pr > F

Model                     6      2243.01335      373.83556      19.95    <.0001
Error                    15       281.13438       18.74229
Corrected Total          21      2524.14773

                  Parameter      Standard
    Variable       Estimate         Error   Type II SS  F Value  Pr > F

    Intercept    -137.49366      29.76445    399.93779    21.34  0.0003
    Forearm         2.59669       1.23820     82.42946     4.40  0.0533
    Bicep          -0.53249       0.86754      7.06097     0.38  0.5485
    Chest           0.35216       0.30398     25.15450     1.34  0.2648
    Neck            0.99038       1.27842     11.24797     0.60  0.4506
    Waist           0.22585       0.21411     20.85393     1.11  0.3082
    Height          1.18808       0.72564     50.24273     2.68  0.1224

                 Bounds on condition number: 7.1209, 178.44
------------------------------------------------------------------------------

                         Backward Elimination: Step 1


        Variable Bicep Removed: R-Square = 0.8858 and C(p) = 5.3767


                             Analysis of Variance

                                     Sum of           Mean
Source                   DF         Squares         Square    F Value    Pr > F

Model                     5      2235.95238      447.19048      24.83    <.0001
Error                    16       288.19535       18.01221
Corrected Total          21      2524.14773

                  Parameter      Standard
    Variable       Estimate         Error   Type II SS  F Value  Pr > F

    Intercept    -139.89599      28.92560    421.32068    23.39  0.0002
    Forearm         2.36003       1.15349     75.40050     4.19  0.0576
    Chest           0.27890       0.27407     18.65317     1.04  0.3240
    Neck            0.66504       1.14049      6.12476     0.34  0.5679
    Waist           0.29663       0.17684     50.67914     2.81  0.1129
    Height          1.13958       0.70713     46.77905     2.60  0.1266
                              The REG Procedure
                               Model: backward
                          Dependent Variable: Mass

                         Backward Elimination: Step 1

                 Bounds on condition number: 5.7147, 98.033
------------------------------------------------------------------------------

                         Backward Elimination: Step 2


        Variable Neck Removed: R-Square = 0.8834 and C(p) = 3.7035


                             Analysis of Variance

                                     Sum of           Mean
Source                   DF         Squares         Square    F Value    Pr > F

Model                     4      2229.82762      557.45690      32.20    <.0001
Error                    17       294.32011       17.31295
Corrected Total          21      2524.14773
```

TABLE 6.10 (continued)

Results of Backward Elimination for Physical Measurements Data

Variable	Parameter Estimate	Standard Error	Type II SS	F Value	Pr > F
Intercept	-136.16141	27.65473	419.70115	24.24	0.0001
Forearm	2.69833	0.97743	131.94313	7.62	0.0134
Chest	0.37687	0.21228	54.56746	3.15	0.0937
Waist	0.33454	0.16124	74.53255	4.31	0.0535
Height	1.01483	0.66079	40.83548	2.36	0.1430

Bounds on condition number: 4.2691, 44.215

Backward Elimination: Step 3

Variable Height Removed: R-Square = 0.8672 and C(p) = 3.8823

Analysis of Variance

Source	DF	Sum of Squares	Mean Square	F Value	Pr > F
Model	3	2188.99214	729.66405	39.19	<.0001
Error	18	335.15559	18.61975		
Corrected Total	21	2524.14773			

The REG Procedure
Model: backward
Dependent Variable: Mass

Backward Elimination: Step 3

Variable	Parameter Estimate	Standard Error	Type II SS	F Value	Pr > F
Intercept	-135.40544	28.67491	415.18526	22.30	0.0002
Forearm	3.60833	0.80616	373.02958	20.03	0.0003
Chest	0.40270	0.21946	62.69545	3.37	0.0831
Waist	0.38661	0.16347	104.14060	5.59	0.0295

Bounds on condition number: 2.7003, 18.964

All variables left in the model are significant at the 0.1000 level.

Summary of Backward Elimination

Step	Variable Removed	Number Vars In	Partial R-Square	Model R-Square	C(p)	F Value	Pr > F
1	Bicep	5	0.0028	0.8858	5.3767	0.38	0.5485
2	Neck	4	0.0024	0.8834	3.7035	0.34	0.5679
3	Height	3	0.0162	0.8672	3.8823	2.36	0.1430

The forward selection procedure enters Forearm, Waist, Chest, and finally Height. The backward elimination method eliminates first Bicep, and then Neck, and finally Height, arriving at a final model that includes only the three explanatory variables, Forearm, Chest, and Waist. The stepwise selection procedure arrives at the same final model as the forward selection procedure for these data; note that this model corresponds to the model with the lowest value of Mallows' C_p criterion in the previous subsection.

TABLE 6.11

Results of Stepwise Regression on Physical Measurements Data

The REG Procedure
Model: stepwise
Dependent Variable: Mass

Stepwise Selection: Step 1

Variable Forearm Entered: R-Square = 0.8078 and C(p) = 7.8915

Analysis of Variance

Source	DF	Sum of Squares	Mean Square	F Value	Pr > F
Model	1	2038.88223	2038.88223	84.03	<.0001
Error	20	485.26550	24.26327		
Corrected Total	21	2524.14773			

Variable	Parameter Estimate	Standard Error	Type II SS	F Value	Pr > F
Intercept	-68.64410	15.58879	470.46866	19.39	0.0003
Forearm	5.13367	0.56002	2038.88223	84.03	<.0001

Bounds on condition number: 1, 1

Stepwise Selection: Step 2

Variable Waist Entered: R-Square = 0.8424 and C(p) = 5.2274

Analysis of Variance

Source	DF	Sum of Squares	Mean Square	F Value	Pr > F
Model	2	2126.29669	1063.14834	50.77	<.0001
Error	19	397.85104	20.93953		
Corrected Total	21	2524.14773			

Variable	Parameter Estimate	Standard Error	Type II SS	F Value	Pr > F
Intercept	-120.27151	29.12382	357.10480	17.05	0.0006
Forearm	4.73173	0.55620	1515.43992	72.37	<.0001
Waist	0.35181	0.17219	87.41446	4.17	0.0552

Bounds on condition number: 1.143, 4.5719

Stepwise Selection: Step 3

The REG Procedure
Model: stepwise
Dependent Variable: Mass

Stepwise Selection: Step 3

Variable Chest Entered: R-Square = 0.8672 and C(p) = 3.8823

Analysis of Variance

Source	DF	Sum of Squares	Mean Square	F Value	Pr > F
Model	3	2188.99214	729.66405	39.19	<.0001
Error	18	335.15559	18.61975		
Corrected Total	21	2524.14773			

TABLE 6.11 (continued)

Results of Stepwise Regression on Physical Measurements Data

Variable	Parameter Estimate	Standard Error	Type II SS	F Value	Pr > F
Intercept	-135.40544	28.67491	415.18526	22.30	0.0002
Forearm	3.60833	0.80616	373.02958	20.03	0.0003
Chest	0.40270	0.21946	62.69545	3.37	0.0831
Waist	0.38661	0.16347	104.14060	5.59	0.0295

Bounds on condition number: 2.7003, 18.964

Stepwise Selection: Step 4

Variable Height Entered: R-Square = 0.8834 and C(p) = 3.7035

Analysis of Variance

Source	DF	Sum of Squares	Mean Square	F Value	Pr > F
Model	4	2229.82762	557.45690	32.20	<.0001
Error	17	294.32011	17.31295		
Corrected Total	21	2524.14773			

Variable	Parameter Estimate	Standard Error	Type II SS	F Value	Pr > F
Intercept	-136.16141	27.65473	419.70115	24.24	0.0001
Forearm	2.69833	0.97743	131.94313	7.62	0.0134
Chest	0.37687	0.21228	54.56746	3.15	0.0937
Waist	0.33454	0.16124	74.53255	4.31	0.0535
Height	1.01483	0.66079	40.83548	2.36	0.1430

Bounds on condition number: 4.2691, 44.215

All variables left in the model are significant at the 0.1500 level.

The REG Procedure
Model: stepwise
Dependent Variable: Mass

Stepwise Selection: Step 4

No other variable met the 0.1500 significance level for entry into the model.

Summary of Stepwise Selection

Step	Variable Entered	Variable Removed	Number Vars In	Partial R-Square	Model R-Square	C(p)	F Value	Pr > F
1	Forearm		1	0.8078	0.8078	7.8915	84.03	<.0001
2	Waist		2	0.0346	0.8424	5.2274	4.17	0.0552
3	Chest		3	0.0248	0.8672	3.8823	3.37	0.0831
4	Height		4	0.0162	0.8834	3.7035	2.36	0.1430

6.4 Checking Model Assumptions: Residuals and Other Regression Diagnostics

A regression analysis should not end without an attempt to check assumptions such as those of constant variance and normality of the error terms. Violation of these assumptions may invalidate conclusions based on the regression analysis. The estimated residuals $r_i = y_i - \hat{y}_i$ play an essential role in diagnosing a fitted model, although because these do not have the same variance (the precision of $\hat{y}_i$ depends on x_i), they are sometimes standardized before use; see Cook and Weisberg (1982) for details. The following diagnostic plots are generally useful when assessing model assumptions:

- Residuals versus fitted values — If the fitted model is appropriate, the plotted points should lie in an approximately horizontal band across the plot. Departures from this appearance may indicate that the functional form of the assumed model is incorrect, or alternatively, that there is nonconstant variance.
- Residuals versus explanatory variables — Systematic patterns in these plots can indicate violations of the constant variance assumption or an inappropriate model form.
- Normal probability plot of the residuals — The plot checks the normal distribution assumptions on which all statistical inference procedures are based.

A further diagnostic that is often very useful is an index plot of the Cook's distances for each observation. This statistic is defined as follows:

$$D_k = \frac{1}{(p+1)s^2} \sum_{i=1}^{n} \left[\hat{y}_{i(k)} - \hat{y}_i \right]^2$$

where $\hat{y}_{i(k)}$ is the fitted value of the ith observation when the kth observation is omitted from the model. The values of D_k assess the impact of the kth observation on the estimated regression coefficients. Values of D_k greater than one are suggestive that the corresponding observation has undue influence on the estimated regression coefficients (see Cook and Weisberg, 1982).

We can obtain all the required plots for the residuals from the final model selected for the physical measurements data (i.e., the one that has the four explanatory variables, Forearm, Chest, Waist, and Height) using the `plot` statement within `proc reg` as follows;

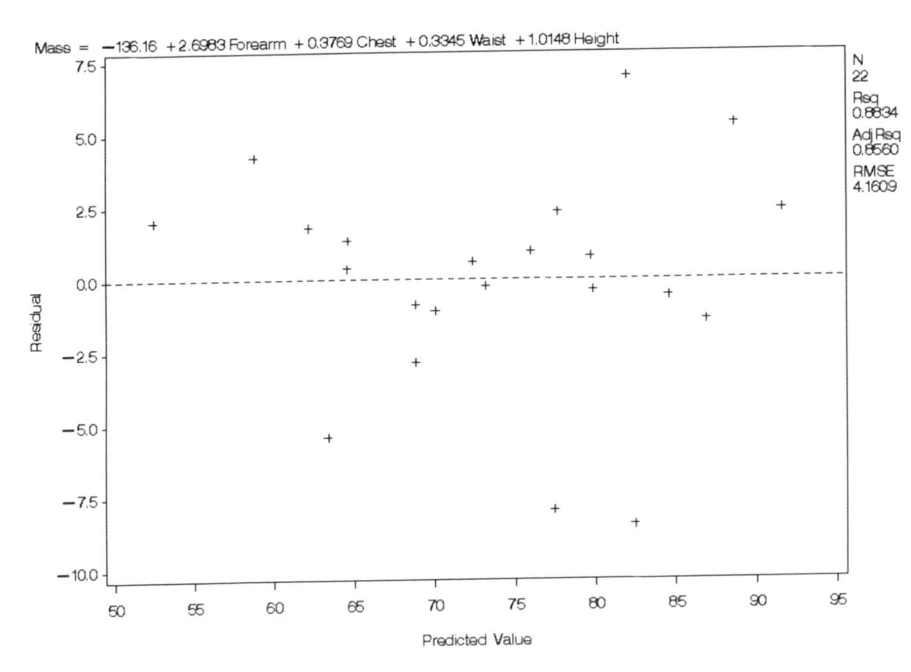

FIGURE 6.5
Plot of residuals against fitted values for the final multiple regression model selected for the physical measurements data.

```
proc reg data=young_man gout=regplots;
  model mass=forearm chest waist height;
  plot r.*(forearm chest waist height) /
 nomodel nostat;
  plot r.*p.;
  plot npp.*r.;
  plot cookd.*obs.;
run;
proc greplay igout=regplots nofs;
%template(nrows=2,ncols=2);
treplay 1:1 2:2 3:3 4:4;
run;
```

The resulting plots are shown in Figure 6.5, Figure 6.6, and Figure 6.7. In this example we also store the plots in a graphics catalog, `regplots`, and replay the plots of the residuals by the predictors in a multipanel plot — see Figure 6.8. With so few data points it is difficult to draw definite conclusions

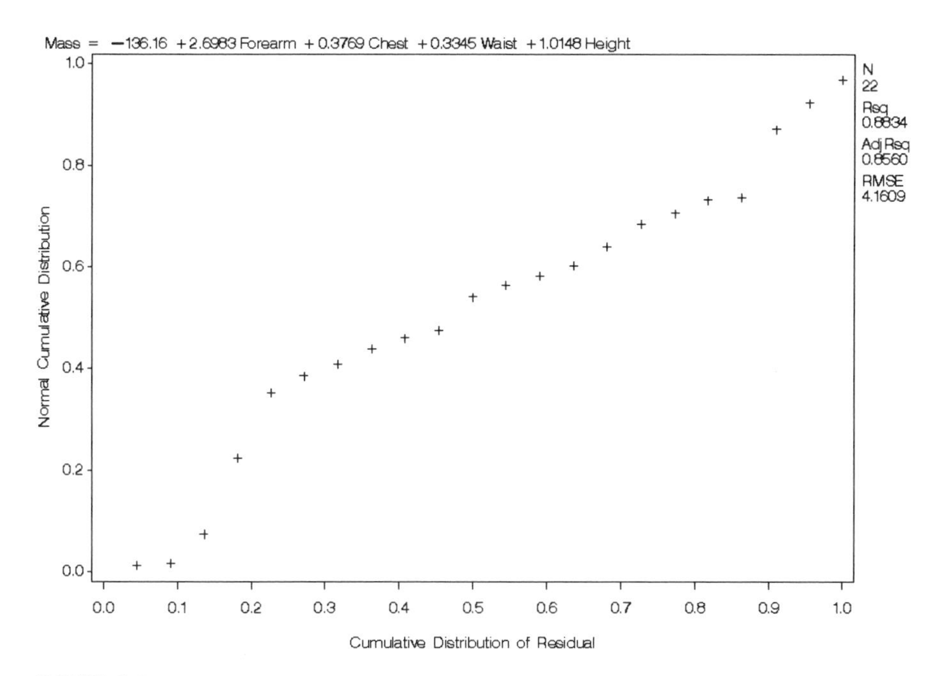

FIGURE 6.6
Normal probability plot of residuals for the final model selected for the physical measurements data.

from these plots. There may be some slight indication of non-normality in Figure 6.6, and observation 11 has a rather high value of Cook's distance but not above the generally recommended 'cause for concern' value of one.

6.5 The General Linear Model

We have so far discussed analysis of variance (ANOVA), analysis of covariance (ANCOVA), and linear regression as though they were separate models. In fact, all of these models are equivalent and can be viewed as special cases of a *general linear model* in which the residuals have a normal distribution with constant variance, σ^2. The only difference between ANOVA , ANCOVA, and linear regression models as described in this and previous chapters is that ANOVA uses categorical explanatory variables, linear regression uses continuous (or binary) explanatory variables, and ANCOVA uses a mixture of the two. But such apparent differences can easily be accommodated by a general formulation in which a continuous response variable is modeled as a linear function of explanatory variables. More will be said of this when we discuss *generalized linear models* in Chapter 8.

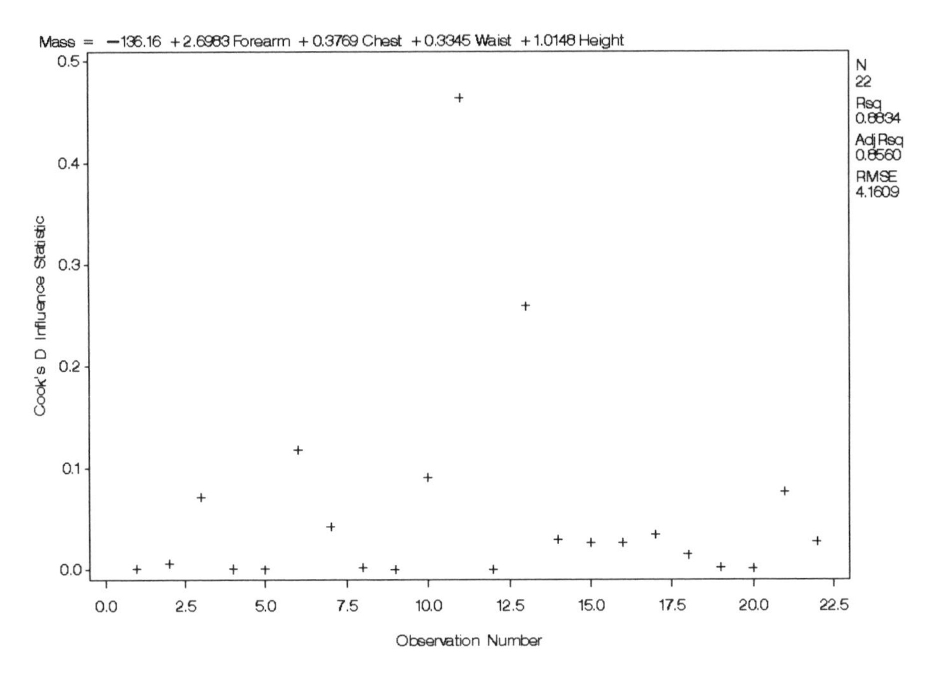

FIGURE 6.7
Plot of Cook's distance for each observation after fitting the chosen model for the physical measurements data.

6.6 Summary

Multiple regression is one of the most used (one is tempted to say overused) statistical techniques. It can be helpful for assessing the relationship between a response variable and a number of explanatory variables, but researchers using the technique should take care to check assumptions using a variety of regression diagnostics, and they should not accept blindly the results of automatic techniques for selecting subsets of explanatory variables. The multiple regression model and the ANOVA and ANCOVA models described in previous chapters are all essentially the same model, one that can be further subsumed into an even more general setting of generalized linear models, as we shall see in the next chapter.

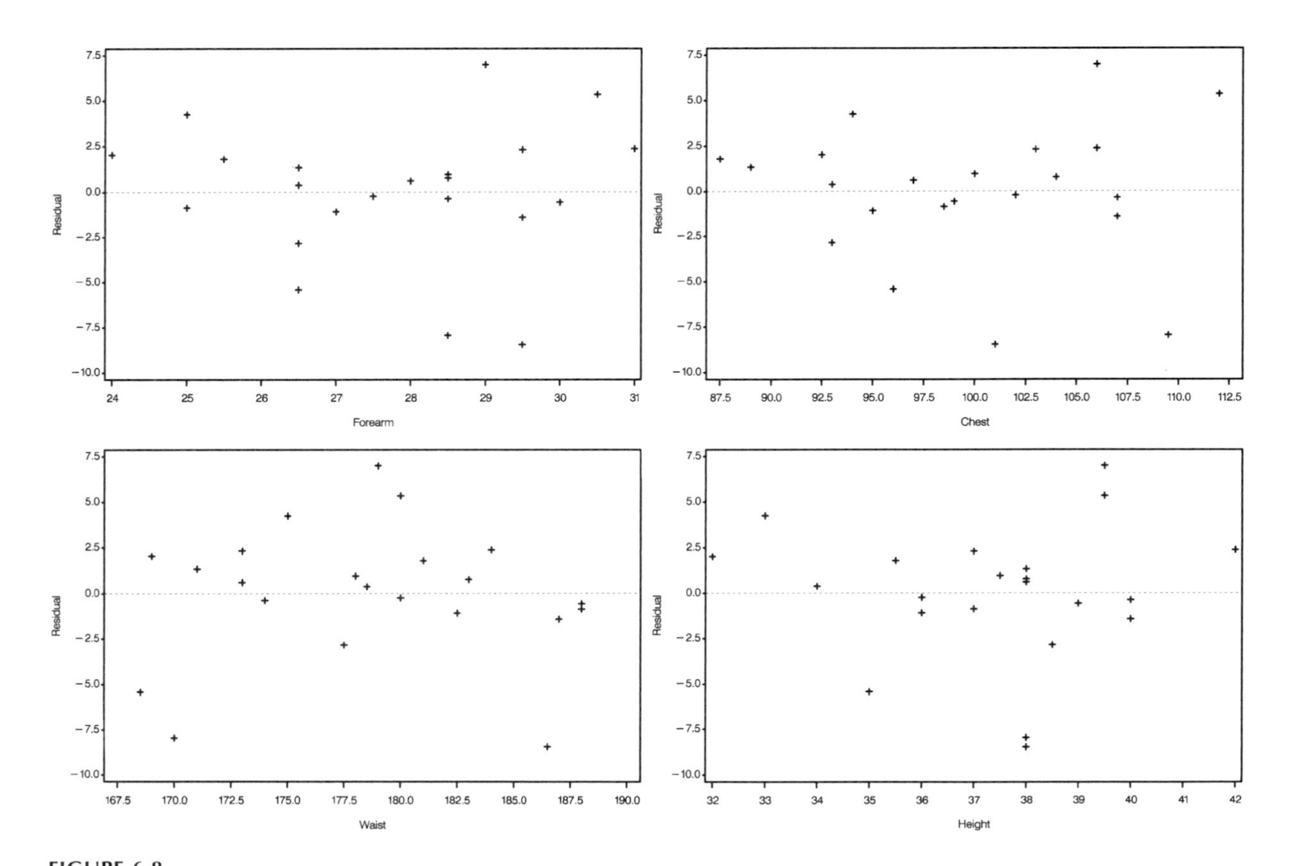

FIGURE 6.8
Multipanel display of residuals against each of the four explanatory variables in the final model for the physical measurements data.

7

Logistic Regression

7.1 Introduction

The multiple regression model as described in the previous chapter assumes that the response variable, y, is continuous and, given the values of the explanatory variables, has a normal distribution with a mean that is a linear function of the explanatory variables and variance σ^2. But in many studies in medicine, the response variable is binary, for example, improved or not improved. In this chapter we examine a suitable model for exploring the effects of explanatory variables on such a response.

7.2 Logistic Regression

In any regression problem the key quantity is the mean or expected value of the response variable given the values of the explanatory variables. In linear regression, the expected value of a response variable, y, is modeled as a linear function of the explanatory variables.

$$E\left(y \mid x_1,\ldots,x_p\right) = \beta_0 + \beta_1 x_1 \ldots + \beta_p x_p$$

For a dichotomous response variable coded 0 and 1, this expected value is simply the probability, π, that the response variable takes the value 1. This could be modelled directly as above, but there are two clear problems:

- The predicted value of the probability, π, must satisfy $0 \leq \pi < 1$, whereas a linear predictor can yield values from minus infinity to plus infinity.
- The observed values of y conditional on the values of the explanatory variables will not now follow a normal distribution with mean π but rather a Bernoulli distribution — see Display 7.1.

Details of how these problems are addressed and overcome in what is known as *logistic regression* are also given in Display 7.1.

DISPLAY 7.1

Logistic Regression

- We have a binary response variable y, and a set of explanatory variables $x_1, x_2, \ldots, x_q$.
- The expected value of y is simply the probability that y takes the value 1, which we will label π — assume that this value corresponds to the occurrence of some event of interest.
- The probability that the event of interest happens, π, should not be modelled directly as a linear function of the explanatory variables since this will not constrain predicted values of π to be in the interval [0, 1]. Instead a suitable transformation of π is modelled.
- The transformation most often used is the *logit* function of the probability given by, $\log \pi / (1 - \pi)$. This leads to the logistic regression model given by

$$\log\text{it}(\pi) = \log \frac{\pi}{1-\pi} = \beta_0 + \beta_1 x_1 + \cdots \beta_p x_p$$

- The logit transformation is chosen since, from a mathematical point-of-view, it is extremely flexible and from a practical point of view leads to meaningful and convenient interpretation as we discuss in the body of the text.
- The logit of a probability is nothing more than the log of the odds of the event of interest, and since its values can range from $-\infty$ to $+\infty$, the first problem of modelling π directly is overcome.
- The logistic regression model can be expressed directly in terms of π as

$$\pi = \frac{\exp(\beta_0 + \beta_1 x_1 + \cdots \beta_p x_p)}{1 + \exp(\beta_0 + \beta_1 x_1 + \cdots \beta_p x_p)}$$

- In a logistic regression model the parameter β_i associated with explanatory variable x_i represents the expected change in the logit when x_i is increased by one unit, conditional on the other explanatory variables remaining the same.
- Interpretation is simpler using $\exp(\beta_i)$, which corresponds to an odds ratio. A confidence interval for the latter is obtained by exponentiation of the upper and lower limits of the corresponding confidence interval of the regression coefficient itself. See examples in the text.

DISPLAY 7.1 (continued)

Logistic Regression

- In linear regression the observed value of the outcome variable is expressed as its expected value given the explanatory variables plus an error term. The error terms are assumed to have a normal distribution with mean zero and a variance that is constant across levels of the explanatory variables.
- With a binary response we can express an observed value in the same way as

$$y = \pi + \varepsilon$$

but here ε can only assume one of two possible values. If $y = 1$ then $\varepsilon = 1 - \pi$ with probability π, and if $y = 0$ then $\varepsilon = -\pi$ with probability $1 - \pi$.

- Consequently ε has a distribution with mean zero and variance equal to $\pi(1 - \pi)$.
- So the conditional distribution of the outcome variable follows what is known as a Bernoulli distribution (which is simply a binomial distribution for a single trial) with probability given by the mean conditional on the explanatory variables; we shall denote this as $\pi(\mathbf{x})$.
- Maximum likelihood is used to estimate the parameters in the logistic regression model; the log-likelihood function is

$$l(\beta; y) = \sum_{i=1}^{n} \left\{ y_i \log\left[\pi(\beta'\mathbf{x}_i)\right] + (1 - y_i)\log\left[1 - \pi(\beta'\mathbf{x}_i)\right] \right\}$$

where $y' = \left[y_1, y_2, \ldots, y_n\right]$ are the n observed values of the dichotomous response variable and $\mathbf{x}_i' = \left[x_{i1}, x_{i2,} \ldots, x_{iq}\right]$ is the vector of values of the explanatory variables associated with the ith observation.

- The log-likelihood is maximized numerically using an iterative algorithm. For details see Collett (2003).
- Logistic regression can also be used when the response is observed as a proportion rather than directly as a binary variable; an example is the proportion of headache-free days on a number of subjects. The appropriate distribution in this case is the binomial distribution with the correct denominator — in the suggested example, the number of days over which headache status has been recorded.

DISPLAY 7.1 (continued)

Logistic Regression

- The lack of fit of a logistic regression model can be measured by a term known as the *deviance*, which is essentially the ratio of the likelihoods of the model of interest to the saturated model that fits the data perfectly (see Collett, 2003, for a full explanation).
- Explicitly, the deviance is defined as

$$D = 2\sum_{i=1}^{n}\left\{y_i \log\left(\frac{y_i}{\hat{y}_i}\right) + (n_i - y_i)\log\left(\frac{n_i - y_i}{n_i - \hat{y}_i}\right)\right\}$$

where $\hat{y}_i$ is the predicted number of events of interest under the current model, i.e., $\hat{y}_i = n_i\hat{\pi}_i$.

- D compares the observed values y_i with their fitted values, $\hat{y}_i$, under the current model.
- Differences in deviance can be used to compare alternative nested logistic regression models. For example

$$\text{Model 1 (Deviance } D_1\text{)}: \log\text{it}(\pi) = \beta_0 + \beta_1 x_1$$

$$\text{Model 2 (Deviance } D_2\text{)}: \log\text{it}(\pi) = \beta_0 + \beta_1 x_1 + \beta_2 x_2 + \beta_3 x_3$$

- The difference in deviance $D_1 - D_2$ reflects the combined effect of explanatory variables x_2 and x_3, and under the hypothesis that these variables have no effect, i.e., β_2 and β_3 are both zero. The difference has an approximate chi-squared distribution with degrees of freedom equal to, in general, the difference in the number of parameters in the two models, in this case 2.
- The deviance or (likelihood ratio) can be used to test that all regression coefficients in a model zero.
- Two other test statistics are available for the same purpose, the score statistic and Wald's test. Both are described in Collett (2003).
- The three tests are asymptotically equivalent but differ in finite samples. The likelihood ratio test is generally considered the most appropriate.

7.3 Two Examples of the Application of Logistic Regression

7.3.1 Psychiatric 'Caseness'

The data shown in Table 7.1 arise from a study of a psychiatric screening questionnaire called the GHQ (General Health Questionnaire; see Goldberg, 1972). Here the question of interest is to determine how the probability of being judged a 'case' is related to gender and GHQ score.

To begin we can read in the data and plot the estimated probability of being a case against GHQ score, identifying males and females on the plot.

```
data ghq;
  input ghq sex $ cases noncases;
  total=cases+noncases;
  prcase=cases/total;
cards;
0       F       4       80
1       F       4       29
2       F       8       15
. . .
8       M       3       1
9       M       2       0
10      M       2       0
;
proc gplot data=ghq;
  plot prcase*ghq=sex;
  symbol1 v=dot i=join;
  symbol2 v=circle i=join l=2;
run;
```

The resulting diagram is shown in Figure 7.1. Clearly the probability of being considered a case increases with increasing GHQ value, but the relationship is not linear and appears to differ for men and women.

To begin we shall ignore gender and fit both a linear regression and a logistic regression to the probability of being a case with GHQ score as the single explanatory variable. First, linear regression:

```
proc reg data=ghq;
  model prcase=ghq;
  output out=rout p=rpred;
run;
```

TABLE 7.1

Psychiatric Caseness Data

GHQ Score	Sex	Number of Cases	Number of Noncases
0	F	4	80
1	F	4	29
2	F	8	15
3	F	6	3
4	F	4	2
5	F	6	1
6	F	3	1
7	F	2	0
8	F	3	0
9	F	2	0
10	F	1	0
0	M	1	36
1	M	2	25
2	M	2	8
3	M	1	4
4	M	3	1
5	M	3	1
6	M	2	1
7	M	4	2
8	M	3	1
9	M	2	0
10	M	2	0

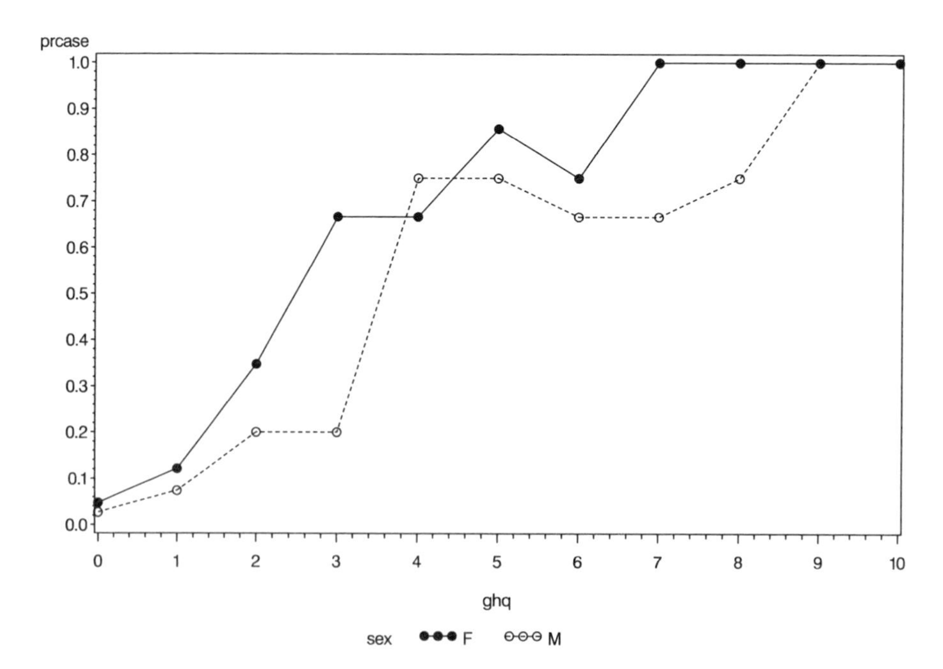

FIGURE 7.1
Plot of probability of being a case against GHQ score identifying males and females.

The output statement creates an output data set that contains all the original variables plus those created by options. The p=rpred option specifies that the predicted values are included in a variable named rpred. The out=rout option specifies the name of the data set to be created.

We then calculate the predicted values from a logistic regression, using proc logistic, in the same way.

```
proc logistic data=ghq;
   model cases/total=ghq;
   output out=lout p=lpred;
run;
```

There are two forms of model statement within proc logistic. This example shows the events/trials syntax, where two variables are specified separated by a slash. The alternative is to specify a single binary response variable before the equal sign.

The two output data sets are combined in a short data step. Because proc gplot plots the data in the order in which they occur, if the points are to be joined by lines it may be necessary to sort the data set into the appropriate order. Both sets of predicted probabilities are to be plotted on the same graph together with the observed values, so three symbol statements are defined to distinguish them.

```
data lrout;
  set rout;
  set lout;
run;
proc sort data=lrout;
  by ghq;
symbol1 i=join v=none l=1;
symbol2 i=join v=none l=2;
symbol3 v=circle;
proc gplot data=lrout;
  plot (rpred lpred prcase)*ghq /overlay;
run;
```

The resulting diagram is shown in Figure 7.2. The problems of using the unsuitable linear regression model become apparent on studying Figure 7.2. Using this model two of the predicted values are greater than one, but the response is a probability constrained to be in the interval (0,1). Additionally, the model provides a very poor fit for the observed data. Using the logistic model, on the other hand, leads to predicted values that are satisfactory in

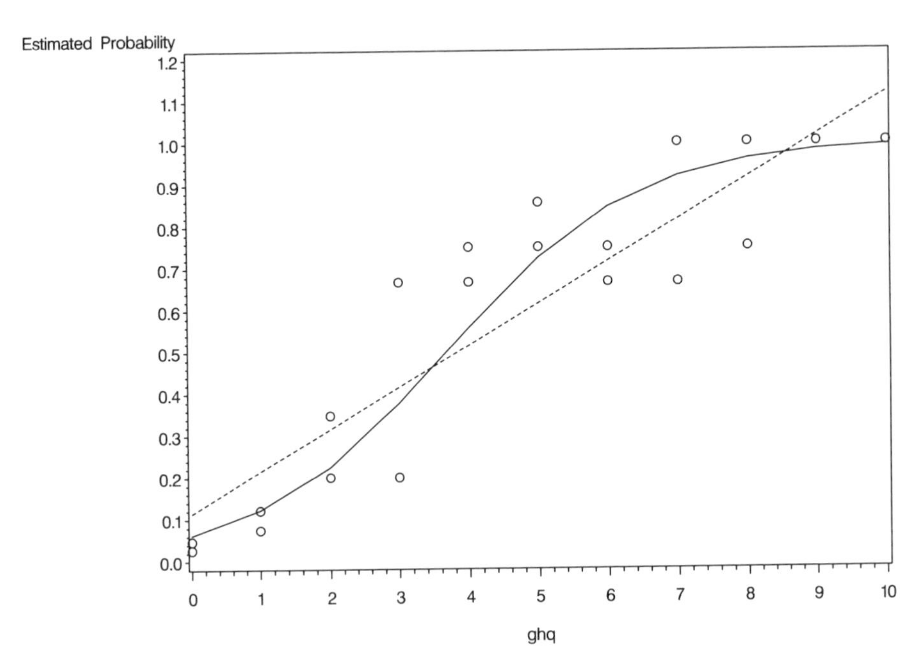

FIGURE 7.2
Predicted probabilities of "caseness" for the GHQ data from fitting linear and logistic regression models.

that they all lie between 0 and 1, and the model clearly provides a better description of the observed data.

Now let us consider a logistic regression model that uses GHQ score, gender, and their interaction as explanatory variables;

```
proc logistic data=ghq;
  class sex;
  model cases/total=sex ghq sex*ghq /
 selection=b details;
run;
```

The model statement now includes `sex ghq` and their interaction. Within `proc logistic` effects are specified in the same way as for `proc glm`, so the specification of this model could have been abbreviated to `sex|ghq`. This example illustrates some features of automatic model selection in `proc logistic`, via backward elimination in this case. Other possibilities are: forward, stepwise and best subsets — specified with `selection= f, s` and `score`, respectively. The `details` option provides effect estimates for each step of the model selection process. The output is shown in Table 7.2. At the first step (step 0), all three effects are entered into the model. From the analysis of effects, neither `sex` nor its interaction with `ghq` would appear to

TABLE 7.2

Results of Fitting Logistic Regression Model That Includes GHQ, Sex, and Sex × GHQ to the GHQ Data

```
                          The LOGISTIC Procedure

                            Model Information

                Data Set                      WORK.GHQ
                Response Variable (Events)    cases
                Response Variable (Trials)    total
                Model                         binary logit
                Optimization Technique        Fisher's scoring


                    Number of Observations Read          22
                    Number of Observations Used          22
                    Sum of Frequencies Read             278
                    Sum of Frequencies Used             278


                             Response Profile

                       Ordered     Binary          Total
                         Value     Outcome     Frequency

                             1     Event              68
                             2     Nonevent          210


                       Backward Elimination Procedure


                          Class Level Information

                                              Design
                         Class     Value     Variables

                         sex       F               1
                                   M              -1

Step  0. The following effects were entered:

Intercept  sex  ghq  ghq*sex


                          Model Convergence Status

                 Convergence criterion (GCONV=1E-8) satisfied.



                          The LOGISTIC Procedure

                           Model Fit Statistics

                                                 Intercept
                                  Intercept            and
                      Criterion        Only     Covariates

                      AIC           311.319        195.780
                      SC            314.947        210.291
                      -2 Log L      309.319        187.780


                  Testing Global Null Hypothesis: BETA=0

          Test                 Chi-Square       DF     Pr > ChiSq

          Likelihood Ratio       121.5390        3         <.0001
          Score                  121.6891        3         <.0001
          Wald                    63.3620        3         <.0001
```

TABLE 7.2 (continued)

Results of Fitting Logistic Regression Model That Includes GHQ, Sex, and Sex × GHQ to the GHQ Data

```
                        Type 3 Analysis of Effects

                                         Wald
                  Effect         DF    Chi-Square     Pr > ChiSq

                  sex             1        0.1367         0.7116
                  ghq             1       63.0651         <.0001
                  ghq*sex         1        2.3023         0.1292


                 Analysis of Maximum Likelihood Estimates

                                       Standard          Wald
Parameter        DF     Estimate          Error    Chi-Square     Pr > ChiSq

Intercept         1      -2.8858         0.3047       89.7226         <.0001
sex        F      1       0.1126         0.3047        0.1367         0.7116
ghq               1       0.7902         0.0995       63.0651         <.0001
ghq*sex    F      1       0.1510         0.0995        2.3023         0.1292



        Association of Predicted Probabilities and Observed Responses

              Percent Concordant      86.4    Somers' D    0.779
              Percent Discordant       8.6    Gamma        0.820
              Percent Tied             5.0    Tau-a        0.289
              Pairs                  14280    c            0.889

                         The LOGISTIC Procedure

                 Analysis of Effects Eligible for Removal

                                              Wald
                 Effect            DF     Chi-Square     Pr > ChiSq

                 ghq*sex            1         2.3023         0.1292

Step  1. Effect ghq*sex is removed:


                        Model Convergence Status

              Convergence criterion (GCONV=1E-8) satisfied.


                          Model Fit Statistics

                                                  Intercept
                                    Intercept           and
                  Criterion              Only    Covariates

                  AIC                 311.319       196.126
                  SC                  314.947       207.009
                  -2 Log L            309.319       190.126


                 Testing Global Null Hypothesis: BETA=0

          Test                  Chi-Square       DF     Pr > ChiSq

          Likelihood Ratio        119.1929        2         <.0001
          Score                   120.1327        2         <.0001
          Wald                     61.9555        2         <.0001
```

TABLE 7.2 (continued)

Results of Fitting Logistic Regression Model That Includes GHQ, Sex, and Sex × GHQ to the GHQ Data

Type 3 Analysis of Effects

Effect	DF	Wald Chi-Square	Pr > ChiSq
sex	1	4.6446	0.0312
ghq	1	61.8891	<.0001

The LOGISTIC Procedure

Analysis of Maximum Likelihood Estimates

Parameter		DF	Estimate	Standard Error	Wald Chi-Square	Pr > ChiSq
Intercept		1	-2.9615	0.3155	88.1116	<.0001
sex	F	1	0.4680	0.2172	4.6446	0.0312
ghq		1	0.7791	0.0990	61.8891	<.0001

Odds Ratio Estimates

Effect	Point Estimate	95% Wald Confidence Limits	
sex F vs M	2.550	1.088	5.974
ghq	2.180	1.795	2.646

Association of Predicted Probabilities and Observed Responses

Percent Concordant	85.8	Somers' D	0.766
Percent Discordant	9.2	Gamma	0.806
Percent Tied	5.0	Tau-a	0.284
Pairs	14280	c	0.883

Residual Chi-Square Test

Chi-Square	DF	Pr > ChiSq
2.3930	1	0.1219

Analysis of Effects Eligible for Removal

Effect	DF	Wald Chi-Square	Pr > ChiSq
sex	1	4.6446	0.0312
ghq	1	61.8891	<.0001

NOTE: No (additional) effects met the 0.05 significance level for removal from the model.

The LOGISTIC Procedure

Summary of Backward Elimination

Step	Effect Removed	DF	Number In	Wald Chi-Square	Pr > ChiSq
1	ghq*sex	1	2	2.3023	0.1292

be significant. A naive approach to model selection might drop sex from the next step, since it is the least significant effect. However, by default proc logistic preserves the hierarchy of effects whereby main effects must be included in a model if the interaction between them is. More generally, higher-order effects will only be retained (or entered) if the lower-order effects which they contain are also present in the model. Hence, in this example, the sex*ghq interaction term is removed from the model in the second step. Fitting the reduced model yields significant main effects for both sex and ghq, and the model selection ends there.

7.3.2 Birthweight of Babies

For our second example of the application of logistic regression, we will use part of the data set given in Hosmer and Lemeshow (1989) collected during a study to identify risk factors associated with giving birth to a low birth-weight baby, defined as weighing less than 2500 g. The risk factors considered were age of the mother, weight of the mother at her last menstrual period, race of mother, and number of physician visits during the first trimester of the pregnancy. The data used are shown in Table 7.3.

The SAS code reading in the data and then fitting the logistic regression model is

```
data lobwgt;
  input id low age lwt race ftv;
cards;
85  0   19  182 2   0
86  0   33  155 3   3
. . . .
82  1   23  94  3   0
83  1   17  142 2   0
84  1   21  130 1   3
;
proc logistic data=lobwgt desc;
  class race / param=ref ref=first;
  model low= age lwt race ftv;
run;
```

Where a binary response variable is used on the model statement, as opposed to the events/trials used for the GHQ data, SAS models the lower of the two response categories as the 'event'. However, it is common practice for a binary response variable to be coded 0,1 with 1 indicating a response, or event, and 0 indicating no response, or a nonevent. In this case the

TABLE 7.3

Low Infant Birthweight Data

ID	LOW	AGE	LWT	RACE	FTV
85	0	19	182	2	0
86	0	33	155	3	3
87	0	20	105	1	1
88	0	21	108	1	2
89	0	18	107	1	0
91	0	21	124	3	0
92	0	22	118	1	1
93	0	17	103	3	1
94	0	29	123	1	1
95	0	26	113	1	0
96	0	19	95	3	0
97	0	19	150	3	1
98	0	22	95	3	0
99	0	30	107	3	2
100	0	18	100	1	0
101	0	18	100	1	0
102	0	15	98	2	0
103	0	25	118	1	3
104	0	20	120	3	0
105	0	28	120	1	1
106	0	32	121	3	2
107	0	31	100	1	3
108	0	36	202	1	1
109	0	28	120	3	0
111	0	25	120	3	2
112	0	28	167	1	0
113	0	17	122	1	0
114	0	29	150	1	2
115	0	26	168	2	0
116	0	17	113	2	1
117	0	17	113	2	1
115	0	24	90	1	1
119	0	35	121	2	1
120	0	25	155	1	1
121	0	25	125	2	0
123	0	29	140	1	2
124	0	19	138	1	2
125	0	27	124	1	0
126	0	31	215	1	2
127	0	33	109	1	1
128	0	21	185	2	2
129	0	19	189	1	2
130	0	23	130	2	1
131	0	21	160	1	0
132	0	18	90	1	0
133	0	18	90	1	0
134	0	32	132	1	4
135	0	19	132	3	0
136	0	24	115	1	2

TABLE 7.3 (continued)

Low Infant Birthweight Data

ID	LOW	AGE	LWT	RACE	FTV
137	0	22	85	3	0
138	0	22	120	1	1
139	0	23	128	3	0
140	0	22	130	1	0
141	0	30	95	1	2
142	0	19	115	3	0
143	0	16	110	3	0
144	0	21	110	3	0
145	0	30	153	3	0
146	0	20	103	3	0
147	0	17	119	3	0
148	0	17	119	3	0
149	0	23	119	3	2
150	0	24	110	3	0
151	0	28	140	1	0
154	0	26	133	3	0
155	0	20	169	3	1
156	0	24	115	3	2
159	0	28	250	3	6
160	0	20	141	1	1
161	0	22	158	2	2
162	0	22	112	1	0
163	0	31	150	3	2
164	0	23	115	3	1
166	0	16	112	2	0
167	0	16	135	1	0
168	0	18	229	2	0
169	0	25	140	1	1
170	0	32	134	1	4
172	0	20	121	2	0
173	0	23	190	1	0
174	0	22	131	1	1
175	0	32	170	1	0
176	0	30	110	3	0
177	0	20	127	3	0
179	0	23	123	3	0
180	0	17	120	3	0
181	0	19	105	3	0
182	0	23	130	1	0
183	0	36	175	1	0
184	0	22	125	1	1
185	0	24	133	1	0
186	0	21	134	3	2
187	0	19	235	1	0
188	0	25	95	1	0
189	0	16	135	1	0
190	0	29	135	1	1
191	0	29	154	1	1
192	0	19	147	1	0

TABLE 7.3 (continued)

Low Infant Birthweight Data

ID	LOW	AGE	LWT	RACE	FTV
193	0	19	147	1	0
195	0	30	137	1	1
196	0	24	110	1	1
197	0	19	184	1	0
199	0	24	110	3	0
200	0	23	110	1	1
201	0	20	120	3	0
202	0	25	241	2	0
203	0	30	112	1	1
204	0	22	169	1	0
205	0	18	120	1	2
206	0	16	170	2	4
207	0	32	186	1	2
208	0	18	120	3	1
209	0	29	130	1	2
210	0	33	117	1	1
211	0	20	170	1	0
212	0	28	134	3	1
213	0	14	135	1	0
214	0	28	130	3	0
215	0	25	120	1	2
216	0	16	95	3	1
217	0	20	158	1	1
218	0	26	160	3	0
219	0	21	115	1	1
220	0	22	129	1	0
221	0	25	130	1	2
222	0	31	120	1	2
223	0	35	170	1	1
224	0	19	120	1	0
225	0	24	116	1	1
226	0	45	123	1	1
4	1	28	120	3	0
10	1	29	130	1	2
11	1	34	187	2	0
13	1	25	105	3	0
15	1	25	85	3	0
16	1	27	150	3	0
17	1	23	97	3	1
18	1	24	128	2	1
19	1	24	132	3	0
20	1	21	165	1	1
22	1	32	105	1	0
23	1	19	91	1	0
24	1	25	115	3	0
25	1	16	130	3	1
26	1	25	92	1	0
27	1	20	150	1	2
28	1	21	200	2	2

TABLE 7.3 (continued)

Low Infant Birthweight Data

ID	LOW	AGE	LWT	RACE	FTV
29	1	24	155	1	0
30	1	21	103	3	0
31	1	20	125	3	0
32	1	25	89	3	1
33	1	19	102	1	2
34	1	19	112	1	0
35	1	26	117	1	0
36	1	24	138	1	0
37	1	17	130	3	0
40	1	20	120	2	3
42	1	22	130	1	1
43	1	27	130	2	0
44	1	20	80	3	0
45	1	17	110	1	0
46	1	25	105	3	1
47	1	20	109	3	0
49	1	18	148	3	0
50	1	18	110	2	0
51	1	20	121	1	0
52	1	21	100	3	4
54	1	26	96	3	0
56	1	31	102	1	1
57	1	15	110	1	0
59	1	23	187	2	1
60	1	20	122	2	0
61	1	24	105	2	0
62	1	15	115	3	0
63	1	23	120	3	0
65	1	30	142	1	0
67	1	22	130	1	1
68	1	17	120	1	3
69	1	23	110	1	0
71	1	17	120	2	2
75	1	26	154	3	1
76	1	20	105	3	3
77	1	26	190	1	0
78	1	14	101	3	0
79	1	28	95	1	2
81	1	14	100	3	2
82	1	23	94	3	0
83	1	17	142	2	0
84	1	21	130	1	3

Note: LOW, 0 = weight of baby > 2500 g, 1 = weight of baby <= 2500 g; AGE, age of mother in years; LWT, weight of mother at last menstrual period; RACE, 1 = white, 2 = black, 3 = other; FTV, number of physician visits in the first trimester.

Source: Hosmer, D.W. and Lemeshow, S., 1989, *Applied Logistic Regression*, Wiley.

seemingly perverse default in SAS will be to model the probability of a nonevent. The `desc` (`descending`) option on the `proc` statement reverses this behaviour.

The `class` statement specifies classification variables, or factors, and these may be numeric or character variables. The options, following the slash, allow a choice of coding; `param=ref` specifies reference cell coding, which is equivalent to dummy variable coding, and `ref=first` specifies that the first category is the reference category. The specification of explanatory effects on the `model` statement is the same as for `proc glm`: with main effects specified by variable names and interactions by joining variable names with asterisks. The bar operator may also be used as an abbreviated way of entering interactions if these are to be included in the model. The results are shown in Table 7.4.

Examining first the three tests that all the regression coefficients in the model are zero, we see that both the likelihood ratio and score tests have associated p-values less than 0.05, but that for Wald's test is a little greater than 0.05. Perhaps the most sensible conclusion to draw is that there is *some* evidence that at least one of the regression coefficients differs from zero, but that this evidence is not particularly strong. Looking now at the regression coefficients associated with each of the *five* explanatory variables (remember that race has been recoded in terms of two dummy variables) suggests that weight of mother at her last menstrual period (LWT) and the first of the dummy variables for race may be the most important predictors of low infant birthweight. For LWT the estimated odds ratio is 0.986 with 95% confidence interval [0.973,0.999] — the interval just excludes the value one at its upper end. So we can conclude that the odds of having a low birthweight baby for mothers with weight (LWT + 1) pounds is between about 97.3 and 99.9% of the odds for mothers with weight LWT pounds. Interpretation in terms of a 1-pound weight difference may not be particularly helpful here, and it is relatively simple to find the results corresponding to a more meaningful weight difference. Suppose for example we want to look at a 10-pound difference. The estimated regression coefficient for such a difference is simply 10 times the original regression coefficient, i.e., $10 \times (-0.0142)$, a value of -0.142. The associated standard error of this value is 10×0.00654, giving 0.0654. This leads to an estimated value of $\exp(-0.142)$ for the odds ratio and a 95% confidence interval for the odds ratio of $[\exp(-0.142 + 1.96 \times 0.0654), \exp(-0.142 - 1.96 \times 0.0654)]$. So for a 10-pound weight difference, the odds of the heavier mothers giving birth to a low birthweight baby is between 76 and 99% the odds of the lighter mothers.

For race the significant dummy variable is that coding the difference between white and black mothers. For the latter the odds of a low birthweight child are estimated to be 2.729 times the corresponding odds for the former. But this apparently large effect needs to be considered in terms of the associated 95% confidence interval of [1.029, 7.240], which is very wide with the lower limit being only a little above 1.

TABLE 7.4

Results from Applying Logistic Regression to Low Birthweight Data

```
                    The LOGISTIC Procedure

                     Model Information

     Data Set                          WORK.LOBWGT
     Response Variable                 low
     Number of Response Levels         2
     Number of Observations            189
     Model                             binary logit
     Optimization Technique            Fisher's scoring


                      Response Profile

            Ordered                          Total
              Value           low        Frequency

                  1             1               59
                  2             0              130

              Probability modeled is low=1.


                  Class Level Information

                                      Design
                                    Variables

              Class      Value        1       2

              race       1            0       0
                         2            1       0
                         3            0       1


                 Model Convergence Status

     Convergence criterion (GCONV=1E-8) satisfied.


                   Model Fit Statistics

                                            Intercept
                            Intercept          and
          Criterion           Only         Covariates

          AIC               236.672          234.573
          SC                239.914          254.023
          -2 Log L          234.672          222.573


          Testing Global Null Hypothesis: BETA=0

 Test                   Chi-Square      DF      Pr > ChiSq

 Likelihood Ratio          12.0991       5          0.0335
 Score                     11.3876       5          0.0442
 Wald                      10.6964       5          0.0577

                  The LOGISTIC Procedure

               Type III Analysis of Effects

                                   Wald
        Effect        DF     Chi-Square     Pr > ChiSq

        age            1         0.4988         0.4800
        lwt            1         4.7428         0.0294
        race           2         4.4108         0.1102
        ftv            1         0.0869         0.7681
```

TABLE 7.4 (continued)

Results from Applying Logistic Regression to Low Birthweight Data

Analysis of Maximum Likelihood Estimates

Parameter		DF	Estimate	Standard Error	Wald Chi-Square	Pr > ChiSq
Intercept		1	1.2953	1.0714	1.4616	0.2267
age		1	-0.0238	0.0337	0.4988	0.4800
lwt		1	-0.0142	0.00654	4.7428	0.0294
race	2	1	1.0039	0.4979	4.0660	0.0438
race	3	1	0.4331	0.3622	1.4296	0.2318
ftv		1	-0.0493	0.1672	0.0869	0.7681

Odds Ratio Estimates

Effect	Point Estimate	95% Wald Confidence Limits	
age	0.976	0.914	1.043
lwt	0.986	0.973	0.999
race 2 vs 1	2.729	1.029	7.240
race 3 vs 1	1.542	0.758	3.136
ftv	0.952	0.686	1.321

Association of Predicted Probabilities and Observed Responses

Percent Concordant	65.1	Somers' D	0.308
Percent Discordant	34.3	Gamma	0.310
Percent Tied	0.6	Tau-a	0.133
Pairs	7670	c	0.654

7.4 Diagnosing a Logistic Regression Model

As with the multiple regression model considered in the previous chapter, fitting a logistic regression model is not complete without checking on model assumptions by examining the properties of some suitably defined 'residuals' or other diagnostics. There are a number of ways in which a fitted logistic model may be inadequate.

- The linear function of the explanatory variables may be inadequate; for example, one or more of the explanatory variables may need to be transformed.
- The logistic transformation of the response probability may not be entirely appropriate, for example, the complementary log-log transformation (see Collett, 2003).
- The data may contain outliers that are not well fitted by the model, or observations with undue impact on the conclusions drawn from the analysis, i.e., influential values.
- The assumption of a binomial distribution may not be correct. For example, with grouped data the observations y_i can only be assumed to have a binomial distribution when the n_i individual observations on which they are based are independent.

DISPLAY 7.2

Residuals for Logistic Regression

- The raw residual for the type of observations modelled by logistic regression is simply $y_i - \hat{y}_i$, where $\hat{y}_i = n_i\pi_i$.
- But for reasons discussed in Collett (2003), these raw residuals are difficult to interpret.
- Consequently, the following residuals are more often used:
  a. Pearson residuals

$$d_i = \frac{y_i - n_i\hat{\pi}_i}{\sqrt{n_i\hat{\pi}_i(1-\hat{\pi}_i)}}$$

  b. Deviance residuals

$$d_i = \text{sign}(y_i - \hat{y}_i)\left[2y_i \log\left(\frac{y_i}{\hat{y}_i}\right) + 2(n - y_i)\log\left(\frac{n - y_i}{n - \hat{y}_i}\right)\right]^{\frac{1}{2}}$$

  where sign is the function that makes d_i positive when $y_i \geq \hat{y}_i$ and negative when $y_i < \hat{y}_i$.
- There are various ways of plotting the residuals that give different insights into the possible model inadequacies. Three possibilities are:
  - Index plot: plot of residuals against observation number. Often useful for detecting outliers.
  - Plot of residuals against the linear predictor. The occurrence of a systematic pattern in the plot suggests the model is incorrect in some way.
  - Plot of residuals against explanatory variables may help to identify whether a variable needs to be transformed.

An extremely comprehensive account of residuals and other diagnostics appropriate for checking each of those assumptions is given in Collett (2003). Here we will demonstrate the use of only the basic residuals, which are described and defined in Display 7.2.

We will illustrate the use of some of the diagnostic plots described in Display 7.2 on the logistic regression model fitted to the birthweight data. The following code gives plots of deviance residuals plotted against the observation number, the fitted probabilities and the explanatory variables. lwt, age, and ftv:

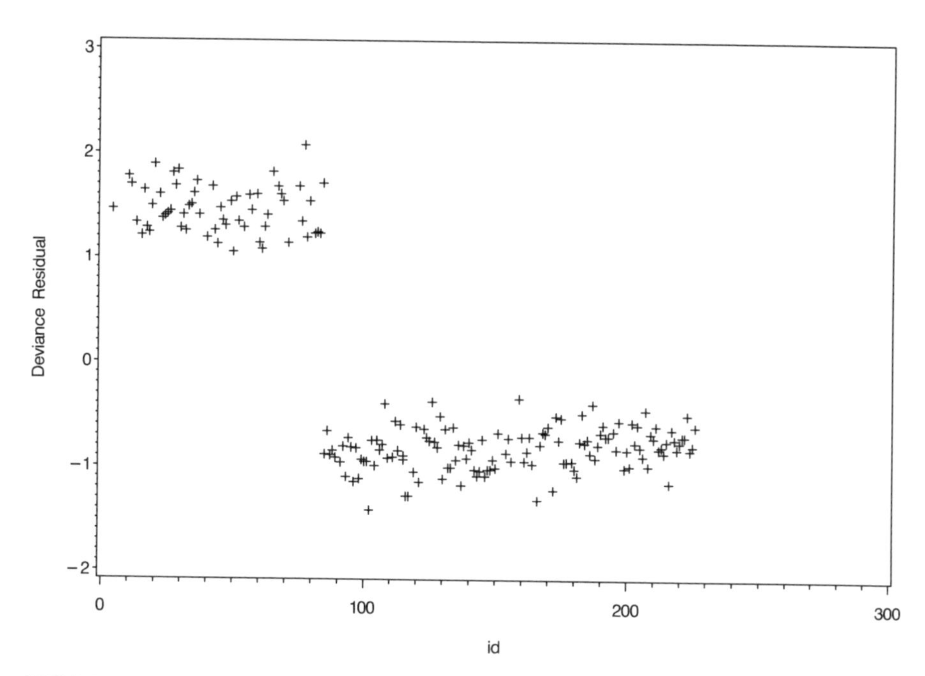

FIGURE 7.3
Deviance residual plotted against ID number for the low birthweight data.

```
proc logistic data=lobwgt desc;
  class race / param=ref ref=first;
  model low=race age lwt ftv;
  output out=lout p=pred resdev=dres;
run;
axis1 label=(a=90);
proc gplot data=lout;
  plot dres*(id pred age lwt ftv) /vaxis=axis1;
run;
```

The `output` statement saves the predicted probabilities and deviance residuals in the `lout` data set. The deviance residuals are then plotted against the predicted probabilities, and the three continuous predictors. The results are shown in Figure 7.3, Figure 7.4, Figure 7.5 , Figure 7.6, and Figure 7.7. The plots of deviance residuals against the linear predictor and each of three of the explanatory variables show no obvious patterns that might suggest the need for say, a quadratic term in any of the variables to be considered, and there are no obvious outliers in the index plot of the residuals. (The distinct separation of points in these plots is entirely due to the binary nature of the data and does not necessarily reflect any problems with the fitted model, although it does make interpretation more difficult.)

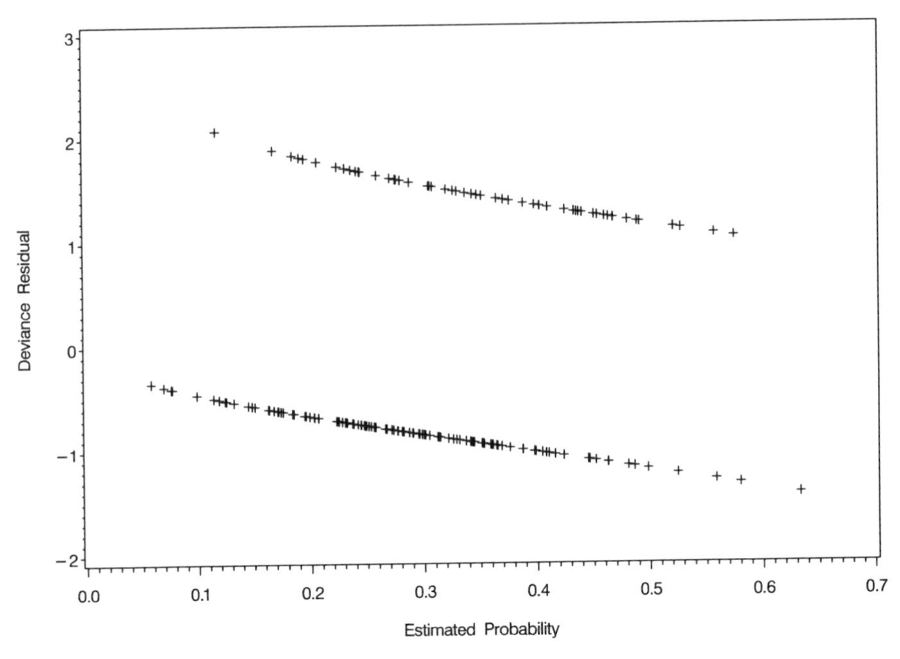

FIGURE 7.4
Deviance residuals plotted against predicted probabilities for the low birthweight data.

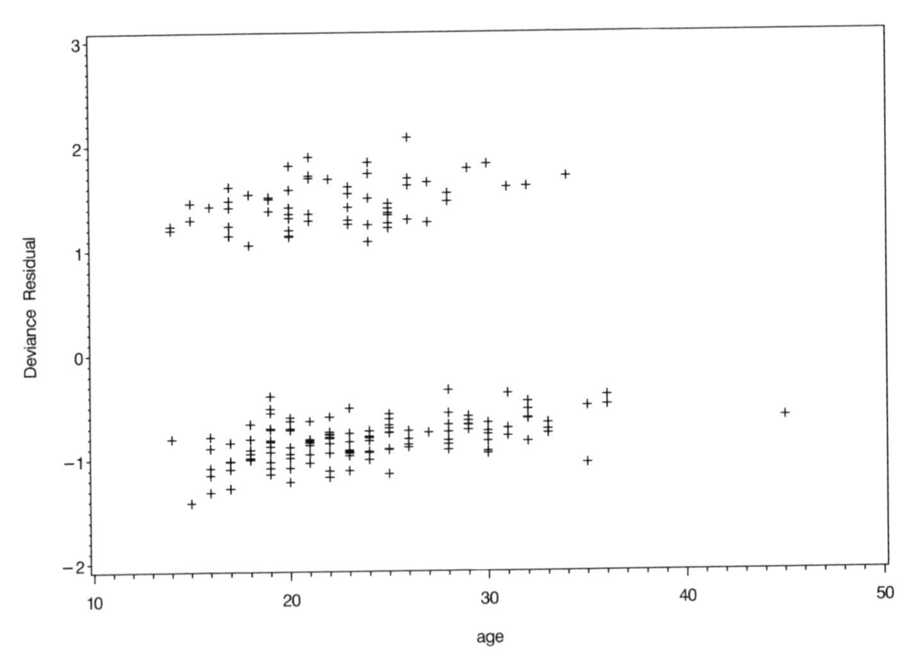

FIGURE 7.5
Deviance residuals plotted against mother's age for the low birthweight data.

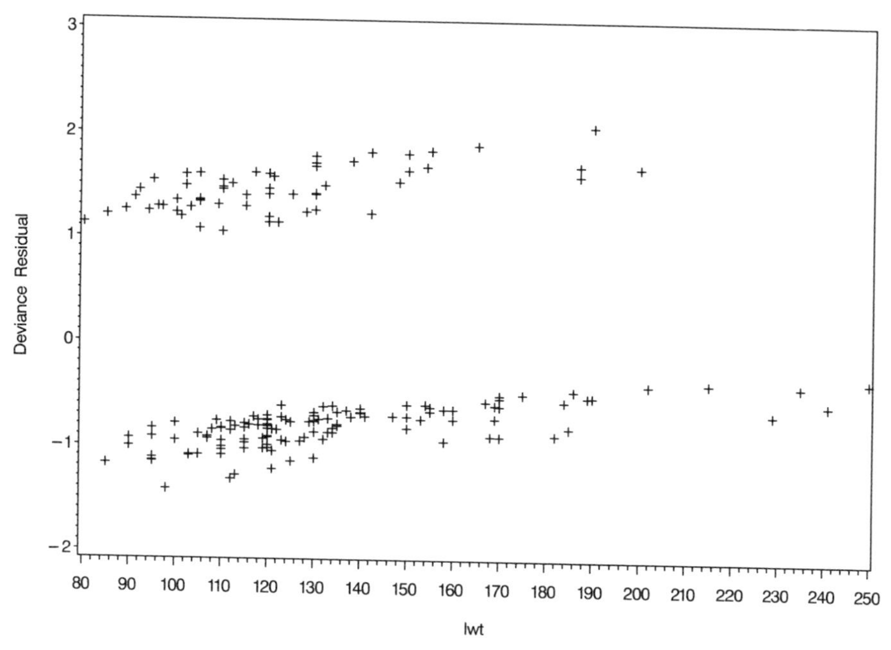

FIGURE 7.6
Deviance residuals plotted against mother's weight for the low birthweight data.

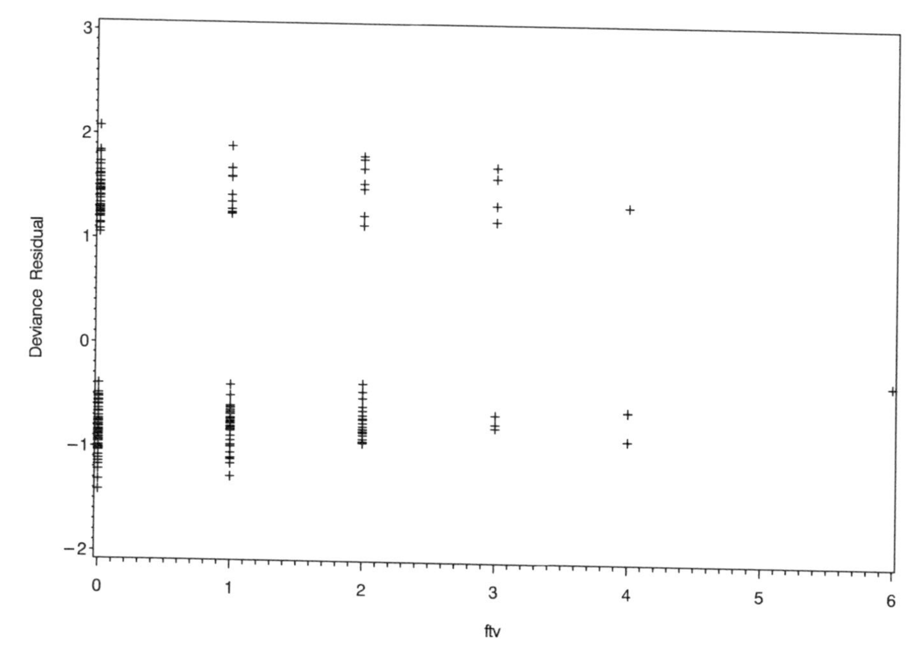

FIGURE 7.7
Deviance residuals plotted against physician visits for the low birthweight data.

TABLE 7.5

1:1 Matched Case-Control Study

		Controls		
		1	0	Total
Cases	1	12	43	55
	0	7	121	128
	Total	19	164	183

Note: 1 = Exposed; 0 = Not exposed.

7.5 Logistic Regression for 1-1 Matched Studies

A frequently used design in medicine is the matched case-control study in which each patient suffering from a particular condition of interest included in the study is matched to one or more people without the condition. The most commonly used matching variables are age, ethnic group, mental status, etc. A design with m controls per case is known as a 1:m matched study. In many cases m will be 1, and it is the 1-1 matched study that we shall concentrate on here.

Table 7.5 illustrates results from a 1-1 matched case-control study. In this study cases of endometrial cancer were matched on age, race, data of admission, and hospital of admission to a suitable control not suffering from cancer, and past exposure to conjugated estrogens of both case and control determined.

The form of the logistic model used for these data involves the probability, $\o_i$, that in matched pair i, for a given value of the explanatory variable, past exposure to conjugated estrogens, x (yes or no), a member of the pair is the case. Specifically, the model is

$$\log\text{it}\left(\o_i\right) = \alpha_i + \beta x$$

The odds that a subject with past exposure ($x = 1$) is a cancer case equal $\exp(\beta)$ times the odds that a subject without past exposure ($x = 0$) is a cancer case.

The model generalizes to the situation where there are p explanatory variables as

$$\log\text{it}\left(\o_i\right) = \alpha_i + \beta_1 x_1 + \cdots \beta_p x_p$$

Typically one x_i is an explanatory variable of real interest, such as past exposure in the example above, with the others being used as a form of statistical control in addition to the variables already controlled by virtue of using them to form matched pairs.

The problem with the model above is that the number of parameters increases at the same rate as the sample size with the consequence that maximum likelihood estimation is no longer viable. We can overcome this problem if we regard the parameters α_i as of little interest and so are willing to forego their estimation. If we do, we can then create a *conditional likelihood function* that will yield maximum likelihood estimators of the coefficients, $\beta_1 \cdots \beta_p$, that are consistent and asymptotically normally distributed. The mathematics behind this are described by Collett (2003), who shows that this conditional logistic regression model can be applied using standard logistic regression software as follows:

- Set the sample size to the number of matched pairs.
- Use as the explanatory variables the differences between corresponding covariate values for each case and control.
- Set the value of the response variable to 1 for all observations.
- Exclude the constant term from the model.

To illustrate this approach we shall apply it to the cancer data in Table 7.5. Exposure to the risk factor, conjugated estrogens, is coded as 1 and nonexposure by 0. We will first need to set all observed response values to 1. And then corresponding to seven of these observations, the single explanatory will take the value –1 (case-control difference in the binary variable denoting exposure), for 43 it will take the value +1, and for (12 + 121) it will take the value 0. The necessary SAS code is

```
data endocal;
  input est num;
  resp=1;
cards;
-1 7
 1 43
 0 133
;
proc logistic data=endocal;
  model resp=est /noint;
  freq num;
run;
```

The `noint` option excludes the intercept term from the model, a feature that is needed for a conditional logistic regression, and the `freq` statement identifies the number of individuals that each observation represents. The results are shown in Table 7.6. The odds that in a matched pair, past exposure to conjugated estrogens has been suffered by the case is estimated to be between 2.8 and 13.7 times the odds that the control has been exposed.

TABLE 7.6

Results of Conditional Logistic Regression Model Fitted to Data in Table 7.5

```
                    The LOGISTIC Procedure
                      Model Information

           Data Set                         WORK.ENDOCA1
           Response Variable                resp
           Number of Response Levels        1
           Number of Observations           3
           Frequency Variable               num
           Sum of Frequencies               183
           Model                            binary logit
           Optimization Technique           Fisher's scoring

                      Response Profile

               Ordered                         Total
                 Value          resp       Frequency

                     1             1             183

               Probability modeled is resp=1.

                  Model Convergence Status

        Convergence criterion (GCONV=1E-8) satisfied.

                    Model Fit Statistics

                             Without           With
               Criterion    Covariates      Covariates

               AIC             253.692         226.873
               SC              253.692         230.083
               -2 Log L        253.692         224.873

           Testing Global Null Hypothesis: BETA=0

   Test                    Chi-Square       DF     Pr > ChiSq

   Likelihood Ratio           28.8184        1         <.0001
   Score                      25.9200        1         <.0001
   Wald                       19.8376        1         <.0001

          Analysis of Maximum Likelihood Estimates

                                       Standard        Wald
Parameter     DF     Estimate          Error     Chi-Square     Pr > ChiSq

est            1       1.8153         0.4076        19.8376         <.0001

                    The LOGISTIC Procedure

                    Odds Ratio Estimates

                          Point           95% Wald
             Effect     Estimate      Confidence Limits

             est           6.143        2.763       13.655

NOTE: Since there is only one response level, measures of association between
      the observed and predicted values were not calculated.
```

7.6 Summary

Logistic regression can be used to model the effects of explanatory variables on a binary response. The model can also be extended to deal with categorical responses with more than two categories and ordinal response variables — see McCullagh (1980) for details. The model can also be adapted for matched case-control data.

8

The Generalized Linear Model

8.1 Introduction

The term "generalized linear model" (GLM) was first introduced in a landmark paper by Nelder and Wedderburn (1972), in which a wide range of seemingly disparate problems of statistical modeling and inference were set in an elegant unifying framework of great power and flexibility. Generalized linear models include all the modeling techniques described in earlier chapter, that is analysis of variance, analysis of covariance, multiple linear regression, and logistic regression, and open up the possibility of other models, for example, *Poisson regression*, that we shall describe in this chapter. A comprehensive account of GLMs is given in McCullagh and Nelder (1989), and a more concise description in Dobson (2001). In the next section we review the main features of such models.

8.2 Generalized Linear Models

The multiple linear regression model described in Chapter 6 has the form

$$y = \beta_0 + \beta_1 x_1 \cdots + \beta_p x_p + \varepsilon$$

The error term, ε, is assumed to have a normal distribution with zero mean and variance, σ^2. An equivalent way of writing the model is as

$$y \sim N\left(\mu, \sigma^2\right)$$

where $\mu = \beta_0 + \beta_1 x_1 + \ldots + \beta_p x_p$. This makes it clear that this model is only suitable for continuous response variables with, conditional on the values of the explanatory variables, a normal distribution with constant variance.

The generalization of such a model made in GLMs consists of allowing the following three assumptions associated with the model to be modified:

- The response variable is normally distributed with a mean determined by the model.
- The mean can be modelled as a linear function of (possibly nonlinear transformations) of the explanatory variables, i.e., the effects of the explanatory variables on the mean are additive.
- The variance of the response variable, given the (predicted) mean, is constant.

In a GLM some transformation of the mean is modelled by a linear function of the explanatory variables, and the distribution of the response variable around its mean (often referred to as the *error distribution*) is generalized usually in a way that fits naturally with a particular transformation. The result is a very wide class of regression models. Display 8.1 summarizes some of the main features of GLMs.

8.3 Applying the Generalized Linear Model

Multiple linear regression (and analysis of variance and analysis of covariance, which as mentioned in Chapter 6 are essentially equivalent to multiple regression) can all be applied via the GLM approach using an identity link function and a normal error distribution. Logistic regression is applied in the GLM framework by using a logit link function and specifying binomial errors. Proc genmod is the main SAS procedure for fitting generalized linear models. Its syntax is broadly similar to that of `proc glm`, with the additional options needed to generalize the linear model. The distribution and the link function are specified on the `model` statement. If the canonical link function is to be used, it is only necessary to specify the distribution. For example the multiple linear regression of the physical measurements data described in Chapter 6 could be applied using `proc genmod` as follows:

```
proc genmod data=young_man;
  model mass=forearm chest waist height / dist=normal
    link=id;
run;
```

The results will be the same as those given in Chapter 6. And the logistic regression model for low birthweight babies described in Chapter 7 would be applied with proc genmod as

DISPLAY 8.1

Generalized Linear Models (GLM)

- Generalized linear models are a general class of models that include many other models as special cases, including analysis of variance, multiple linear regression, and logistic regression.
- The three essential components of a GLM are
  a. A linear predictor, η, formed from the explanatory variables

$$\eta = \beta_0 + \beta_1 x_1 + \beta_2 x_2 \cdots + \beta_p x_p = \beta' x$$

  b. A transformation of the mean, μ, of the response variable called the *link function*, $g(\mu)$. In a GLM it is $g(\mu)$ that is modelled by the linear predictor

$$g(\mu) = \eta$$

  In multiple linear regression and analysis of variance, the link function is the identity function. Other link functions include the log, logit, probit, inverse, and power transformations, although the log and logit are those most commonly met in practice. The logit link, for example, is the basis of logistic regression.

  c. The distribution of the response variable given its mean μ is assumed to be a distribution from the *exponential family;* this has the form

$$f(y;\theta,\phi) = \exp\left\{\left(y\theta - b(\theta)\right) / a(\phi) + c(y,\phi)\right\}$$

  For some specific functions a, b, and c and parameters θ and ϕ.

- For example, in linear regression, a normal distribution is assumed with mean μ and constant variance σ^2. This can be expressed via the exponential family as follows:

$$f(y;\theta,\phi) = \frac{1}{\sqrt{(2\pi\sigma^2)}} \exp\left\{-(y-\mu)^2 / 2\sigma^2\right\}$$

$$= \exp\left\{\left(y\mu - \mu^2/2\right)/\sigma^2 - \frac{1}{2}\left(y^2/\sigma^2 + \log\left(2\pi\sigma^2\right)\right)\right\}$$

DISPLAY 8.1 (continued)

Generalized Linear Models

so that $\theta = \mu, b(\theta) = \theta^2/2, \phi = \sigma^2$ and $a(\phi) = \phi$. Other distributions in the exponential family include the binomial, Poisson, gamma, inverse Gaussian, and exponential distributions.

- Particular link functions in GLMs are generally associated with particular error distributions, for example, the identity link with the Gaussian distribution, the logit with the binomial, and the log with the Poisson.
- The choice of probability distribution determines the relationships between the variance of the response variable (conditional on the explanatory variables) and its mean. This relationship is known as the *variance function*, denoted $V(\mu)$.
- For the Gaussian distribution, $V(\mu) = \sigma^2$, the variance is not a function of the mean and so can be estimated freely. For the Poisson distribution, however, the variance equals the mean, $V(\mu) = \mu$, so the variance is constrained and cannot be estimated freely. More will be said about the variance function in the text.
- The models are estimated by maximizing the joint likelihood of the observed responses given the parameters of the model and the explanatory variables. This generally requires iterative algorithms. See McCullagh and Nelder (1989) for details.

```
proc genmod data=lobwgt desc;
  class race;
  model low=race age lwt ftv / dist=b link=logit;
run;
```

However, in this section we concentrate on describing the use of some less commonly applied link functions and error distributions. We begin with an account of Poisson regression.

8.3.1 Poisson Regression

The Poisson regression model is useful for response variables that are counts or frequencies and for which it is reasonable to assume an underlying Poisson distribution, i.e.,

$$\Pr(y) = \frac{\mu^y e^{-\mu}}{y!} \quad y = 0, 1, 2 \ldots$$

TABLE 8.1

Bladder Cancer Data

Time	X	n
2	0	1
3	0	1
6	0	1
8	0	1
9	0	1
10	0	1
11	0	1
13	0	1
14	0	1
16	0	1
21	0	1
22	0	1
24	0	1
26	0	1
27	0	1
7	0	2
13	0	2
15	0	2
18	0	2
23	0	2
20	0	3
24	0	4
1	1	1
5	1	1
17	1	1
18	1	1
25	1	1
18	1	2
25	1	2
4	1	3
19	1	4

Note: $X = 0$ tumour < 3cm; $X = 1$ tumour > 3 cm.

Source: Seeber, G.U.H. (1998): P. Armitage, T. Colton, Eds., *Encyclopedia of Biostatistics*, Wiley.

For explaining the relationship between the mean of a Poisson variable and some explanatory variables of interest, the appropriate link function is the log since this guarantees positive fitted values as required.

To illustrate the use of Poisson regression we shall apply it to the data shown in Table 8.1, taken from Seeber (1989). The data arise from 31 male patients who have been treated for superficial bladder cancer and give the number of recurrent tumours during a particular time period after removal of the primary tumour, as well as the size of the primary tumour (whether smaller or larger than 3 cm).

Before coming to the analysis of the data in Table 8.1, we first need to introduce the idea of a *Poisson process*, in which the waiting times between successive events of interest (the tumours in this case) are independent and exponentially distributed with common mean, $1/\lambda$ (say). Then the number of events that occur up to time t has a Poisson distribution with mean $\mu = \lambda t$. Here the parameter of real interest is the rate at which events occur, λ, and for a single explanatory variable, x, we can adopt a Poisson regression approach starting with the model

$$\log \lambda = \beta_0 + \beta_1 x$$

to examine the dependence of λ on x. This model can be written in terms of μ as

$$\log \mu = \beta_0 + \beta_1 x + \log t$$

which allows it to be fitted within the GLM framework. In this model log t is a variable in the model whose regression coefficient is fixed at unity, and is usually known as an *offset*.

To read in the data and apply the Poisson regression model here requires the following SAS code:

```
data bladder;
  input time x n;
  logtime=log(time);
cards;
20  1
30  1
...
251 2
41  3
191 4
;
proc genmod data=bladder;
  model n=x / offset=logtime dist=p;
run;
```

The data step reads in the data and calculates the log of the waiting time to be used as the offset in the analysis. The offset is specified on the `model` statement.

The results are shown in Table 8.2. There is no evidence that size of primary tumour is associated with number of recurrent tumours.

As a second example of Poisson regression we shall apply the method to the data shown in Table 8.3, taken from Piantadosi (1997). The data arise

TABLE 8.2

Results from Fitting a Poisson Regression Model to the Bladder Cancer Data in Table 8.1

```
                         The GENMOD Procedure

                          Model Information

                 Data Set                    WORK.BLADDER
                 Distribution                     Poisson
                 Link Function                        Log
                 Dependent Variable                     n
                 Offset Variable                  logtime
                 Observations Used                     31

               Criteria For Assessing Goodness Of Fit

         Criterion                 DF          Value        Value/DF

         Deviance                  29        25.4189          0.8765
         Scaled Deviance           29        25.4189          0.8765
         Pearson Chi-Square        29        38.5938          1.3308
         Scaled Pearson X2         29        38.5938          1.3308
         Log Likelihood                     -33.3234

     Algorithm converged.


                    Analysis Of Parameter Estimates

                                Standard     Wald 95% Confidence       Chi-
  Parameter    DF    Estimate      Error           Limits            Square    Pr > ChiSq

  Intercept     1     -2.3394     0.1768     -2.6859     -1.9929     175.13        <.0001
  x             1      0.2292     0.3062     -0.3709      0.8293       0.56        0.4541
  Scale         0      1.0000     0.0000      1.0000      1.0000

NOTE: The scale parameter was held fixed.
```

from a study of Familial Adenomatous Polyposis (FAP), an autosomal dominant genetic defect that predisposes those affected to develop large numbers of polyps in the colon which, if untreated, may develop into colon cancer. Patients with FAP were randomly assigned to receive an active drug treatment or a placebo. The response variable was the number of colonic polyps at 3 months after starting treatment. Additional covariates of interest were number of polyps before starting treatment, gender, and age.

These data can be read in and a Poisson regression model fitted using the following SAS code:

```
data fap;
  input male treat base_n age r_n;
cards;
01  7   17  6
00  77  20  67
....
01  10  23  6
01  20  22  5
11  12  42  8
;
```

TABLE 8.3

FAP Data

Sex	Treatment	Baseline Count of Polyps	Age	Number of Polyps at 3 Months
0	1	7	17	6
0	0	77	20	67
1	1	7	16	4
0	0	5	18	5
1	1	23	22	16
0	0	35	13	31
0	1	11	23	6
1	0	12	34	20
1	0	7	50	7
1	0	318	19	347
1	1	160	17	142
0	1	8	23	1
1	0	20	22	16
1	0	11	30	20
1	0	24	27	26
1	1	34	23	27
0	0	54	22	45
1	1	16	13	10
1	0	30	34	30
0	1	10	23	6
0	1	20	22	5
1	1	12	42	8

Note: Sex: 0 = female, 1 = male; Treatment: 0 = placebo, 1 = active.
Source: Piantadosi, S., 1997, *Clinical Trials: A Methodologic Perspective*, Wiley.

```
proc genmod data=fap;
  model r_n=male treat base_n age / dist=p;
run;
```

The results are shown in Table 8.4. All the covariates appear to be significant predictors of number of polyps at 3 months, although the conditional nature of the estimated regression coefficients makes this straightforward interpretation of the p-values somewhat suspect (see Chapter 6).

The regression coefficients become easier to interpret if they (and the confidence limits) are exponentiated. So, for example, the exponentiated confidence interval for the gender regression coefficient is [1.07, 1.65]. For treatment the corresponding interval is [0.60, 0.88]; consequently, patients receiving the active treatment are estimated to have between 60 and 88% the number of polyps at 3 months as those receiving the placebo. One aspect of the fitted model for these data, namely the value of the deviance divided by degrees of freedom, has implications for the appropriateness of the model, which we shall take up in Section 8.5.

TABLE 8.4

Results of Fitting a Poisson Regression Model to the FAP Data in Table 8.3

The GENMOD Procedure

Model Information

Data Set	WORK.FAP
Distribution	Poisson
Link Function	Log
Dependent Variable	r_n
Observations Used	22

Criteria For Assessing Goodness Of Fit

Criterion	DF	Value	Value/DF
Deviance	17	186.7304	10.9841
Scaled Deviance	17	186.7304	10.9841
Pearson Chi-Square	17	186.0802	10.9459
Scaled Pearson X2	17	186.0802	10.9459
Log Likelihood		2946.0059	

Algorithm converged.

Analysis Of Parameter Estimates

Parameter	DF	Estimate	Standard Error	Wald 95% Confidence Limits		Chi-Square	Pr > ChiSq
Intercept	1	3.3610	0.1882	2.9922	3.7298	319.09	<.0001
male	1	0.2814	0.1111	0.0637	0.4991	6.42	0.0113
treat	1	-0.3183	0.0984	-0.5112	-0.1254	10.46	0.0012
base_n	1	0.0089	0.0004	0.0081	0.0097	479.32	<.0001
age	1	-0.0264	0.0073	-0.0408	-0.0120	12.95	0.0003
Scale	0	1.0000	0.0000	1.0000	1.0000		

NOTE: The scale parameter was held fixed.

8.3.2 Regression with Gamma Errors

Some of the counts in the polyp data in Table 8.2 are extremely large, indicating that the distribution of counts is very skew. Consequently the data might be better modelled by allowing for this with the use of a *gamma distribution* (defined in Everitt, 2002). Since gamma variables are positive, a log link function will again be used, and the SAS code to fit the model is now:

```
proc genmod data=fap;
  model r_n=male treat base_n age / dist=g link=log;
run;
```

In this example we specify both the link function and the error distribution on the `model` statement, as the log link is not the canonical link for the gamma distribution.

The results are shown in Table 8.5. The gender regression coefficient is now no longer significant at the 5% level, but the p values associated with the other regression coefficients are largely unchanged.

TABLE 8.5

Results from Fitting a Model with Gamma Errors to the FAP Data

```
                          The GENMOD Procedure

                           Model Information

                    Data Set                  WORK.FAP
                    Distribution                 Gamma
                    Link Function                  Log
                    Dependent Variable             r_n
                    Observations Used               22


                Criteria For Assessing Goodness Of Fit

        Criterion                 DF           Value        Value/DF

        Deviance                  17          7.5870          0.4463
        Scaled Deviance           17         23.1875          1.3640
        Pearson Chi-Square        17          5.6485          0.3323
        Scaled Pearson X2         17         17.2629          1.0155
        Log Likelihood                      -80.1699

Algorithm converged.


                   Analysis Of Parameter Estimates

                          Standard      Wald 95%              Chi-
Parameter  DF  Estimate      Error   Confidence Limits      Square   Pr > ChiSq

Intercept   1    3.0155     0.5048    2.0260     4.0049      35.68       <.0001
male        1    0.5093     0.2940   -0.0668     1.0854       3.00       0.0832
treat       1   -0.8358     0.2591   -1.3437    -0.3280      10.40       0.0013
base_n      1    0.0132     0.0027    0.0079     0.0186      23.46       <.0001
age         1   -0.0223     0.0186   -0.0588     0.0142       1.44       0.2306
Scale       1    3.0562     0.8759    1.7428     5.3595

NOTE: The scale parameter was estimated by maximum likelihood.
```

8.4 Residuals for GLMs

As with multiple regression and logistic regression, it is important when fitting GLMs to look at suitable residuals to assess assumptions. Two residuals useful in assessing fitted GLMs are described in Display 8.2. They are essentially equivalent to those described in the previous chapter on logistic regression.

To illustrate the use of residuals for assessing GLMs we shall calculate the Pearson residuals for both the Poisson regression model and the gamma errors model fitted to the FAP data. A probability plot will be used in each case to display the residuals. To do this we rerun the two models adding an `output` statement to save the Pearson (Chi) residuals and then use `proc univariate` for the probability plot, suppressing the printed output with the `noprint` option.

```
proc genmod data=fap;
  model r_n=male treat base_n age / dist=p;
  output out=pout reschi=rs;
```

DISPLAY 8.2

Residuals for GLMs

- The *deviance residuals* are defined as

$$r_i^D = \text{sign}(y_i - \hat{\mu}_i)\sqrt{d_i}$$

where d_i is the contribution of the ith subject to the deviance, with total deviance given by

$$D = \sum_i \left(r_i^D\right)^2.$$

- The *Pearson residuals* are defined as the contribution of the ith subject to the Pearson X^2 statistic,

$$r_i^P = \frac{(y_i - \hat{\mu}_i)}{\sqrt{V(\hat{\mu}_i)}}$$

so that the $X^2 = \sum \left(r_i^P\right)^2$

- Both the Pearson and deviance statistics can be used for detecting observations not well fitted by the model. The deviance residuals are more commonly used because their distribution tends to be closer to normal than that of the Pearson residuals.

```
run;
proc univariate data=pout noprint;
  var rs;
  probplot rs / normal;
run;
proc genmod data=fap;
  model r_n=male treat base_n age / dist=g link=log;
  output out=gout reschi=rs;
run;
proc univariate data=gout noprint;
  var rs;
  probplot rs / normal;
run;
```

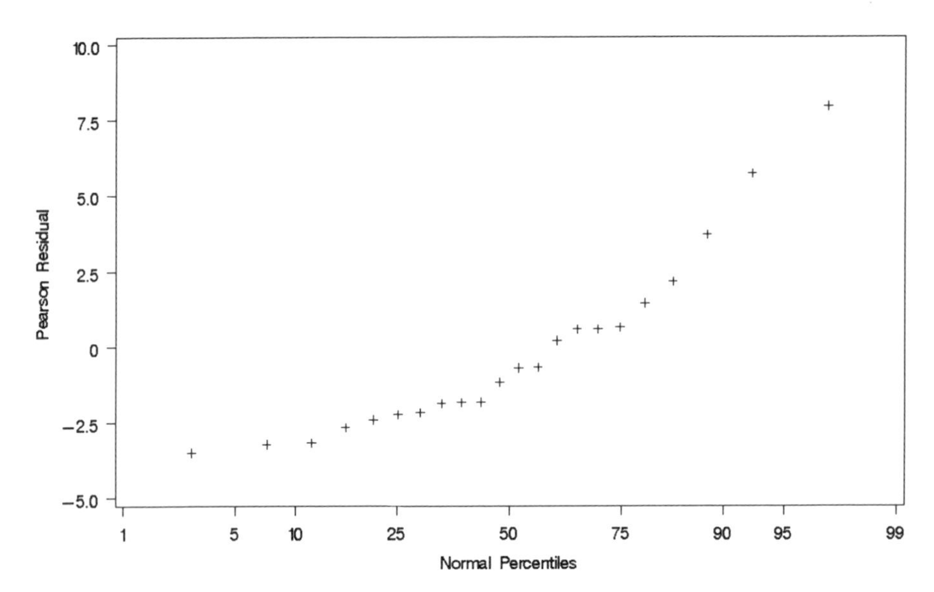

FIGURE 8.1
Normal probability plot of Pearson residuals from the Poisson regression model for the polyp data.

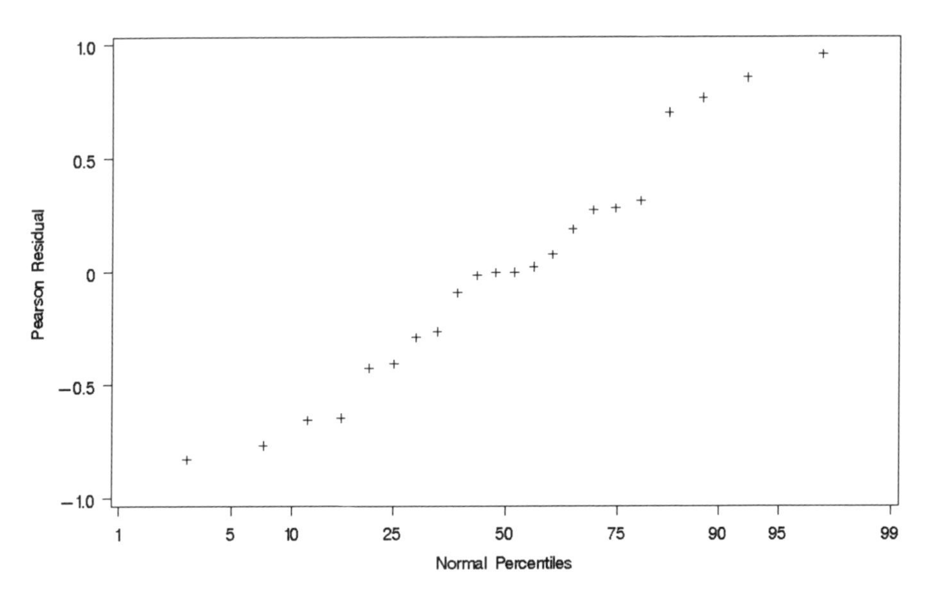

FIGURE 8.2
Normal probability plot of Pearson residuals from the gamma regression model for the polyp data.

The probability plots are shown in Figure 8.1 and Figure 8.2. The plot associated with the Poisson regression shows a clear departure from linearity, with several very large residuals. The plot associated with the gamma errors model appears to be far more satisfactory. The problems with the Poisson model are taken up on the next section.

8.5 Overdispersion

An important aspect of generalized linear models that thus far we have largely ignored is the variance function, $V(\mu)$, that captures how the variance of a response variable depends upon its mean. The general form of the relationship is

$$\text{Var}(\text{response}) = \phi V(\mu)$$

where ϕ is a constant and $V(\mu)$ specifies how the variance depends on the mean μ. For the error distributions considered previously this general form becomes:

1. Normal: $V(\mu) = 1, \phi = \sigma^2$; here the variance does not depend on the mean.
2. Binomial: $V(\mu) = \mu(1-\mu), \phi = 1$.
3. Poisson: $V(\mu) = \mu; \phi = 1$.

In the case of a Poisson variable we see that the mean and variance are equal, and in the case of a binomial variable where the mean is the probability of the occurrence of the event of interest, π, the variance is $\pi(1-\pi)$.

Both the Poisson and binomial distributions have variance functions that are completely determined by the mean. There is no free parameter for the variance since in applications of the generalized linear model with binomial or Poisson error distributions the dispersion parameter, ϕ, is defined to be one (see previous results for logistic and Poisson regression). But in some applications this becomes too restrictive to fully account for the empirical variance in the data; in such cases it is common to describe the phenomenon as *overdispersion*. For example, if the response variable is the proportion of family members who have been ill in the past year, observed in a large number of families, then the individual binary observations that make up the observed proportions are likely to be correlated rather than independent. This nonindependence can lead to a variance that is greater (less) than that on the assumption of binomial variability. And observed counts often exhibit larger variance than would be expected from the Poisson assumption, a fact noted by Greenwood and Yule over 80 years ago (Greenwood and Yule, 1920). Greenwood and Yule's suggested solution to the problem was a model in which μ was a random variable with a gamma distribution leading to a *negative binomial distribution* for the count.

There are a number of strategies for accommodating overdispersion but here we concentrate on a relatively simple approach that retains the use of the binomial or Poisson error distributions as appropriate but allows estimation of a value of ϕ from the data rather than defining it to be unity for these distributions. The estimate is usually the residual deviance divided by its degrees of freedom, exactly the method used with Gaussian models. Parameter estimates remain the same but parameter standard errors are increased by multiplying them by the square root of the estimated dispersion parameter. This process can be carried out manually, or almost equivalently the overdispersed model can be formally fitted using a procedure known as *quasilikelihood*; this allows estimation of model parameters without fully knowing the error distribution of the response variable — see McCullagh and Nelder (1989) for full technical details of the approach.

When fitting generalized linear models with binomial or Poisson error distributions, overdisperson can often be spotted by comparing the residual deviance with its degrees of freedom. For a well-fitting model the two quantities should be approximately equal. If the deviance is far greater than the degrees of freedom, overdispersion may be indicated. In Table 8.4, for example, we see that the ratio of deviance to degrees of freedom is nearly 11, clearly indicating an overdispersion problem. Consequently we will now refit the Poisson model with the `scale=d` option, which uses the square root of the deviance divided by its degrees of freedom as the scale parameter.

```
proc genmod data=fap;
  model r_n=male treat base_n age /  dist=p scale=d;
  output out=pout reschi=rs;
run;
```

The results are shown in Table 8.6. Comparing these with the results in Table 8.4, we see that the estimated regression coefficients are the same, but their standard errors are now much greater, with the consequence that only the coefficient of baseline polyps count remains significant. Gender, treatment, and age are no longer found to be significant predictors of 3-month polyp count.

8.6 Summary

Generalized linear models provide a very powerful and flexible framework for the application of regression models to medical data. Some familiarity with the basis of such models might allow medical researchers to consider more realistic models for their data rather than to rely solely on linear and logistic regression.

TABLE 8.6

Results of Fitting Overdispersed Poisson Model to FAP Data

The GENMOD Procedure

Model Information

Data Set	WORK.FAP
Distribution	Poisson
Link Function	Log
Dependent Variable	r_n
Observations Used	22

Criteria For Assessing Goodness Of Fit

Criterion	DF	Value	Value/DF
Deviance	17	186.7304	10.9841
Scaled Deviance	17	17.0000	1.0000
Pearson Chi-Square	17	186.0802	10.9459
Scaled Pearson X2	17	16.9408	0.9965
Log Likelihood		268.2054	

Algorithm converged.

Analysis Of Parameter Estimates

Parameter	DF	Estimate	Standard Error	Wald 95% Confidence Limits		Chi-Square	Pr > ChiSq
Intercept	1	3.3610	0.6236	2.1388	4.5832	29.05	<.0001
male	1	0.2814	0.3681	-0.4400	1.0028	0.58	0.4445
treat	1	-0.3183	0.3261	-0.9575	0.3209	0.95	0.3291
base_n	1	0.0089	0.0013	0.0063	0.0115	43.64	<.0001
age	1	-0.0264	0.0243	-0.0741	0.0213	1.18	0.2776
Scale	0	3.3142	0.0000	3.3142	3.3142		

NOTE: The scale parameter was estimated by the square root of DEVIANCE/DOF.

9

Generalized Additive Models

9.1 Introduction

The multiple regression model described in Chapter 6 and the generalized linear model featured in Chapter 8 can accommodate nonlinear functions of the explanatory variables, for example, quadratic or cubic terms, if these are thought to be necessary to provide an adequate fit. In this chapter, however, we consider some alternative and generally more flexible statistical methods for modelling nonlinear relationships between a response variable and one or more explanatory variables. The main component of these methods, known as *generalized additive models* (GAMs), is the fitting of a "smooth" relationship between the response and each explanatory variable by means of a *scatterplot smoother* (see Chapter 4 and Section 9.2). GAMs are useful where:

- The relationship between the variables is expected to be of complex form not easily fitted by standard linear or nonlinear models.
- There is no *a priori* reason for using a particular model.
- We would like the data themselves to suggest the appropriate functional form for the relationship between an explanatory variable and the response.

Such models should be regarded as philosophically closer to the concepts of exploratory data analysis, in which the form of any functional relationship emerges from a set of data, rather than arising from a theoretical construct. In the health sciences, this can be especially useful because it reflects the uncertainty of knowledge regarding the mechanisms that determine disease and its prognosis.

Since the building blocks of the GAM approach are scatterplot smoothers, these are described in the next section.

9.2 Scatterplot Smoothers

The scatterplot is an excellent first exploratory graph to study the dependence of two variables. An important second exploratory graph adds a curve to the scatterplot to help us better perceive the pattern of dependence. Most readers will be familiar with adding a parametric curve, such as a simple linear or polynomial regression fit, but there are nonparametric alternatives that are perhaps less familiar but which can often be more useful, since many bivariate data sets are too complex to be described by a simple parametric family. Perhaps the simplest of these alternatives is a *locally weighted regression* or *loess* fit, first suggested by Cleveland (1979) and introduced in Chapter 4. In essence this approach assumes that the variables x and y are related by the equation

$$y_i = g(x_i) + \varepsilon_i \tag{9.1}$$

where g is a 'smooth' function and the ε_i are random variables with mean zero and constant scale. Values $\hat{y}_i$ used to 'estimate' the y_i at each x_i, are found by fitting polynomials using weighted least squares with large weights for points near to x_i and small weights otherwise. So smoothing takes place essentially by local averaging of the y-values of observations having predicted values close to a target value.

Two parameters control the shape of a loess curve; the first is a smoothing parameter, α, with larger values leading to smoother curves — typical values are π to 1. The second parameter, λ, is the degree of certain polynomials that are fitted by the method; λ can take values 1 or 2. In any specific application, the choice of the two parameters must be based on a combination of judgment and of trial and error. Residual plots may be helpful, however, in judging a particular combination of values.

We shall illustrate the use of locally weighted regression on the data shown in Table 9.1, which gives the oxygen uptake and the expired ventilation of a number of subjects performing a standard exercise task. Within SAS locally weighted regression can be performed with `proc loess` or `proc gam`. Although `proc loess` has more options for choosing the parameters of the locally weighted regression, `proc gam` fits a wider range of generalised additive models and so is used here. (The use of `proc loess` was illustrated in Chapter 4.)

```
data oxygen;
input id o2uptake expired;
cards;
 1   574      21.9
 2   592      18.6
 3   664      18.6
```

TABLE 9.1

Oxygen Uptake and Expired Ventilation in 53 Subjects

	Oxygen Uptake	Expired Ventilation
1	574	21.9
2	592	18.6
3	664	18.6
4	667	19.1
5	718	19.2
6	770	16.9
7	927	18.3
8	947	17.2
9	1020	19.0
10	1096	19.0
11	1277	18.6
12	1323	22.8
13	1330	24.6
14	1599	24.9
15	1639	29.2
16	1787	32.0
17	1790	27.9
18	1794	31.0
19	1874	30.7
20	2049	35.4
21	2132	36.1
22	2160	39.1
23	2292	42.6
24	2312	39.9
25	2475	46.2
26	2489	50.9
27	2490	46.5
28	2577	46.3
29	2766	55.8
30	2812	54.5
31	2893	63.5
32	2957	60.3
33	3052	64.8
34	3151	69.2
35	3161	74.7
36	3266	72.9
37	3386	80.4
38	3452	83.0
39	3521	86.0
40	3543	88.9
41	3676	96.8
42	3741	89.1
43	3844	100.9
44	3878	103.0
45	4002	113.4
46	4114	111.4
47	4152	119.9
48	4252	127.2
49	4290	126.4
50	4331	135.5

TABLE 9.1 (continued)

Oxygen Uptake and Expired Ventilation in 53 Subjects

	Oxygen Uptake	Expired Ventilation
51	4332	138.9
52	4390	143.7
53	4393	144.8

```
....
52  4390    143.7
53  4393    144.8
;
proc gam data=oxygen;
  model expired=loess(o2uptake) / method=gcv;
  output out=gamout pred;
run;
proc gplot data=gamout;
  plot (expired p_expired)*o2uptake /overlay;
symbol1 i=none v=dot;
symbol2 i=join v=none;
run;
```

The first point to notice about the syntax of `proc gam` is that the specification of predictors on the `model` statement is different from procedures covered in previous chapters. The name of the predictor variable is enclosed in parentheses and prefixed with a keyword indicating the type of smoother to be employed. The keyword `param` is used for variables that are *not* to be smoothed but entered as parametric linear predictors; `loess` is used for a locally weighted regression; `spline` for a cubic smoothing *spline* (described later in the chapter, and `spline2` for a thin plate smoothing spline, which is a multivariate version of the *cubic spline* (again see later in the chapter — Display 9.1). Parametric effects must be specified before smoothed effects and must be included in the same set of parentheses, where there are more than one. Parametric effects can be categorical but in that case must also be named on a `class` statement. For smoothed effects the degree of smoothing can be specified for each in terms of its effective number of parameters (analogous to the number of parameters in a parametric fit — see Display 9.1) or degrees of freedom. For example,

```
model expired = loess(o2uptake,df=6);
```

Alternatively, the `method=gcv` option on the `model` statement can be used to select a degree of smoothing using generalized cross validation. The

DISPLAY 9.1

Fitting a Cubic Spline Scatterplot Smoother

- The smooth curve $f(x)$ that summarizes the dependence of a response variable y on an explanatory variable x is fitted by minimizing

$$\sum_{i=1}^{n}\left[y_i - f(x_i)\right]^2 + \lambda \int f''(x)^2\,dx \qquad (1)$$

where $f''(x)$ is the second derivative of $f(x)$ with respect to x.
- The first term represents the sum of squares criterion used in least squares. The integral in the second term, $\int f''(x)^2\,dx$, measures the departure from linearity of f (for linear f, the term is zero), and λ is a non-negative smoothing parameter. It governs the tradeoff between the goodness-of-fit to the data and the degree of smoothness of f. Larger values of λ force f to be smoother.
- For any value of λ, the solution to (1) is a cubic spline — a piecewise cubic polynomial with pieces joined at the unique observed values x_i of the explanatory variable.
- The 'effective number of parameters' (analogous to the number of parameters in a parametric fit) or degrees of freedom of a cubic spline smoother is generally used to specify its smoothness, rather than λ directly. A numerical search is then used to determine the value of λ corresponding to the required degrees of freedom.
- Roughly, the complexity of a cubic spline is about the same as a polynomial of degree one less than the degrees of freedom. But the cubic spline smoother 'spreads out' its parameters in a more even way and, hence, is much more flexible than is polynomial regression.
- The above account follows that given in Hastie and Tibshirani, 1990.

`dist=` option on the `model` statement specifies the distribution. `Gaussian` is the default, and other possibilities are `binomial`, `binary`, `gamma`, `igaussian (inverse Gaussian)`, or `poisson`.

The `output` statement creates the `gamout` data set, which contains the variables used in the model plus predicted values, specified using the keyword `pred`. (The `id` statement can be used to copy additional variables to

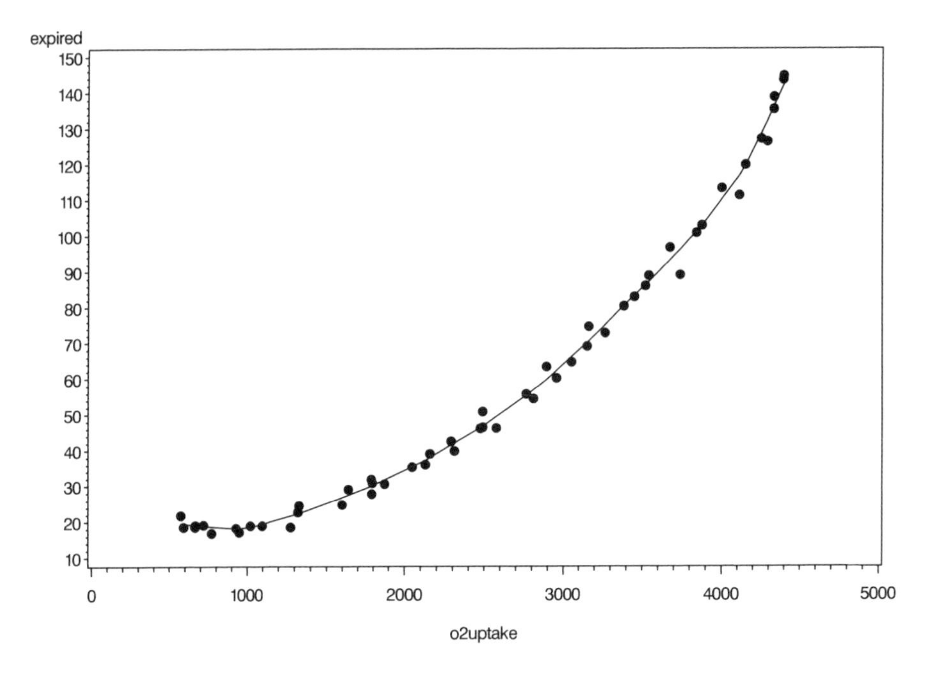

FIGURE 9.1
Plot of oxygen uptake data showing fitted locally weighted regression curve.

the output data set.) There are predicted values for each smoothed effect and overall predicted values. These are automatically named by prefixing the original variable name with `p_`, so the `gamout` data set contains both `p_expired` and `p_o2uptake`.

A plot of the data and the overall predicted values is shown in Figure 9.1.

We can compare this result to results from fitting parametric regressions that include various polynomial functions.

```
proc glm data=oxygen;
  model expired=o2uptake|o2uptake|o2uptake|o2uptake;
  output out=glmout p=pred;
run;
proc gplot data=glmout;
 plot (expired expired pred)*o2uptake /overlay;
symbol1 i=rq v=dot;
symbol2 i=rc v=none l=2;
symbol3 i=join v=none l=3;
run;
```

Quadratic and cubic functions can be overlaid on a scatterplot using the regression interpolation option on the `symbol` statement. For higher-degree

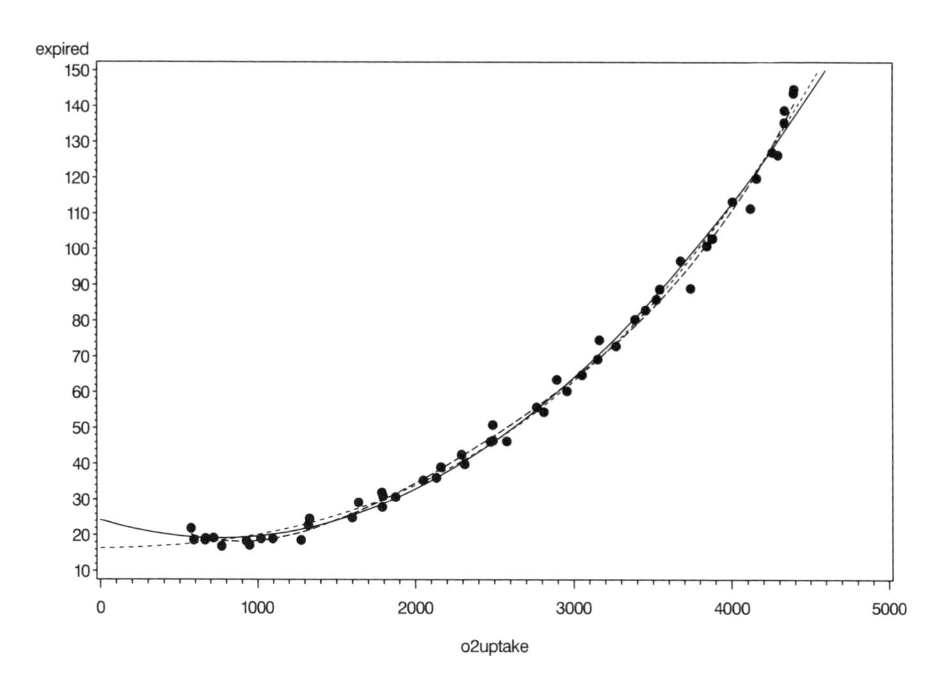

FIGURE 9.2
Plot of oxygen uptake data showing quadratic, cubic, and quartic polynomial fits.

polynomials, we need to fit the model using a regression procedure and save the predicted values. This example illustrates both methods. First, the `glm` step fits a quartic function of oxygen uptake and saves the predicted values. `Proc glm` is more convenient than `proc reg` as the polynomial function can be directly specified, rather than having to compute new variables. The predicted values are then plotted, along with two plots of the original data, each using the regression interpolation. The first symbol statement fits a quadratic regression (`i=rq`), the second a cubic (`i=rc`), and the three plots are overlaid. Naturally, the regression interpolation option can be used to fit linear regression (`i=rl`). It also has options for confidence limits. The regression equations that it uses are given in the log.

The resulting plot is shown in Figure 9.2. Here the locally weighted regression and the polynomial give very similar fits.

A more difficult challenge for the locally weighted regression approach is provided by the data shown in Table 9.2; these are monthly deaths from bronchitis, emphysema, and asthma in the U.K. from 1974 to 1979 for both men and women.

First we read these data in as follows:

```
data respdeaths;
 retain obs 0;
 input year @;
```

TABLE 9.2

Monthly Deaths from Bronchitis, Emphysema, and Asthma in the U.K. from 1974 to 1979 for Both Men and Women

	Jan.	Feb.	Mar.	Apr.	May	Jun.	Jul.	Aug.	Sep.	Oct.	Nov.	Dec.
1974	3035	2552	2704	2554	2014	1655	1721	1524	1596	2074	2199	2512
1975	2933	2889	2938	2497	1870	1726	1607	1545	1396	1787	2076	2837
1976	2787	3891	3179	2011	1636	1580	1489	1300	1356	1653	2013	2823
1977	2996	2523	2540	2520	1994	1964	1691	1479	1596	1877	2032	2484
1978	2899	2990	2890	2379	1933	1734	1617	1495	1440	1777	1970	2745
1979	2841	3535	3010	2091	1667	1589	1518	1348	1392	1619	1954	2633

```
  do month=1 to 12;
  input deaths @;
  output;
  obs=obs+1;
  end;
cards;
1974 3035 2552 2704 2554 2014 1655 1721 1524 1596 2074 2199 2512
1975 2933 2889 2938 2497 1870 1726 1607 1545 1396 1787 2076 2837
1976 2787 3891 3179 2011 1636 1580 1489 1300 1356 1653 2013 2823
1977 2996 2523 2540 2520 1994 1964 1691 1479 1596 1877 2032 2484
1978 2899 2990 2890 2379 1933 1734 1617 1495 1440 1777 1970 2745
1979 2841 3535 3010 2091 1667 1589 1518 1348 1392 1619 1954 2633
run;
```

The `retain` statement specifies a variable whose values are to be kept from the previous iteration of the data step and sets its initial value to zero. Then the year is read in with the trailing @ holding the line for further data to be read. The do loop then reads the number of deaths for each month and writes out an observation. With a single trailing @, the data line is released at the end of the data step iteration.

Now we fit a model using locally weighted regressions with two components, one for year and one for month.

```
proc gam data=respdeaths;
  model deaths=loess(year) loess(month)/ method=gcv;
  id obs;
  output out=respout all;
run;
proc gplot data=respout;
  plot (deaths p_deaths)*obs /overlay;
symbol1 i=none v=dot;
symbol2 i=join v=none;
run;
```

The code is very similar to that given earlier. The obs variable is needed for the subsequent plot, so the id statement is used to add it to the respout data set. The output statement also uses the all keyword to request all available statistics.

The plot of the observed data and the fitted locally weighted regression are shown in Figure 9.3. The characteristic cyclic nature of the data has been modelled reasonably accurately by the fitted curve.

When the model contains more than one smoothed effect, separate plots of the additive fit of each are useful in assessing their functional form. The plots, referred to in SAS as *component plots*, are produced as follows:

```
proc sort data=respout; by month; run;
proc gplot data=respout gout=addfits;
  plot (p_month uclm_month lclm_month)*month /overlay;
symbol1 i=join v=none;
symbol2 i=join l=2 r=2;
run;
proc sort data=respout; by year; run;
proc gplot data=respout gout=addfits;
  plot (p_year uclm_year lclm_year)*year /overlay;
run;
%panelplot(igout=addfits,ncols=2);
```

The all keyword on the output statement has added confidence limits to the respout data set as well as the predicted values. There are overall predicted values with confidence limits and partial predictions with confidence limits for each smoothed effect. These are automatically named by prefixing the name of the variable with p_, lclm_, and uclm_. The result is shown in Figure 9.4.

In the left-hand panel we see more clearly the pattern of winter excess of respiratory deaths, whereas the year-to-year change has a weak linear form with wide confidence limits. In fact a formal test of of the two components shows that the effect of year is nonsignificant. (Such tests will be described later in the chapter.)

An alternative smoother that can often usefully be applied to bivariate data is some form of *spline function*. (A spline is a term for a flexible strip of metal or rubber used by a draftsman to draw curves.) Spline functions are polynomials within intervals of the x-variable that are connected across different values of x. Figure 9.5, for example, shows a linear spline function, i.e., a piecewise linear function, of the form

$$f(x) = \beta_0 + \beta_1 X + \beta_2 (X-a)_+ + \beta_3 (X-b)_+ + \beta_4 (X-c)_+ \tag{9.2}$$

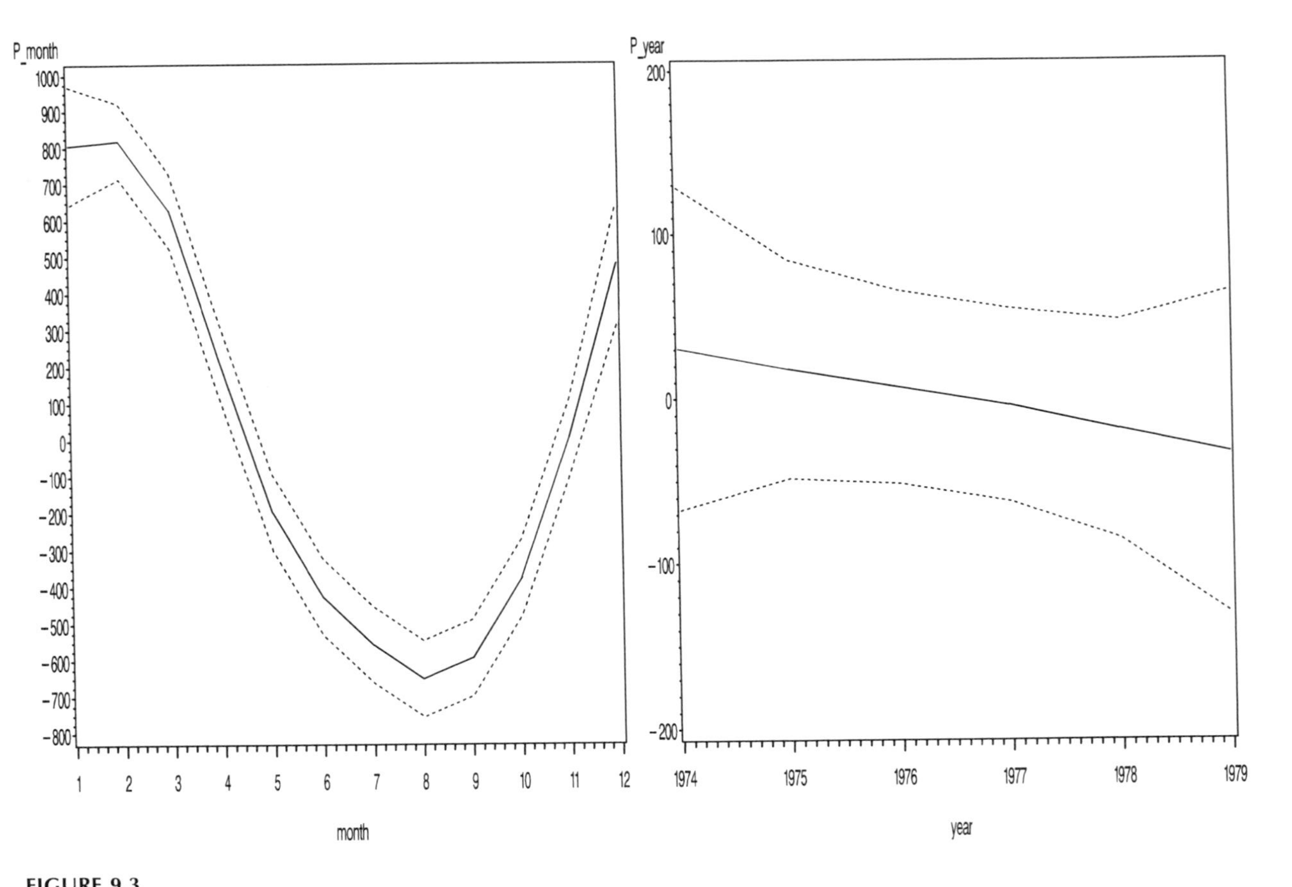

FIGURE 9.3
Plot of monthly deaths from bronchitis showing fitted locally weighted regression.

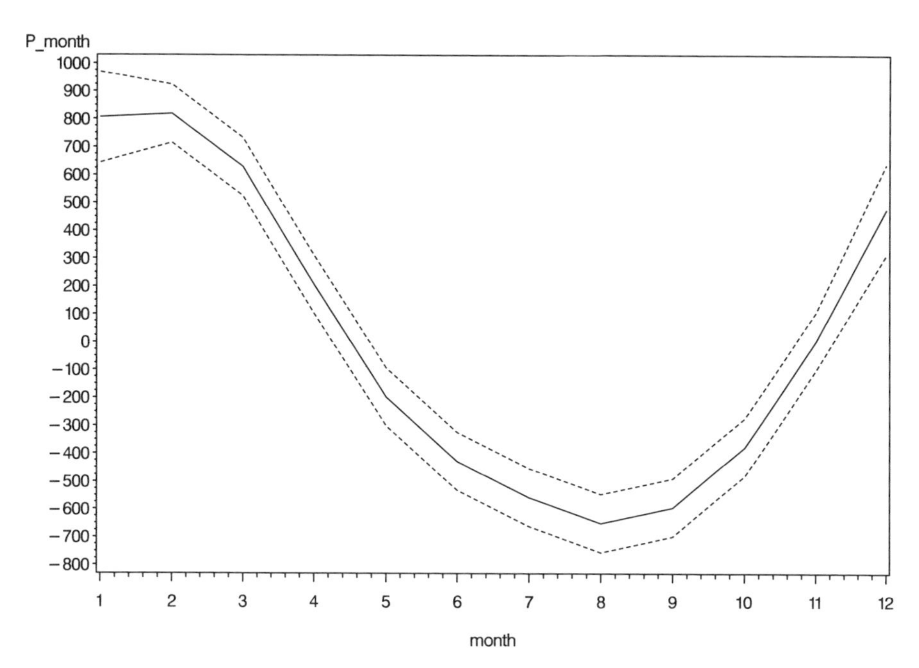

FIGURE 9.4
Component plots for the locally weighted regression model for the bronchitis data.

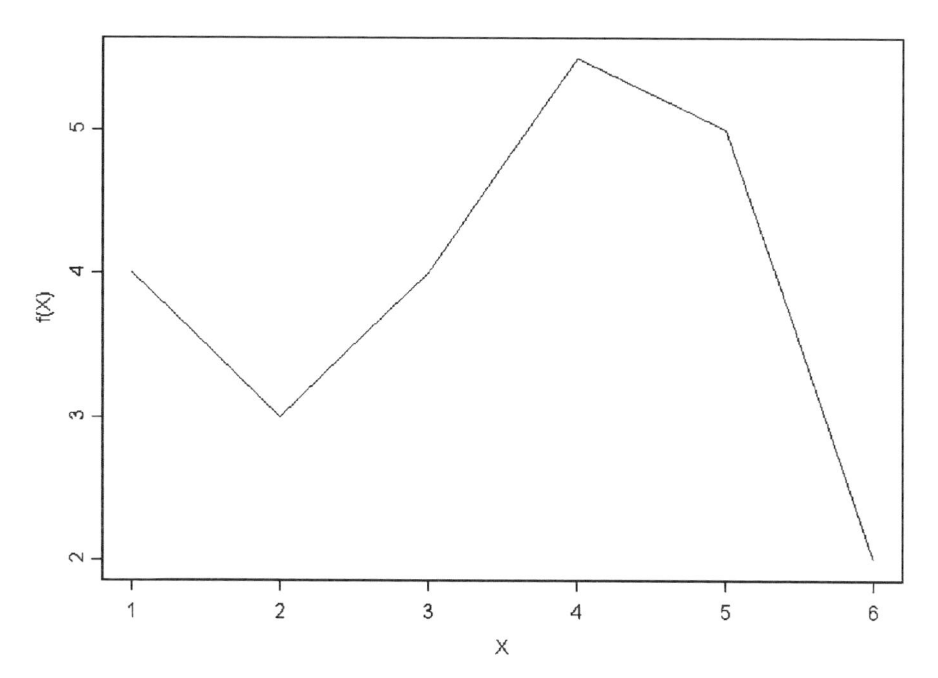

FIGURE 9.5
A linear spline function with knots at a = 1, b = 4, c = 5.

$$\text{where } (u)_+ = u \quad u > 0$$
$$= 0 \quad u \le 0$$

The interval endpoints, *a*, *b*, and *c*, are called *knots*. The number of knots can vary according to the amount of data available for fitting the function.

The linear spline is simple and can approximate some relationships, but it is not smooth and so will not fit highly curved functions well. The problem is overcome by using piecewise polynomials — in particular, cubics — which have been found to have nice properties with good ability to fit a variety of complex relationships. The result is a cubic spline, which is described more formally in Display 9.1.

As mentioned earlier, `proc gam` can also fit spline smoothers, and very similar results to those shown above for the two-component locally weighted regression fit for the bronchitis data can be obtained by changing the model statement to

```
model deaths=spline(year) spline(month)/ method=gcv;
```

For exploratory analysis of bivariate data, spline smoothers are also available as an interpolation option on the `symbol` statement. We can illustrate this by fitting spline smoothers to the overall sequence of the respiratory deaths data.

```
proc gplot data=respdeaths;
  plot (deaths deaths deaths)*obs /overlay;
symbol1 i=sm20 v=dot l=1;
symbol2 i=sm40 v=none l=2;
symbol3 i=sm60 v=none l=3;
run;
```

The number that follows `i=sm` determines the degree of smoothness. It can range from 0 (no smoothing) to 99. The number can be followed by an `s`, as in `i=sm20s`, which presorts the data by the x axis values. The results are shown in Figure 9.6. The solid line (`i=sm20`) and dotted line (`i=sm40`) both suggest the cyclical pattern, whereas the greater degree of smoothing shown by the dashed line (`i=sm60`) misses it.

9.3 Additive and Generalized Additive Models

In a linear regression model there is a dependent variable, *y*, and a set of explanatory variables, $x_1, \cdots, x_q$, and the model assumed is

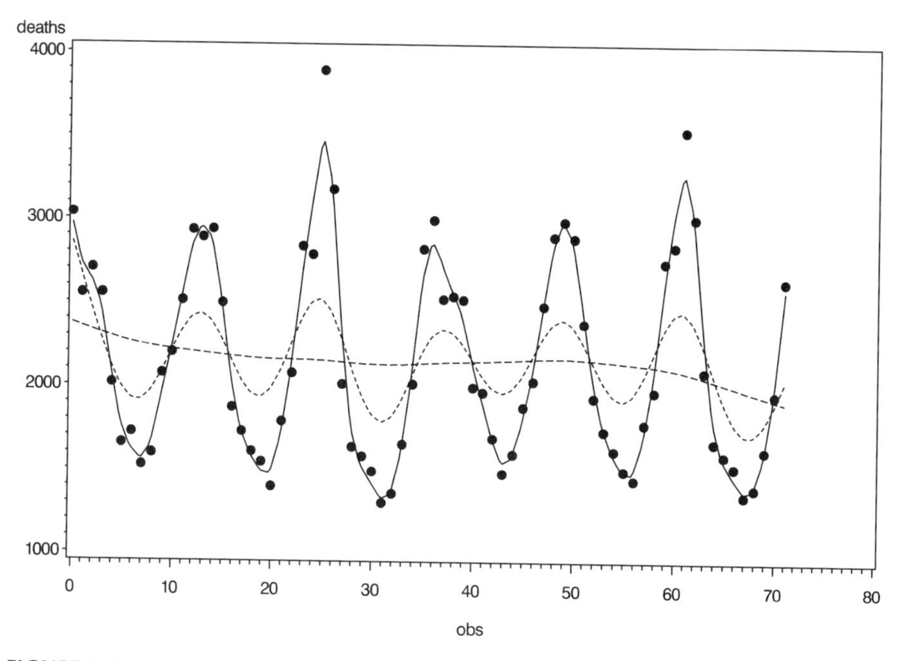

FIGURE 9.6
Spline smoothers fitted to the bronchitis data.

$$y = \beta_0 + \sum_{j=1}^{q} \beta_j x_j + \varepsilon \tag{9.3}$$

Additive models replace the linear function, $\beta_j x_j$, by a smooth nonparametric function to give

$$y = \beta_0 + \sum_{j=1}^{q} g_j(x_j) + \varepsilon \tag{9.4}$$

where g_i can be one of the scatterplot smoothers described in the previous section, or, if the investigator chooses, a linear function for particular x_j. Models can therefore include a mixture of linear and smooth functions if necessary.

A generalized additive model arises from Equation (9.4) in the same way as a generalized linear model arises from a multiple regression model, namely that some function of the expectation of the response variable is now modelled by a sum of nonparametric functions. So, for example, the logistic additive model is

$$\operatorname{logit}\left[\Pr(y=1)\right] = \beta_0 + \sum_{j=1}^{q} g_j(x_j) \tag{9.5}$$

Fitting a generalized additive model involves what is known as a *backfitting algorithm*. The smooth functions g_i are fitted one at a time by taking the residuals.

$$y - \sum_{k \neq j} g_k(x_k) \tag{9.6}$$

and fitting them against x_j using one of the scatterplot smoothers described in Section 9.2. The process is repeated until it converges. Linear terms in the model are fitted by least squares. Full details are given in Chambers and Hastie (1993).

Various tests are available to assess the nonlinear contributions of the fitted smoothers, and generalized additive models can be compared with, say, linear models fitted to the same data by means of likelihood ratio tests often set out in an analysis of deviance table (cf. Table 5.5). In this process the fitted smooth curve is assigned an estimated equivalent number of degrees of freedom. For full details again see Chambers and Hastie (1993).

9.4 Examples of the Application of GAMs

Our first example will involve applying a generalized additive model to the data shown in Table 9.3. These data are given in Hastie and Tibshirani (1990) and come from a study of the factors affecting patterns of insulin-dependent diabetes mellitus in children (Socket et al., 1987). The objective was to investigate the dependence of the level of serum C-peptide on various other factors in order to understand the patterns of residual insulin secretion. The response measure to be used is the logarithm of C-peptide concentration at diagnosis, and the two explanatory variables are age and base deficit, a measure of acidity.

We begin by reading in the data and examining scatterplots of log (peptide) against age and against base.

```
data diabetes;
input id age base peptide;
logpeptide=log10(peptide);
cards;
1  5.2-8.14.8
2  8.8-16.14.1
....
41 13.2-1.94.6
```

TABLE 9.3

Insulin-Dependent Diabetes in Children

Subject	Age	Base Deficit	Peptide
1	5.2	–8.1	4.8
2	8.8	–16.1	4.1
3	10.5	–0.9	5.2
4	10.6	–7.8	5.5
5	10.4	–29.0	5.0
6	1.8	–19.2	3.4
7	12.7	–18.9	3.4
8	15.6	–10.6	4.9
9	5.8	–2.8	5.6
10	1.9	–25.0	3.7
11	2.2	–3.1	3.9
12	4.8	–7.8	4.5
13	7.9	–13.9	4.8
14	5.2	–4.5	4.9
15	0.9	–11.6	3.0
16	11.8	–2.1	4.6
17	7.9	–2.0	4.8
18	11.5	–9.0	5.5
19	10.6	–11.2	4.5
20	8.5	–0.2	5.3
21	11.1	–6.1	4.7
22	12.8	–1.0	6.6
23	11.3	–3.6	5.1
24	1.0	–8.2	3.9
25	14.5	–0.5	5.7
26	11.9	–2.0	5.1
27	8.1	–1.6	5.2
28	13.8	–11.9	3.7
29	15.5	–0.7	4.9
30	9.8	–1.2	4.8
31	11.0	–14.3	4.4
32	12.4	–0.8	5.2
33	11.1	–16.8	5.1
34	5.1	–5.1	4.6
35	4.8	–9.5	3.9
36	4.2	–17.0	5.1
37	6.9	–3.3	5.1
38	13.2	–0.7	6.0
39	9.9	–3.3	4.9
40	12.5	–13.6	4.1
41	13.2	–1.9	4.6
42	8.9	–10.0	4.9
43	10.8	–13.5	5.1

Source: Hastie, T.J. and Tibshirani, R.J., 1990, *Generalized Additive Models*, CRC/Chapman & Hall.

```
42  8.9-10.04.9
43 10.8-13.55.1
run;
proc gplot data=diabetes gout=logpep;
   plot (logpeptide logpeptide)*age /overlay;
   plot (logpeptide logpeptide)*base /overlay;
   symbol1 i=rl v=dot;
   symbol2 i=sm50s v=none;
run;
%panelplot(igout=logpep,ncols=2);
```

We use log10 of the peptide value, following Hastie and Tibshirani. Log peptide is then plotted against age and base, superimposing on each the associated linear regression and a spline smooth. Note that the use of the s suffix on i=sm50s option enables both plots to be generated in a single step. The results are shown in Figure 9.7. In both plots there appears to be at least some evidence of a departure from linearity, although this is stronger for age than base deficit.

To begin we fit a generalized additive model to these data using locally weighted regression fits for both age and base.

```
ods html;
ods graphics on;
proc gam data=diabetes plots(clm commonaxes);
  model logpeptide=loess(age) loess(base) /
method=gcv;
run;
ods graphics off;
ods html close;
```

In this example, we use ods graphics to generate the component plots. First we specify the type of output to be html (pdf and rtf are other useful options). We could also specify a file to store the output; the sashtml file in the current directory is the default. We then switch ods graphics on, run proc gam, switch ods graphics off, and close the html output file. The plots are automatically generated, but the plots option on the proc statement is used to specify options. Here we have specified confidence bands and common vertical axes for the plots. The plots are shown in Figure 9.8 and the procedure output in Table 9.4.

The results shown in Table 9.4 confirm the need for a nonlinear function for age, but it appears there is not a strong case for fitting a nonlinear term for base. The plot of the fitted functions in Figure 9.8 shows the wide standard error limits for the base curve.

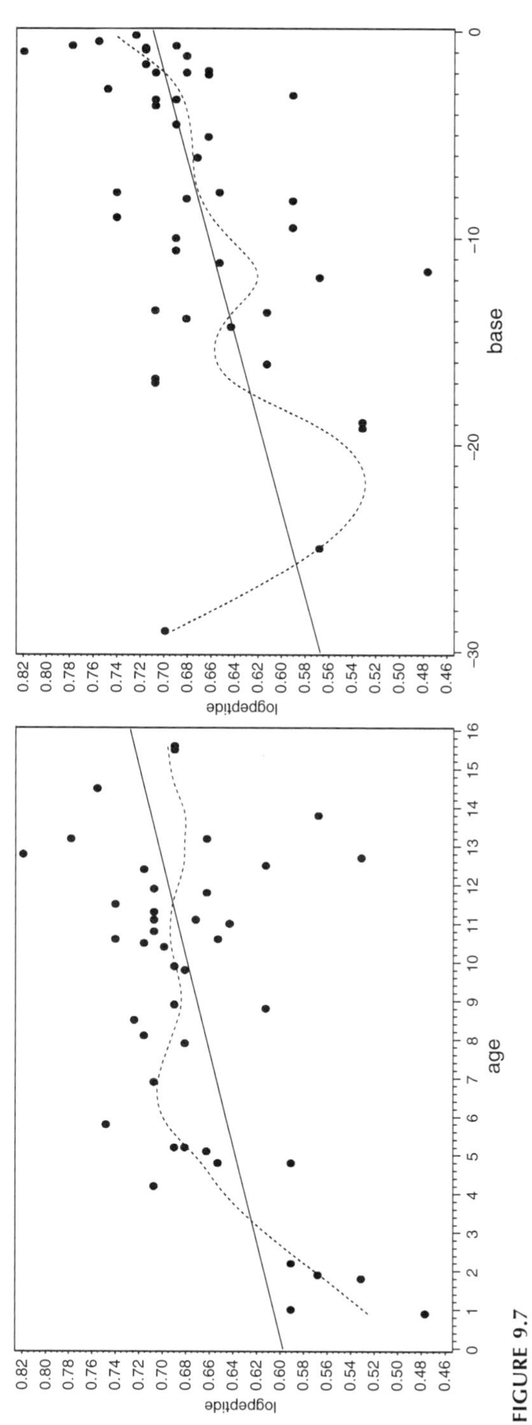

FIGURE 9.7
Plots of log peptide against base and age for insulin dependence data, showing linear and spline fits.

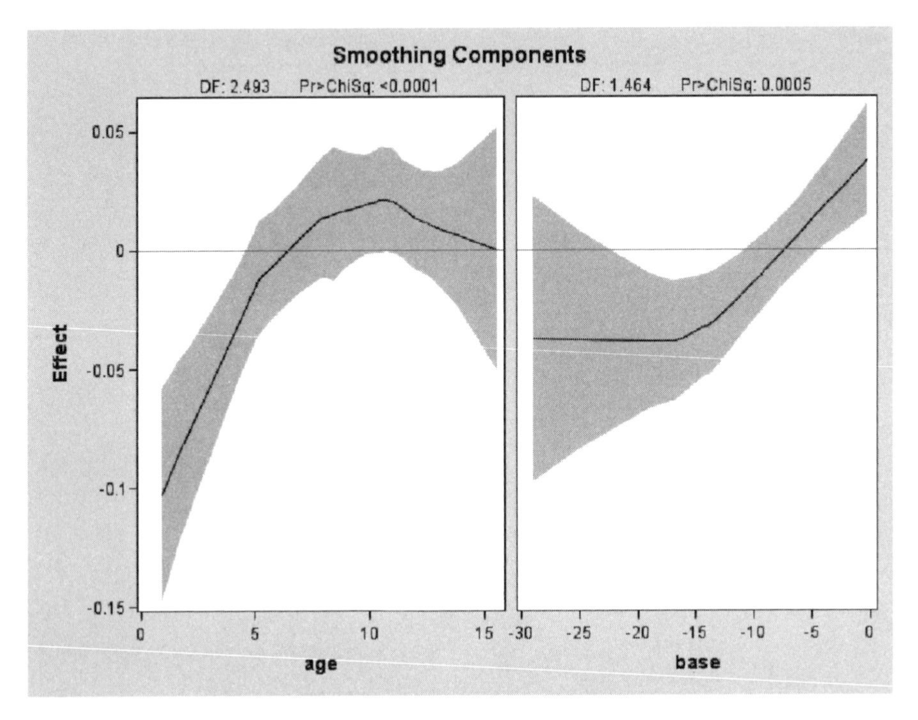

FIGURE 9.8
Fitted functions for age and base deficit.

We now fit a model which includes a locally weighted regression fit for age but a linear term for base; the results are given in Table 9.5. A comparison of this model with the one described above shows that allowing for possible nonlinearity of base contributes very little to the model.

Finally, we can compare the fit of the model with a locally weighted regression term for age and a linear term for base, with a multiple regression model which includes linear effects only for both explanatory variables. This leads to the results for the comparison shown below.

	Terms	Resid DF	RSS	Test	DF	SS	F	Pr(F)
Model 1	Age + base	40	0.1261					
Model 2	Lo(age) + base	39.14	0.1016	1v2	0.86	0.0245	10.97	0.003

Allowing for nonlinearity in age contributes significantly to the model. We could, of course allow for this nonlinearity in the classical way, by including say a quadratic term for age, but it is the fitting of the GAM models that has identified the need for such a term.

The next data set we shall consider is shown in Table 9.6. These data relate to air pollution in 41 U.S. cities. For each city a binary variable is recorded to indicate whether the annual mean concentration of sulphur dioxide is

TABLE 9.4

Results of Fitting a GAM to the Insulin Dependence Data with Spline Functions for Both Age and Base

```
                    The GAM Procedure
              Dependent Variable: logpeptide
      Smoothing Model Component(s): loess(age) loess(base)

                  Summary of Input Data Set

          Number of Observations                  43
          Number of Missing Observations           0
          Distribution                      Gaussian
          Link Function                     Identity

            Iteration Summary and Fit Statistics

  Final Number of Backfitting Iterations                  5
  Final Backfitting Criterion                  3.200717E-10
  The Deviance of the Final Estimate           0.0904097049

The local score algorithm converged.

                  Regression Model Analysis
                     Parameter Estimates

                Parameter         Standard
Parameter        Estimate            Error    t Value    Pr > |t|

Intercept         0.67118          0.00743      90.28      <.0001

                  Smoothing Model Analysis
            Fit Summary for Smoothing Components

                                                                  Num
                  Smoothing                                    Unique
Component         Parameter             DF            GCV         Obs

Loess(age)         0.639535       2.493208    0.000059834          43
Loess(base)        1.000000       1.464229    0.000055703          43

                  Smoothing Model Analysis
                    Analysis of Deviance

                                   Sum of
Source                  DF        Squares    Chi-Square    Pr > ChiSq

Loess(age)         2.49321       0.054911       23.1052        <.0001
Loess(base)        1.46423       0.032338       13.6072        0.0005
```

below 30 micrograms per cubic metre or equal to or above this value. Also recorded are six other variables, two of which relate to human ecology and four to climate. (The data are given in Sokal and Rohlf, 1981, and in Hand, et al., 1994.)

We will use this example to illustrate how GAM models may uncover a relationship that could easily be overlooked if the data were analysed using logistic regression. A naïve approach using logistic regression might conclude that none of the six predictor variables are related to sulphur dioxide concentration. However, some exploratory plots suggest the possibility of nonlinear relationships. We concentrate on two of the six variables, population size and average rainfall.

TABLE 9.5

Results from Fitting a GAM with Spline Function for Age and a Linear Term for Base to the Insulin Dependence Data

```
                         The GAM Procedure
                   Dependent Variable: logpeptide
               Regression Model Component(s): base
             Smoothing Model Component(s): loess(age)

                      Summary of Input Data Set

             Number of Observations                    43
             Number of Missing Observations             0
             Distribution                        Gaussian
             Link Function                       Identity


               Iteration Summary and Fit Statistics

    Final Number of Backfitting Iterations                    5
    Final Backfitting Criterion                    3.820507E-10
    The Deviance of the Final Estimate             0.1016161029


  The local score algorithm converged.


                    Regression Model Analysis
                       Parameter Estimates

                  Parameter        Standard
   Parameter       Estimate           Error     t Value     Pr > |t|

   Intercept        0.70064         0.01189       58.95       <.0001
   base             0.00362         0.00110        3.28       0.0022


                     Smoothing Model Analysis
               Fit Summary for Smoothing Components

                                                                   Num
                   Smoothing                                    Unique
 Component         Parameter              DF            GCV        Obs

 Loess(age)         0.779070        1.857962    0.000064782         43


                     Smoothing Model Analysis
                       Analysis of Deviance

                                       Sum of
 Source                      DF       Squares     Chi-Square    Pr > ChiSq

 Loess(age)             1.85796      0.051817        19.9595        <.0001
```

```
data usair;
  input city $16. hiso2 temperature factories
population windspeed rain rainydays;
cards;
Phoenix             0  70.3   213   582  6.0  7.05   36
Little Rock         0  61.0    91   132  8.2 48.52  100
. . . .
Seattle             0  51.1   379   531  9.4 38.79  164
```

```
Charleston          1  55.2    35    71  6.5 40.75  148
Milwaukee           0  45.7   569   717 11.8 29.07  123
;
proc sort data=usair;
  by hiso2;
run;
proc boxplot data=usair gout=boxplots;
 plot (population rain)*hiso2 /boxstyle=schematicid;
 id city;
run;
%panelplot(igout=boxplots,nrows=2);
```

We begin with some boxplots constructed using the previous code. The `schematicid` boxstyle produces a schematic plot where the whiskers only extend to observations within 1.5 times the interquartile range of the upper and lower quartiles. Observations beyond this are plotted separately and identified by the `id` variable, `city` in this case. The resulting plot is shown in Figure 9.9. This shows that Chicago is an outlier in population size, and it is dropped from the analysis.

The spline smoothing plot introduced earlier can also be useful with binary data.

```
data usair;
  set usair;
  if city=:'Chicago' then delete;
run;
symbol1 i=sm70s v='|' f=roman;
proc gplot data=usair gout=smplots;
 plot hiso2*(population rain);
run;
%panelplot(igout=smplots,nrows=2);
```

The `v` and `f` (`font`) options on the `symbol` statement plot the data values as ticks at 0 and 1. Figure 9.10 shows the resulting plots, both of which suggest nonlinear relationships. We now fit a logistic model with a spline smooth of average rainfall.

```
ods rtf;
ods graphics on;
proc gam data=usair;
```

TABLE 9.6

Air Pollution Data

city	hiso2	temperature	factories	population	windspeed	rain	rainydays
Phoenix	0	70.3	213	582	6.0	7.05	36
Little Rock	0	61.0	91	132	8.2	48.52	100
San Francisco	0	56.7	453	716	8.7	20.66	67
Denver	0	51.9	454	515	9.0	12.95	86
Hartford	1	49.1	412	158	9.0	43.37	127
Wilmington	1	54.0	80	80	9.0	40.25	114
Washington	0	57.3	434	757	9.3	38.89	111
Jacksonville	0	68.4	136	529	8.8	54.47	116
Miami	0	75.5	207	335	9.0	59.80	128
Atlanta	0	61.5	368	497	9.1	48.34	115
Chicago	1	50.6	3344	3369	10.4	34.44	122
Indianapolis	0	52.3	361	746	9.7	38.74	121
Des Moines	0	49.0	104	201	11.2	30.85	103
Wichita	0	56.6	125	277	12.7	30.58	82
Louisville	1	55.6	291	593	8.3	43.11	123
New Orleans	0	68.3	204	361	8.4	56.77	113
Baltimore	1	55.0	625	905	9.6	41.31	111
Detroit	1	49.9	1064	1513	10.1	30.96	129
Minneapolis	0	43.5	699	744	10.6	25.94	137
Kansas City	0	54.5	381	507	10.0	37.00	99
St. Louis	1	55.9	775	622	9.5	35.89	105
Omaha	0	51.5	181	347	10.9	30.18	98
Albuquerque	0	56.8	46	244	8.9	7.77	58
Albany	1	47.6	44	116	8.8	33.36	135
Buffalo	0	47.1	391	463	12.4	36.11	166
Cincinnati	0	54.0	462	453	7.1	39.04	132
Cleveland	1	49.7	1007	751	10.9	34.99	155
Columbus	0	51.5	266	540	8.6	37.01	134
Philadelphia	1	54.6	1692	1950	9.6	39.93	115
Pittsburgh	1	50.4	347	520	9.4	36.22	147
Providence	1	50.0	343	179	10.6	42.75	125
Memphis	0	61.6	337	624	9.2	49.10	105
Nashville	0	59.4	275	448	7.9	46.00	119
Dallas	0	66.2	641	844	10.9	35.94	78
Houston	0	68.9	721	1233	10.8	48.19	103
Salt Lake City	0	51.0	137	176	8.7	15.17	89
Norfolk	1	59.3	96	308	10.6	44.68	116
Richmond	0	57.8	197	299	7.6	42.59	115
Seattle	0	51.1	379	531	9.4	38.79	164
Charleston	1	55.2	35	71	6.5	40.75	148
Milwaukee	0	45.7	569	717	11.8	29.07	123

```
  model hiso2=spline(rain,df=2) /dist=binary;
  output out=gamout p;
run;
ods graphics off;
ods rtf close;
```

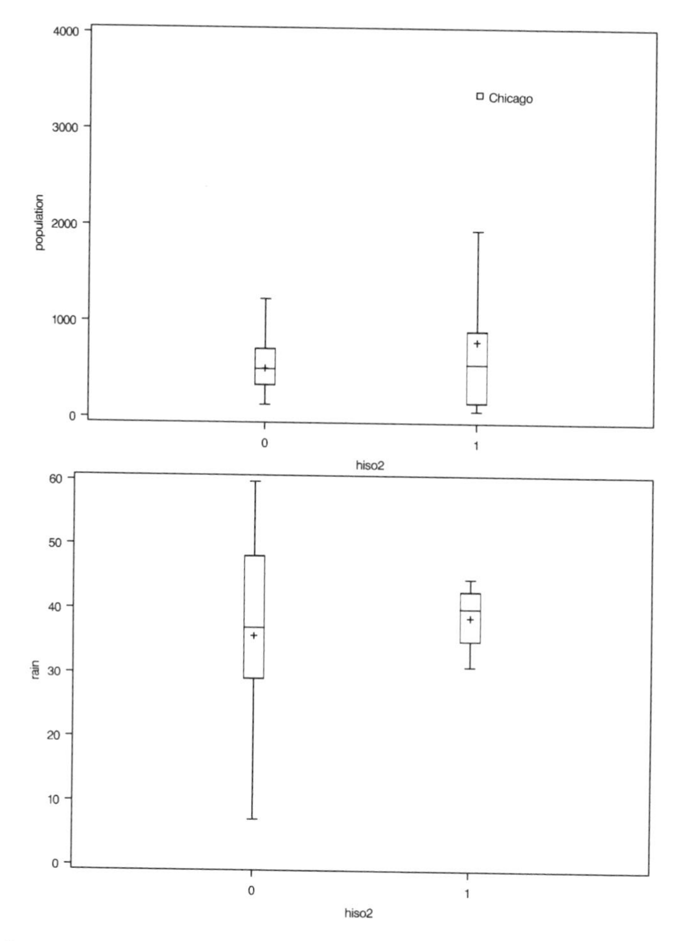

FIGURE 9.9
Boxplots for average rainfall and population size for the air pollution data.

The `dist=` option on the `model` statement specifies that the outcome is binary. The degree of smoothing for spline smooth of rain is set to two degrees of freedom. In the case of a spline smooth one of these degrees of freedom is allocated to the linear component. ODS graphics are used to generate the component plot, which is shown in Figure 9.11. The `output` statement with the `p` option saves the predicted values in the `gamout` dataset. The output is shown in Table 9.7. There we see that the linear component is not significant but the nonlinear smooth is. The predicted values (`p_hiso2`) in the output data set are the log odds of a high SO_2 value. The predicted probabilities can be calculated and plotted as follows.

```
data gamout;
  set gamout;
  odds=exp(P_hiso2);
  pred=odds/(1+odds);
```

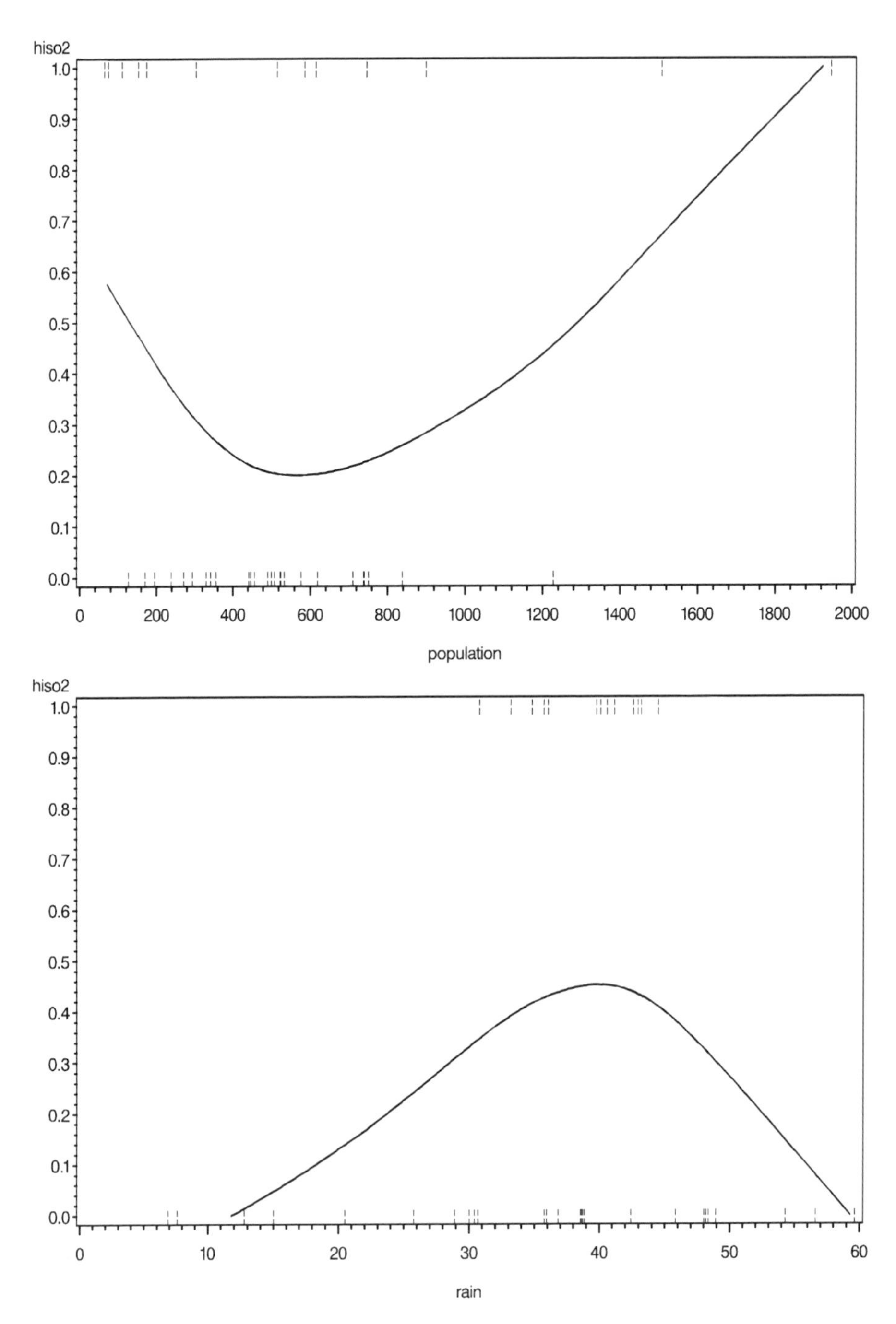

FIGURE 9.10
Plots of average rainfall and population size against high SO_2 for the U.S. air pollution data.

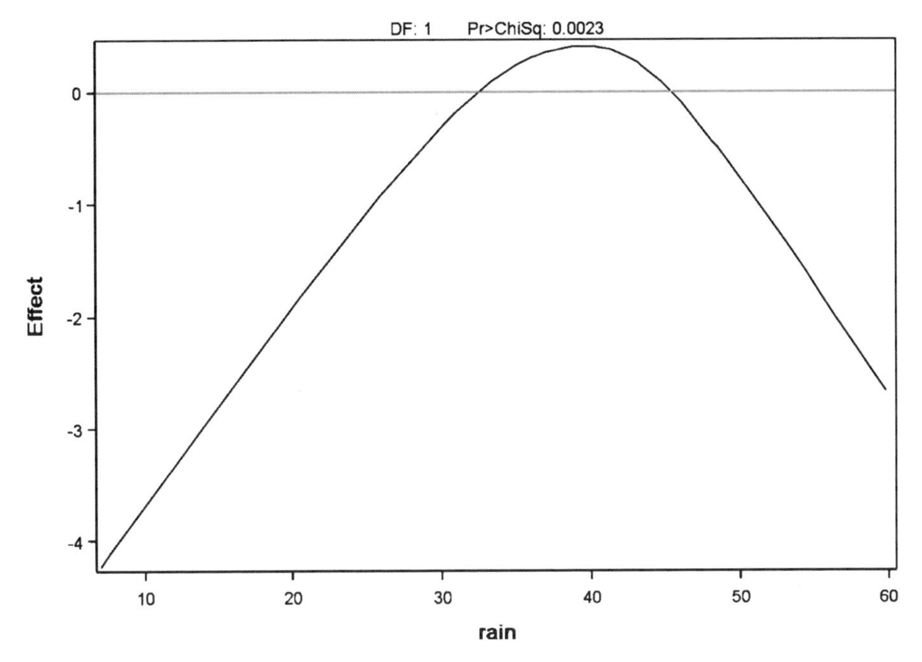

FIGURE 9.11
Fitted function for average rainfall for the air pollution data.

```
run;
goptions reset=symbol;
proc gplot data=gamout;
 plot pred*rain;
run;
```

The resulting plot is shown in Figure 9.12.

9.5 Summary

Generalized additive models provide a useful addition to the tools available for exploring the relationship between a response variable and a set of explanatory variables. Such models allow possible nonlinear terms in the latter to be uncovered, and perhaps then to be modelled in terms of more familiar low-degree polynomials. The GAM model can deal with nonlinearity in covariates that are not the main interest in a study and 'adjust' for those effects appropriately.

TABLE 9.7

Results from Fitting a GAM to the Air Pollution Data

```
                         The GAM Procedure
                     Dependent Variable: hiso2
            Smoothing Model Component(s): spline(rain)

                     Summary of Input Data Set

            Number of Observations                    40
            Number of Missing Observations             0
            Distribution                        Binomial
            Link Function                          Logit


                Iteration Summary and Fit Statistics

    Number of local score iterations                          17
    Local score convergence criterion               8.619374E-10
    Final Number of Backfitting Iterations                     1
    Final Backfitting Criterion                     6.0284857E-9
    The Deviance of the Final Estimate              40.425572907


  The local score algorithm converged.


                      Regression Model Analysis
                         Parameter Estimates

                     Parameter       Standard
  Parameter           Estimate          Error    t Value    Pr > |t|

  Intercept           -0.85734        2.05467      -0.42      0.6789
  Linear(rain)         0.00886        0.05190       0.17      0.8654


                      Smoothing Model Analysis
                Fit Summary for Smoothing Components

                                                                     Num
                 Smoothing                                        Unique
Component        Parameter            DF             GCV             Obs

Spline(rain)      0.999899      1.000000       29.622066              40


                      Smoothing Model Analysis
                        Analysis of Deviance

                                           Sum of
 Source                    DF             Squares    Chi-Square    Pr > ChiSq

 Spline(rain)         1.00000            9.312978        9.3130        0.0023
```

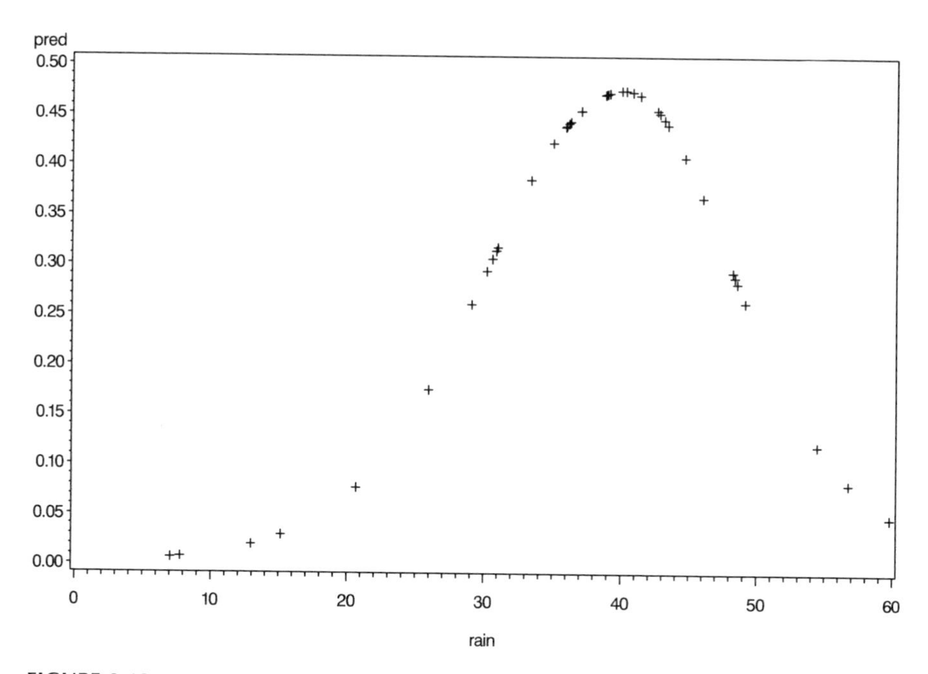

FIGURE 9.12
Predicted values of probability of a high SO_2 value plotted against average rainfall for the U.S. air pollution data.

10

Nonlinear Regression Models

10.1 Introduction

The regression techniques described in previous chapters have involved modelling the response variable, or some transformation of the response variable, as a linear function of the explanatory variables of interest. The term 'linear' here refers to the parameters rather than to the explanatory variables themselves so, for example, a model such as

$$y = \beta_0 + \beta_1 x_1 + \beta_2 x_2^2 + \beta_3 x_1 x_2 + \beta_4 x_3^2 + \varepsilon$$

is a linear model.

In this chapter we will consider regression models that are *nonlinear* with respect to at least one of their parameters, for example,

$$y = \beta_1 e^{\beta_2 x_1} + \beta_3 e^{\beta_4 x_2} + \beta_5 \log(x_3) + \varepsilon$$

Some nonlinear models can, by taking a suitable transformation, be made linear; the logistic regression model described in Chapter 7 is an example. (The process of transformation is not necessarily straightforward, however, since both the expectation function and the disturbance term are transformed, possibly invalidating the assumption of constant variance and normality required for the usual linear regression approach. Linearization should only be used when the transformed data are adequately described by a model with an additive normal error. See Kolkiewicz, 2005, for more details.) In this chapter, however, we shall concentrate, in the main, on models that cannot be linearized, the so-called *intrinsically nonlinear models.*

10.2 Nonlinear Regression

In contrast to linear models, in nonlinear models it is not possible to write down an explicit expression for the least squares estimators of the parameters; estimation of the parameters is, consequently, more complex. A brief account of estimation for nonlinear regression models is given in Display 10.1.

DISPLAY 10.1

Estimating the Parameters in Nonlinear Models

- Assume the model to be fitted is $y_i = f(\mathbf{x}_i;\boldsymbol{\theta}) + \varepsilon_i$, where $\mathbf{x}_i' = [x_{i1}, x_{i2}, \cdots x_{ip}]$ is the vector of explanatory variable values for the ith observation, y_i is the corresponding response, $\boldsymbol{\theta}' = [\theta_1, \theta_2, \cdots, \theta_k]$ is a vector of parameters, and ε_i is a residual term generally assumed to be independent of other error terms and to have a $N(0, \sigma^2)$ distribution.

- In a nonlinear model the expected value of the variable given the explanatory variables normally distributed with a mean that is a nonlinear function of the explanatory variables and a constant variance σ^2.
- The sum of squares function, S, given by

$$S(\theta) = \sum_{i=1}^{n} \left[y_i - f(\mathbf{x}_i;\boldsymbol{\theta}) \right]^2$$

provides the basis of estimation, and the least-squares estimator of θ is the value of θ minimizing S.
- One way of finding such an estimator directly is to use a minimization technique such as steepest descent, Gauss–Newton, or Marquardt's method (see Everitt, 1987) to minimize S numerically with respect to θ.
- Alternatively, differentiating S with respect to each of the θ_i in turn and setting the resulting expressions to zero yields the set of simultaneous equations

$$\sum_{i=1}^{n} \left[\{ y_i - f(\mathbf{x}_i;\boldsymbol{\theta}) \} \left(\frac{\partial f}{\partial \theta_j} \right)_{\boldsymbol{\theta}=\hat{\boldsymbol{\theta}}} \right] = 0 \quad (j = 1, \cdots, k)$$

DISPLAY 10.1 (continued)

Estimating the Parameters in Nonlinear Models

- In general, an iterative numerical method is needed to solve these equations.
- The optimisation procedures used to find parameter estimates in nonlinear models require initial values. Two possibilities listed by Krzanowski (1998) are as follows:
  a. Use knowledge of the parameters to estimate initial values from a plot of the data.
  b. Fit a regression to the nearest 'linear' approximation of the model, and use the resulting parameter estimates as initial values.
- An estimate of σ^2 is provided by $S(\hat{\theta})/n$.
- In nonlinear models, the parameter estimates will not in general be linear combinations of the observations y_i, so even assuming normality of the y_i, the covariance matrix of θ will no longer be $(\mathbf{X}'\mathbf{X})^{-1}\sigma^2$ (see Chapter 6).
- If we assume normality of the y_i, then the least-squares estimators are also maximum likelihood ones, so we can obtain approximate standard errors of the $\hat{\theta}_i$ from asymptotic properties of maximum likelihood estimators, i.e., from the matrix of second derivatives of the log-likelihood.
- More about standard errors and confidence intervals for the parameters in nonlinear models can be found in Huet et al. (2004).

10.3 Some Examples of Nonlinear Regression Models

Our first example of the application of a nonlinear model will involve the data shown in Table 10.1, taken from Krzanowski (1998). These data were obtained from a radioimmunoassay experiment in which a standard solution was diluted to a number of concentrations and the absorbance was measured at each concentration. A model used widely in radioimmunoassay work is the four-parameter logistic model given by

$$y_i = \alpha + \frac{\beta - \alpha}{1 + (x_i/\gamma)^{-\delta}} + \varepsilon \quad (i = 1 \cdots n)$$

where α, β, γ, and δ are the four parameters.

TABLE 10.1

Results of Radioimmunoassay Experiment

Concentration	Absorbance
10,000	0.880
10,000	0.784
5,000	0.776
5,000	0.769
2,500	0.622
2,500	0.614
1,250	0.500
1,250	0.488
625	0.347
625	0.356
312	0.263
312	0.260
156	0.192
156	0.173
78	0.125
78	0.138
39	0.070
39	0.064
20	0.050
20	0.044
10	0.029
10	0.029
5	0.018
5	0.018

Source: Krzanowski, W.J. and Marriott, F.H.C., 1995, *Multivariate Analysis,* Pt 2, Arnold. With permission.

Initial values for α, β, and γ can be found from a plot of absorbance against log (concentration). The required SAS code is

```
data assay;
 input conc absorb;
 logconc=log(conc);
cards;
10000   0.880
10000   0.784
....
5       0.018
5       0.018
;
proc gplot data=assay;
  plot absorb*logconc;
run;
```

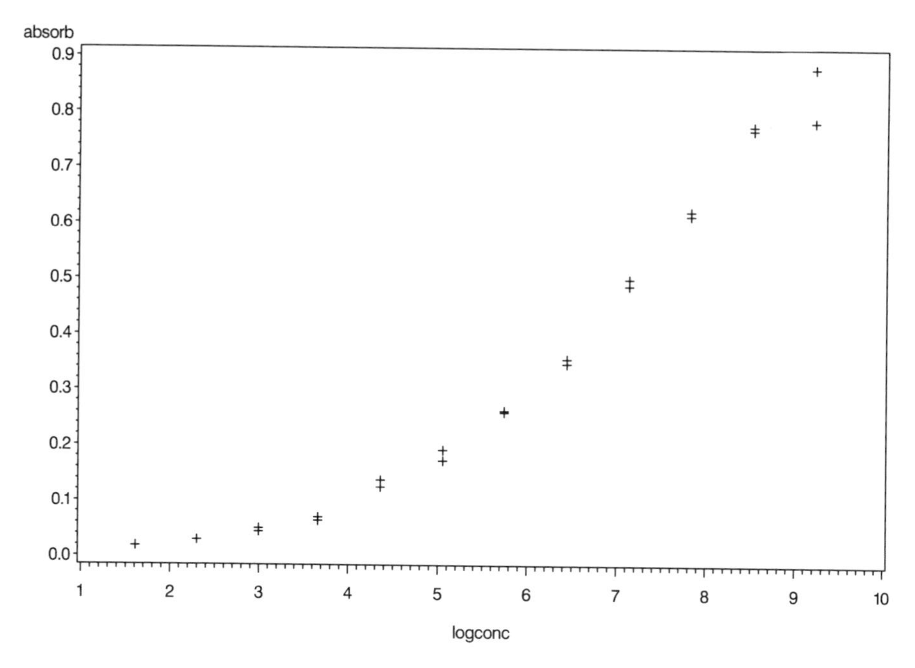

FIGURE 10.1
Plot of absorbance against log concentration.

The resulting plot is shown in Figure 10.1. The initial value for α is the intercept, 0.0, that for β the asymptote, 0.9, and γ is the value of concentration when $y = \frac{1}{2}(\alpha + \beta)$, leading to the value 1096.

An initial estimate of δ can be found from the slope of the approximate straight line given by plotting

$$\log\left[\frac{\text{absorption} - \alpha}{\beta - \text{absorption}}\right] \text{against log (concentration)}$$

using the initial values of α and β found previously. The code required to get this additional plot is

```
data assay;
  set assay;
  logratio=log(absorb/(.9-absorb));
run;
proc gplot data=assay;
  plot logratio*logconc;
  symbol1 i=r v=plus;
run;
```

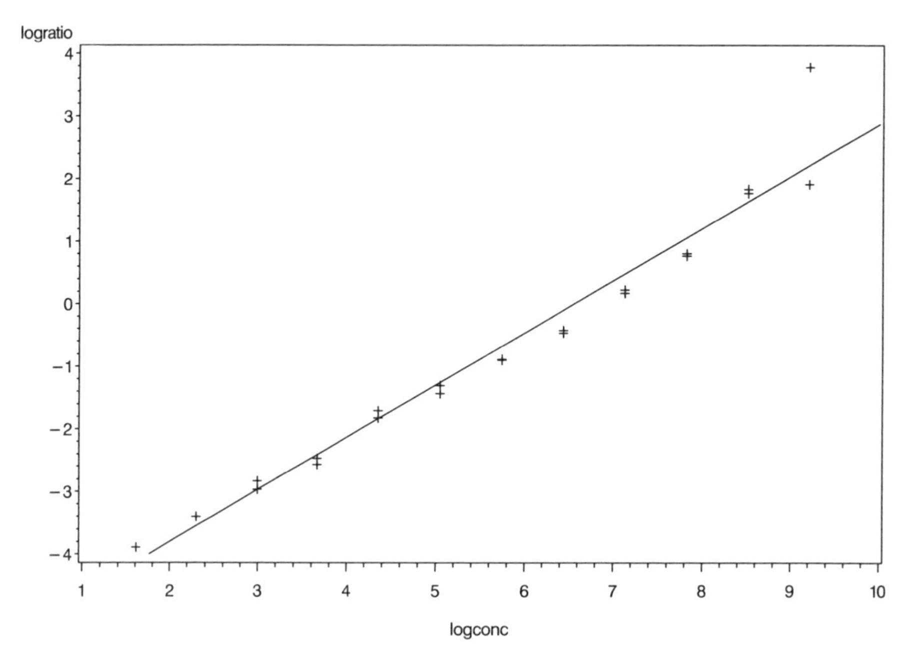

FIGURE 10.2
Plot for finding initial value of δ.

The regression interpolation option (`i=r`) on the symbol statement calculates and plots the regression line at the same time as plotting the data. The regression equation is given in the SAS log and suggests an initial value of δ of 0.7. The plot is shown in Figure 10.2.

We can use SAS `proc nlin` to estimate the parameters of the model as follows;

```
proc nlin data=assay;
  parms alpha=0 beta=.9 gamma=1096 delta=.7;
  model absorb=alpha + (beta-alpha)/(1 + (conc/
gamma)**-delta);
  output out=nlout p=pr;
run;
```

`Proc nlin` estimates the parameters of a nonlinear model by least squares or weighted least squares, using steepest descent, Newton, Gauss–Newton, or Marquardt's method (see, for example, Everitt, 1987). Gauss–Newton is the default. The parameters of the model are specified and given starting values in the `parms` or `parameters` statement. A range of starting values can be given for each parameter. The `output` statement saves the predicted values in the `nlout` data set.

TABLE 10.2

Parameter Estimates for Radioimmunoassay Data

The NLIN Procedure
Dependent Variable absorb
Method: Gauss-Newton

Iterative Phase

Iter	alpha	beta	gamma	delta	Sum of Squares
0	0	0.9000	1096.0	0.7000	0.0481
1	-0.00078	1.0859	1612.9	0.6835	0.00862
2	0.00251	1.0737	1577.0	0.7096	0.00827
3	0.00252	1.0737	1578.6	0.7106	0.00827
4	0.00254	1.0737	1578.3	0.7108	0.00827
5	0.00254	1.0737	1578.3	0.7108	0.00827

NOTE: Convergence criterion met.

Estimation Summary

Method	Gauss-Newton
Iterations	5
R	1.16E-6
PPC(alpha)	0.000021
RPC(alpha)	0.00017
Object	3.9E-10
Objective	0.008272
Observations Read	24
Observations Used	24
Observations Missing	0

Source	DF	Sum of Squares	Mean Square	F Value	Approx Pr > F
Model	3	1.9151	0.6384	1543.43	<.0001
Error	20	0.00827	0.000414		
Corrected Total	23	1.9234			

Parameter	Estimate	Approx Std Error	Approximate 95% Confidence Limits	
alpha	0.00254	0.0140	-0.0266	0.0317
beta	1.0737	0.0697	0.9283	1.2191
gamma	1578.3	308.4	934.9	2221.7
delta	0.7108	0.0645	0.5762	0.8453

The NLIN Procedure

Approximate Correlation Matrix

	alpha	beta	gamma	delta
alpha	1.0000000	-0.6443702	-0.4804066	0.8137671
beta	-0.6443702	1.0000000	0.9665607	-0.9158663
gamma	-0.4804066	0.9665607	1.0000000	-0.8398692
delta	0.8137671	-0.9158663	-0.8398692	1.0000000

The least-squares estimates of the four parameters and their standard errors are shown in Table 10.2. The fitted curve and the observed values can be graphed using

```
proc gplot data=nlout;
  plot (absorb pr)* conc/overlay;
```

```
  symbol1 v=plus;
  symbol2 i=join v=none;
run;
```

This leads to Figure 10.3. Clearly, the model provides an excellent fit for these data.

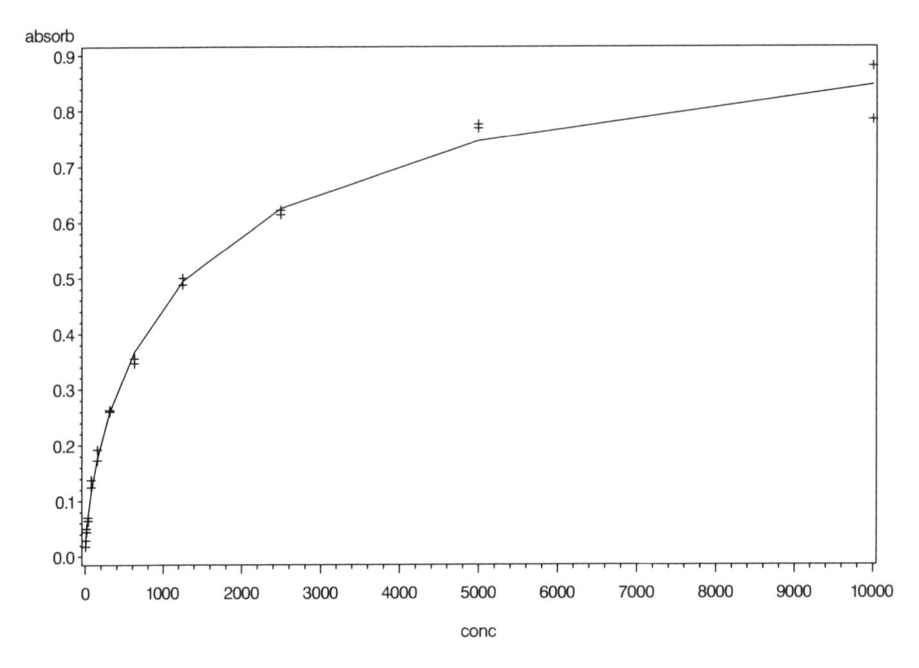

FIGURE 10.3
Observed and fitted radioimmunoassay data.

As a second example of fitting a nonlinear model we shall use the data shown in Table 10.3, taken with permission from Huet et al. (2004). These data arise from a radioimmunological assay (RIA) of cortisol. First, we can plot the observed responses as functions of the logarithm of the dose. In this experiment, the response has been observed for zero dose and for infinite dose. We shall represent these doses by values –3 and +2 on the plot, which can be constructed using the following SAS code;

```
data cortisol;
input dose @;
select(dose);
  when(0) logdose=-3;
  when(9999)logdose=2;
  otherwise logdose=log10(dose);
end;
```

TABLE 10.3

Data for the Calibration Curve of an RIA of Cortisol

Dose (ng/0.1ml)	Response (c.p.m.)			
0	2868	2785	2849	2805
0	2779	2588	2701	2752
0.02	2615	2651	2506	2498
0.04	2474	2573	2378	2494
0.06	2152	2307	2101	2216
0.08	2114	2052	2016	2030
0.1	1862	1935	1800	1871
0.2	1364	1412	1377	1304
0.4	910	919	855	875
0.6	702	701	689	696
0.8	586	596	561	562
1	501	495	478	493
1.5	392	358	399	394
2	330	351	343	333
4	250	261	244	242
∞	131	135	134	133

Source: Huet, S. et al., 2004, *Statistical Tools for Nonlinear Regression: A Practical Guide with R and S-PLUS Examples.* Springer.

```
do i=1 to 4;
 input resp @;
 output;
end;
input;
cards;
0       2868    2785    2849    2805
0       2779    2588    2701    2752
0.02    2615    2651    2506    2498
....
4       250     261     244     242
9999            131     135     134 133
;
proc gplot data=cortisol;
  plot resp*logdose;
run;
```

The data step first reads in the value of `dose`, with the trailing `@` holding the data line for further input. `Logdose` is derived using a `select` group. These are simpler to use than nested `if then` and `else` statements when there are several alternatives to deal with. Then an iterative `do` group reads in four values of the response variable, writing out an observation for each

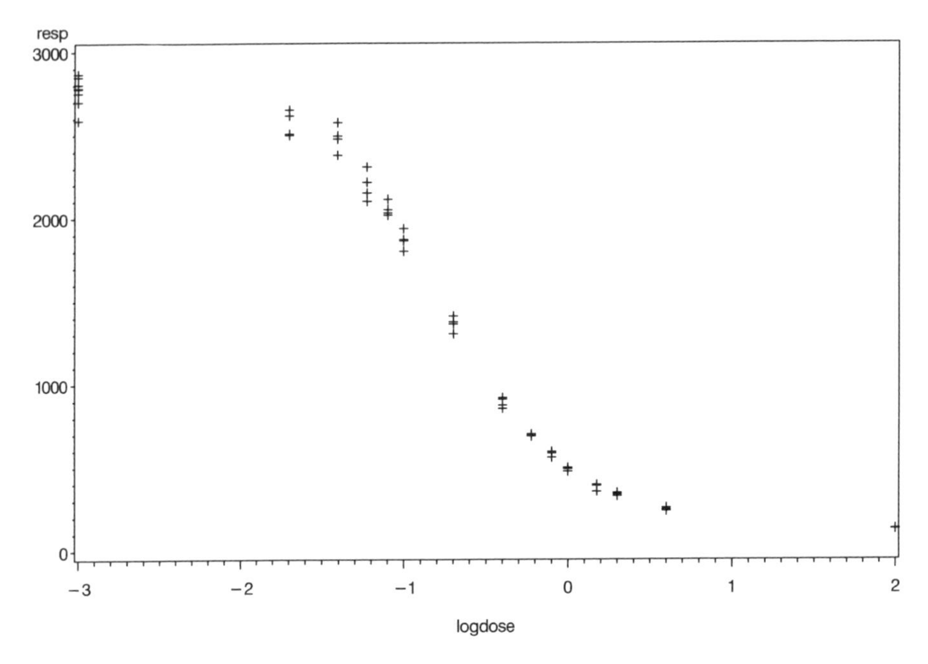

FIGURE 10.4
Cortisol example: observed responses (in c.p.m.) versus the log dose.

via the `output` statement. At each iteration the dataline is held for further values to be read. After the `do` group has completed, the subsequent `input` statement releases the dataline, so that the next line of data can be read. The resulting plot is shown in Figure 10.4.

The model generally used to describe the variations of the response versus the log dose is the generalized logistic function, which depends on five parameters, the first two, θ_1 and θ_2, are the lower asymptote — the response for a theoretical infinite dose, and the upper asymptote — the response for a null dose. The other three parameters describe the shape of the decrease of the curve. Explicitly, the model is

$$f(x,\theta) = \theta_1 + \frac{\theta_2 - \theta_1}{\left[1 + \exp(\theta_3 + \theta_4 x)\right]^{\theta_5}}$$

where x is log dose.

For this example, there are repeated observations for each dose. If we calculate the variances of these repeated observations using `proc means`

```
proc means data=cortisol var n;
  class dose;
  var resp;
  output out=variances var=var_resp;
run;
```

```
The MEANS Procedure
Analysis Variable : resp
               N
Dose         Obs          Variance       N
-------------------------------------------
   0           8           7921.27       8
0.02           4           5947.00       4
0.04           4           6428.25       4
0.06           4           7888.67       4
0.08           4           1873.33       4
 0.1           4           3051.33       4
 0.2           4           2024.25       4
 0.4           4       896.9166667       4
 0.6           4        35.3333333       4
 0.8           4       306.9166667       4
   1           4        95.5833333       4
 1.5           4       350.9166667       4
   2           4        92.2500000       4
   4           4        72.9166667       4
9999           4         2.9166667       4
-------------------------------------------
```

we see immediately that the usual assumption that the variance of the response does not depend on dose is not valid here. In such cases it is natural to favour observations with small variances by weighting the sum of squares function used in estimation. Consequently, here we shall estimate the five parameters using a weighted sum of squares of the form

$$S(\theta) = \sum_{i=1}^{k} \sum_{j=1}^{n_i} \frac{\left[y_{ij} - f(x_i, \theta)\right]^2}{s_i^2}$$

where y_{ij} is the jth observed response for log dose x_i, k is the number of doses, and s_i^2 is the empirical variance for the ith dose.

Here we shall take θ_1 as 100 and θ_2 as 2500 (see Figure 10.1). Each of the other three parameters will be given an initial value of one. We can fit the generalized logistic model using the following code:

```
data cortisol;
  merge cortisol(in=in1) variances;
  by dose;
  if in1;
run;
```

```
proc nlin data=cortisol;
  parms theta1=100 theta2=2500 theta3=1 theta4=1 theta
5=1;
  model resp=theta1 + (theta2-theta1)/
((1+exp(theta3+theta4*logdose))**theta5);
  _weight_=1/var_resp;
  output out=nlout p=pr;
run;
```

The proc means step saved the variances for each dose level in the dataset variances. We now add these to the cortisol data set by merging them in. Normally, it is advisable to sort both data sets on the matching variable before merging, particularly with larger data sets, where it is not so easy to verify the results. The variances data set contains an additional observation with a missing value of dose, and this is dropped from the resulting data set by the subsetting if statement.

The proc nlin step is similar to the earlier example with the addition of the statement that sets the special variable _weight_ equal to the reciprocal of the observed variance for each dose. The results are shown in Table 10.4. A plot of the fitted and observed values, omitting the point for infinite dose, is obtained as follows:

```
proc gplot data=nlout;
  plot (resp pr)*dose/overlay;
  symbol1 v=plus;
  symbol2 i=join v=none;
  where dose<9999;
run;
```

The resulting plot is shown in Figure 10.5. Again the fit of the model to the observations is very good.

10.4 Summary

Nonlinear models often occur in particular areas of medicine. Parameter estimation is generally more difficult than for their linear cousins although some apparently nonlinear models can be transformed relatively simply into linear form.

TABLE 10.4

Results of Fitting the Generalized Logistic Function to the Cortisol Data

The NLIN Procedure
Dependent Variable resp
Method: Gauss-Newton

Iterative Phase

Iter	theta1	theta2	theta3	theta4	theta5	Weighted SS
0	100.0	2500.0	1.0000	1.0000	1.0000	26010.3
1	98.6050	2489.1	1.0617	1.0227	0.9621	25999.2
2	97.8213	2482.9	1.0982	1.0366	0.9410	25939.3
3	96.9053	2475.5	1.1424	1.0536	0.9163	25878.1
4	95.8537	2466.8	1.1955	1.0746	0.8879	25818.9
5	94.6752	2456.9	1.2587	1.1002	0.8557	25765.8
6	93.3954	2445.6	1.3334	1.1312	0.8200	25722.1
7	92.0643	2433.1	1.4204	1.1687	0.7813	25688.9
8	90.7626	2419.8	1.5206	1.2134	0.7402	25662.7
9	89.6060	2405.9	1.6342	1.2664	0.6980	25632.3
10	88.7449	2392.1	1.7612	1.3282	0.6557	25576.6
11	88.3564	2379.0	1.9007	1.3997	0.6146	25464.0
12	88.6280	2367.3	2.0514	1.4811	0.5757	25254.1
13	89.7327	2357.7	2.2115	1.5725	0.5401	24902.6
14	91.7981	2351.0	2.3784	1.6736	0.5083	24367.4
15	97.9561	2344.1	2.7197	1.8935	0.4534	24001.6
16	113.7	2355.7	3.2593	2.2876	0.3937	22914.9
17	164.8	2467.2	4.3526	3.3115	0.3446	17520.2
18	167.1	2691.7	3.5780	3.4821	0.4900	5596.9
19	127.6	2756.0	3.1960	3.2385	0.5871	161.7
20	125.8	2759.0	3.1453	3.2208	0.6094	63.9088
21	125.8	2759.2	3.1363	3.2158	0.6116	63.7408
22	125.8	2759.2	3.1362	3.2157	0.6117	63.7408

NOTE: Convergence criterion met.

Estimation Summary

Method	Gauss-Newton
Iterations	22
Subiterations	37
Average Subiterations	1.681818
R	2.153E-6
PPC(theta5)	7.434E-7
RPC(theta5)	0.000063
Object	3.083E-7
Objective	63.74082
Observations Read	64
Observations Used	64
Observations Missing	0

The NLIN Procedure

Source	DF	Sum of Squares	Mean Square	F Value	Approx Pr > F
Model	4	72206.6	18051.6	16709.0	<.0001
Error	59	63.7408	1.0804		
Corrected Total	63	72270.3			

Parameter	Estimate	Approx Std Error	Approximate 95% Confidence Limits	
theta1	125.8	1.2385	123.3	128.2
theta2	2759.2	29.8754	2699.4	2819.0
theta3	3.1362	0.2107	2.7145	3.5579
theta4	3.2157	0.1538	2.9079	3.5235
theta5	0.6117	0.0416	0.5284	0.6949

TABLE 10.4 (continued)

Results of Fitting the Generalized Logistic Function to the Cortisol Data

Approximate Correlation Matrix

	theta1	theta2	theta3	theta4	theta5
theta1	1.0000000	0.1332359	-0.5568222	-0.4624458	0.5696169
theta2	0.1332359	1.0000000	-0.4594839	-0.6110276	0.5169039
theta3	-0.5568222	-0.4594839	1.0000000	0.9691613	-0.9964423
theta4	-0.4624458	-0.6110276	0.9691613	1.0000000	-0.9738140
theta5	0.5696169	0.5169039	-0.9964423	-0.9738140	1.0000000

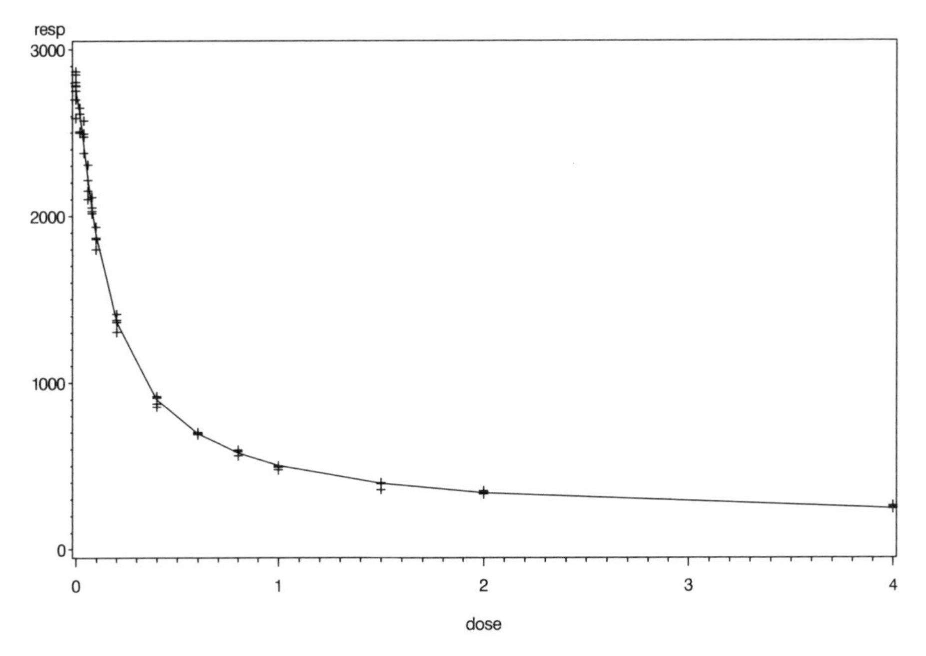

FIGURE 10.5
Plot of observed and fitted values for the cortisol data.

11

The Analysis of Longitudinal Data I

11.1 Introduction

Longitudinal data arise when participants in a study are measured on the same variable (or variables) on several different occasions. Such data arise frequently in medical investigations, particularly from clinical trials. Longitudinal data can be analyzed in a variety of ways, ranging from the simple to the relatively complex. In this chapter we concentrate on the former, leaving the latter until Chapter 12 and Chapter 13.

11.2 Graphical Displays of Longitudinal Data

Graphical displays of data are often useful for exposing patterns in the data, particularly when these are unexpected; this might be of great help in suggesting which class of models might be most sensibly applied in the later, more formal analysis. According to Diggle et al. (1994), there is no single prescription for making effective graphical displays of longitudinal data, although they do offer the following simple guidelines:

- Show as much of the relevant raw data as possible, rather than only data summaries.
- Highlight aggregate patterns of potential scientific interest.
- Identify both cross-sectional and longitudinal patterns.
- Try to make the identification of unusual individuals or unusual observations simple.

A number of graphical displays that can be useful in the preliminary assessment of longitudinal data from clinical trials will now be illustrated using the data shown in Table 11.1 (taken from Davis, 2002). Forty male subjects were randomly assigned to one of two treatment groups, and each patient had his Brief Psychiatric Rating Scale (BPRS) factor measured before treatment (week 0) and at weekly intervals for 8 weeks.

TABLE 11.1

BPRS Measurements from 40 Subjects

		Week								
Treatment	**Subject**	**0**	**1**	**2**	**3**	**4**	**5**	**6**	**7**	**8**
1	1	42	36	36	43	41	40	38	47	51
	2	58	68	61	55	43	34	28	28	28
	3	54	55	41	38	43	28	29	25	24
	4	55	77	49	54	56	50	47	42	46
	5	72	75	72	65	50	39	32	38	32
	6	48	43	41	38	36	29	33	27	25
	7	71	61	47	30	27	40	30	31	31
	8	30	36	38	38	31	26	26	25	24
	9	41	43	39	35	28	22	20	23	21
	10	57	51	51	55	53	43	43	39	32
	11	30	34	34	41	36	36	38	36	36
	12	55	52	49	54	48	43	37	36	31
	13	36	32	36	31	25	25	21	19	22
	14	38	35	36	34	25	27	25	26	26
	15	66	68	65	49	36	32	27	30	37
	16	41	35	45	42	31	31	29	26	30
	17	45	38	46	38	40	33	27	31	27
	18	39	35	27	25	29	28	21	25	20
	19	24	28	31	28	29	21	22	23	22
	20	38	34	27	25	25	27	21	19	21
2	1	52	73	42	41	39	38	43	62	50
	2	30	23	32	24	20	20	19	18	20
	3	65	31	33	28	22	25	24	31	32
	4	37	31	27	31	31	26	24	26	23
	5	59	67	58	61	49	38	37	36	35
	6	30	33	37	33	28	26	27	23	21
	7	69	52	41	33	34	37	37	38	35
	8	62	54	49	39	55	51	55	59	66
	9	38	40	38	27	31	24	22	21	21
	10	65	44	31	34	39	34	41	42	39
	11	78	95	75	76	66	64	64	60	75
	12	38	41	36	27	29	27	21	22	23
	13	63	65	60	53	52	32	37	52	28
	14	40	37	31	38	35	30	33	30	27
	15	40	36	55	55	42	30	26	30	37
	16	54	45	35	27	25	22	22	22	22
	17	33	41	30	32	46	43	43	43	43
	18	28	30	29	33	30	26	36	33	30
	19	52	43	26	27	24	32	21	21	21
	20	47	36	32	29	25	23	23	23	23

Source: Davis, C.S., 2002, *Statistical Methods for the Analysis of Repeated Measurements*, Springer. With permission.

Data sets for longitudinal and repeated measures data may be structured in two ways. In the first form there is one observation per subject (typically per person), and the repeated measurements are held in separate variables. We shall refer to this form as the 'wide' form. Alternatively, there may be a separate observation for each measurement occasion, with variables indicating which subject and occasion it belongs to. This is the 'long' form of the data set. Usually both forms will be needed. The wide form is useful for calculating summary measures, whereas the long form is needed for plots and the type of analyses covered in the next chapter.

We begin by reading in the data in the 'wide' format.

```
data bprs;
  input id x0-x8;
  group=1;
  if _n_>20 then group=2;
  id=100*group+id;
cards;
1   42  36  36  43  41  40  38  47  51
2   58  68  61  55  43  34  28  28  28
....
20  38  34  27  25  25  27  21  19  21
1   52  73  42  41  39  38  43  62  50
2   30  23  32  24  20  20  19  18  20
....
20  47  36  32  29  25  23  23  23  23
;
```

The subjects are numbered consecutively within treatment groups. The SAS automatic variable _n_ is used to assign them to groups and a unique id variable is calculated. We then reformat the data set to the long form.

```
data bprsl;
  set bprs;
  array xs {*} x0-x8;
  do week=0 to 8;
    bprs=xs{week+1};
    weekgroup=week+(group/10);
    output;
  end;
  keep id group week weekgroup bprs;
run;
```

The key elements of the data step needed to do this are the `array` statement, the iterative `do` group, and the `output` statement. These were introduced in

Chapter 5, in which we dealt with the equivalent situation where each line of raw data contained values for several subjects. To recap briefly, the `array` statement declares a shorthand alias, `xs`, for the variables `x0` to `x8`. The iterative `do` statement repeats the subsequent statements, up to the corresponding `end` statement, a number of times with the index variable changing at each repetition. In this instance, there are nine repetitions with the index variable, `week`, taking values 0, 1, 2, ... 8. The elements of an array are always numbered from 1, so we need to add 1 to `week`. The `output` statement writes out an observation to the data set being created with the current values of all variables. As this is between the `do` statement and the `end` statement, nine observations are created for every one read in. The `weekgroup` variable is created for use later.

Having reformatted the data, we can plot the values for all 40 men, differentiating between the treatment groups.

```
proc gplot data=bprsl;
  plot bprs*week=id /nolegend;
  symbol1 i=join v=none r=20;
  symbol2 i=join v=none l=2 r=20;
run;
```

Including `r=20` on each `symbol` statement specifies that each symbol definition is to be repeated 20 times, as there are 20 subjects in each group. The second symbol definition used `l(linetype)=2` to distinguish the subjects of the second group. The resulting diagram is shown in Figure 11.1. This simple graph makes a number of features of the data readily apparent. First, the BPRS values of almost all the men decrease over the 8 weeks of the study. Second, the men who have higher BPRS values at the beginning tend to have higher values throughout the study. This phenomenon is generally referred to as *tracking*. Third, substantial individual differences exist, and variability appears to decrease with time.

The tracking phenomenon can be seen more clearly in a plot of the standardized values of each observation, i.e., the values obtained by subtracting the relevant occasion mean from the original observation and then dividing by the corresponding visit standard deviation. The following code produces Figure 11.2.

```
proc sort data=bprsl;
 by week;
run;
proc stdize data=bprsl out=bprslz method=std;
  var bprs;
  by week;
run;
```

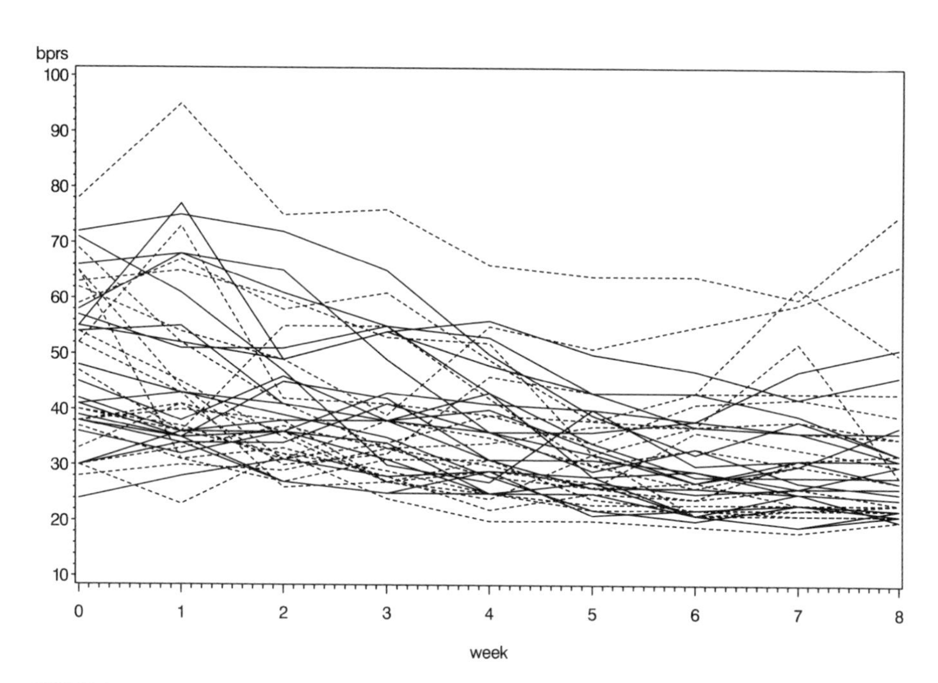

FIGURE 11.1
Individual response profiles by treatment group for the BPRS data.

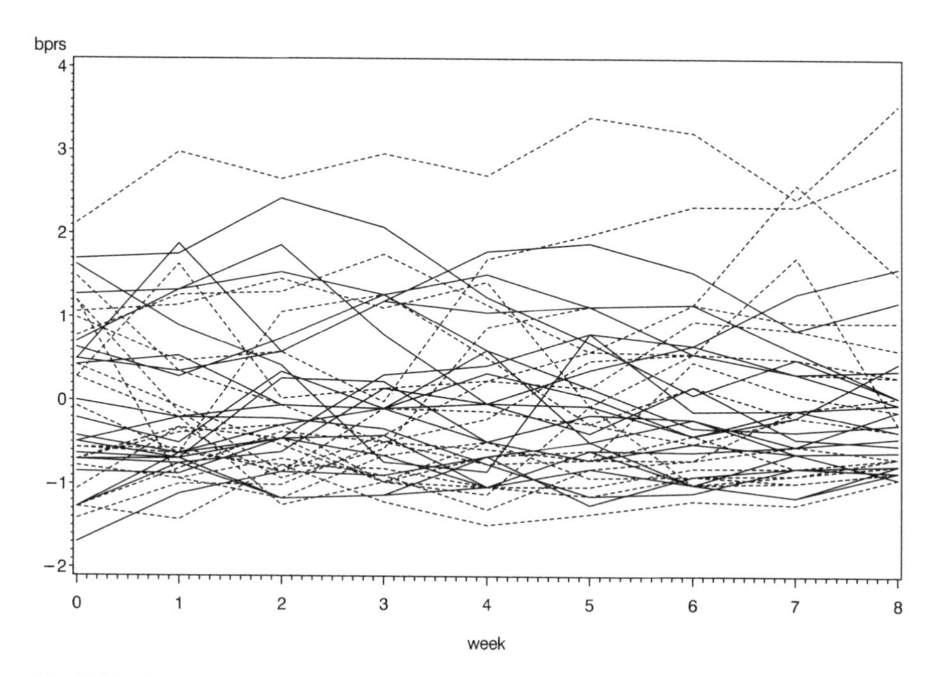

FIGURE 11.2
Individual response profiles for the BPRS data after standardization.

```
proc gplot data=bprslz;
  plot bprs*week=id /nolegend;
run;
```

The data are first sorted by week. Proc stdize with the method=std option and the by week statement then standardises within each measurement occasion. The var bprs statement specifies the variable to be standardised — the default is for all numeric variables to be. The standardised values are saved in the data set bprslz. Because symbol statements are global, the two symbol definitions set up earlier are still current.

With large numbers of observations, graphical displays of individual response profiles are of little use, and investigators then commonly produce graphs showing average profiles for each treatment group along with some indication of the variation of the observations at each time point. Such a graph can be constructed by using the i=std interpolation on the symbol statement, as follows.

```
goptions reset=symbol;
proc gplot data=bprsl;
  plot bprs*week=group;
  symbol1 i=stdm1j;
  symbol2 i=stdm1j l=2;
run;
```

The goptions statement resets symbol definitions to their default. This is recommended when redefining symbols that have already been used in the same session, or program. The std option plots means and standard deviations for data where there are multiple values of y for each x value. Appending m, as we have done, specifies that the standard error of the mean is to be used instead of the standard deviation. We have also specified 1 standard error, where one, two, or three are possible with two as the default. The j suffix results in the means being joined, and as before the second group has a different linetype.

The result is Figure 11.3. There is considerable overlap in the mean profiles of the two treatment groups suggesting that there is little difference between the two groups with respect to the mean BPRS values.

A possible alternative to plotting the mean profiles as in Figure 11.3 is to graph side-by-side boxplots of the observations at each time point.

```
goptions reset=symbol;
proc gplot data=bprsl;
  plot bprs*weekgroup=group /nolegend;
  symbol1 i=box v=plus;
```

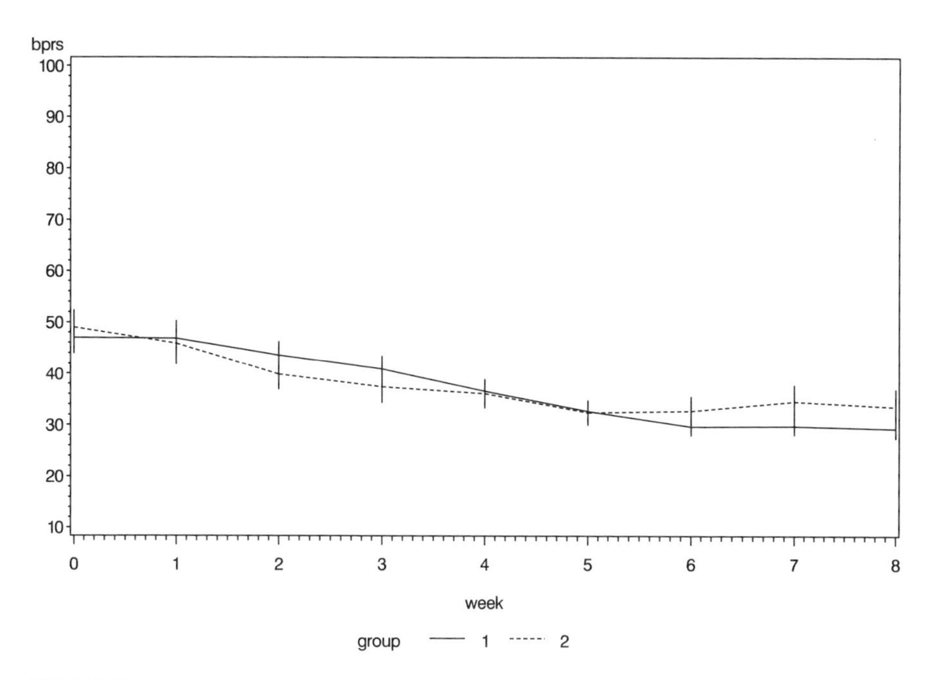

FIGURE 11.3
Mean response profiles for the two treatment groups in the BPRS data.

```
    symbol2 i=box v=star;
  run;
```

This makes use of the `weekgroup` variable defined earlier and the `box` interpolation option. The box covers the interquartile range with a tick at the median, and the whiskers extend to the furthest point within 1.5 interquartile ranges of the box. Plotting symbols are defined for the points that lie beyond this. The length of the whiskers can be controlled by suffixing a centile in the range 00 to 25: `box00` extends them to the most extreme points, `box05` to the most extreme points between the 5th and 95th centiles, and `box25` produces none, as the box itself extends from the 25th to the 75th centile.

The resulting plot is shown in Figure 11.4. The plot suggests the presence of some possible "outliers" at a number of time points and indicates the general decline in BPRS values over the 8 weeks of the study.

11.3 Summary Measure Analysis of Longitudinal Data

According to Matthews (2005), 'the use of summary measures is one of the most important and straightforward methods for the analysis of longitudinal

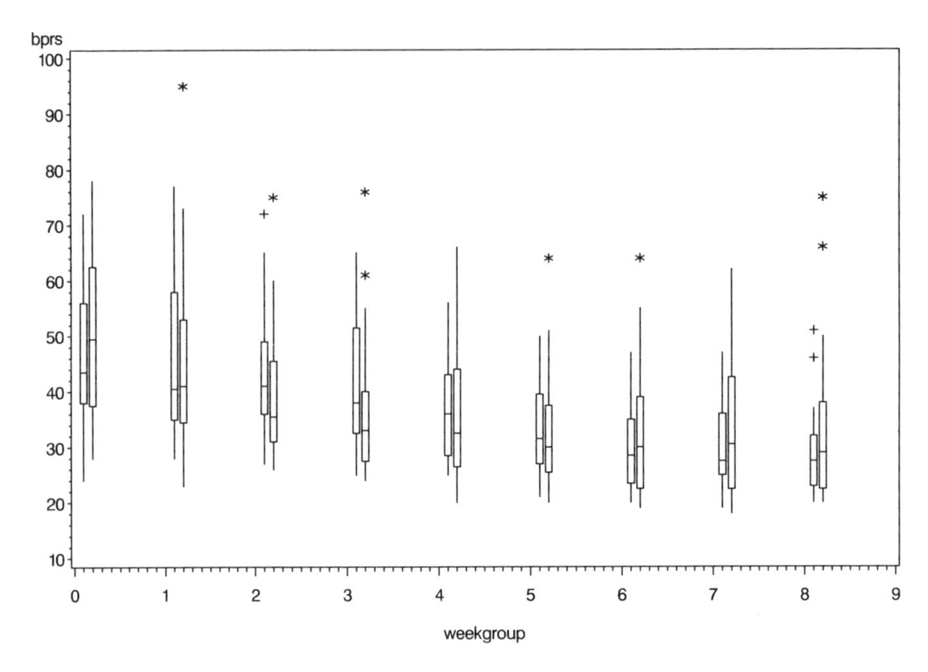

FIGURE 11.4
Boxplots for the BPRS data.

data. The method operates by transferring the repeated measurements made on the ith individual in the study, $x_i' = [x_{i1} \ldots x_{iT}]$, into a single value that captures some essential feature of the patient's response over time (see later). Analysis then proceeds by applying standard univariate methods to the summary measures from the sample of patients (see later examples). The approach has been in use for many years, and is described in Oldham (1962), Yates (1982), and Matthews et al. (1990). It is often referred to by its alternative name, *response feature analysis.*

11.3.1 Choosing Summary Measures

The key step to a successful summary measure analysis of longitudinal data is the choice of a relevant summary measure. The chosen measure needs to be relevant to the particular questions of interest in the study and in the broader scientific context in which the study takes place. In some longitudinal studies, more than a single summary measure might be deemed relevant or necessary, in which case the problem of combined inference may need to be addressed. More often in practice, however, it is likely that the different measures will deal with substantially different questions, so that each will have a notional interpretation in its own right. In most investigations, the decision over what summary measure to use needs to be made before the data are collected.

TABLE 11.2

Possible Summary Measures

Type of Data	Question of Interest	Summary Measure
Peaked	Is overall value of outcome variable the same in different groups?	Overall mean (equal time intervals) or area under curve (unequal intervals)
Peaked	Is maximum (minimum) response different between groups?	Maximum (minimum) value
Peaked	Is time to maximum (minimum) response different between groups?	Time to maximum (minimum) response
Growth	Is rate of change of outcome different between groups?	Regression coefficient
Growth	Is eventual value of outcome different between groups?	Final value of outcome or difference between last and first values or percentage change between first and last values
Growth	Is response in one group delayed relative to the other?	Time to reach a particular value (e.g., a fixed percentage of baseline)

A wide range of possible summary measures has been proposed. Those given in Table 11.2, for example, were suggested by Matthews et al. (1990). Frison and Pocock (1992) argue that the average response to treatment over time is often likely to be the most relevant summary statistic in treatment trials. In some cases the response on a particular visit may be chosen as the summary statistic of most interest, but this must be distinguished from the generally flawed approach that separately analyses the observations at each and every time point.

11.3.2 Applying the Summary Measure Approach

As our first example of the summary measure approach, it will be applied to the posttreatment values of the BPRS in Table 11.1. The mean of weeks 1 to 8 will be the chosen summary measure. We first calculate this measure and then look at boxplots of the measure for each treatment group.

```
data bprs;
 set bprs;
 mnbprs=mean(of x1-x8);
run;
proc boxplot data=bprs;
plot mnbprs*group /boxstyle=schematic;
run;
```

When a variable list is to be used with the `mean` function it must be preceded by `of`.

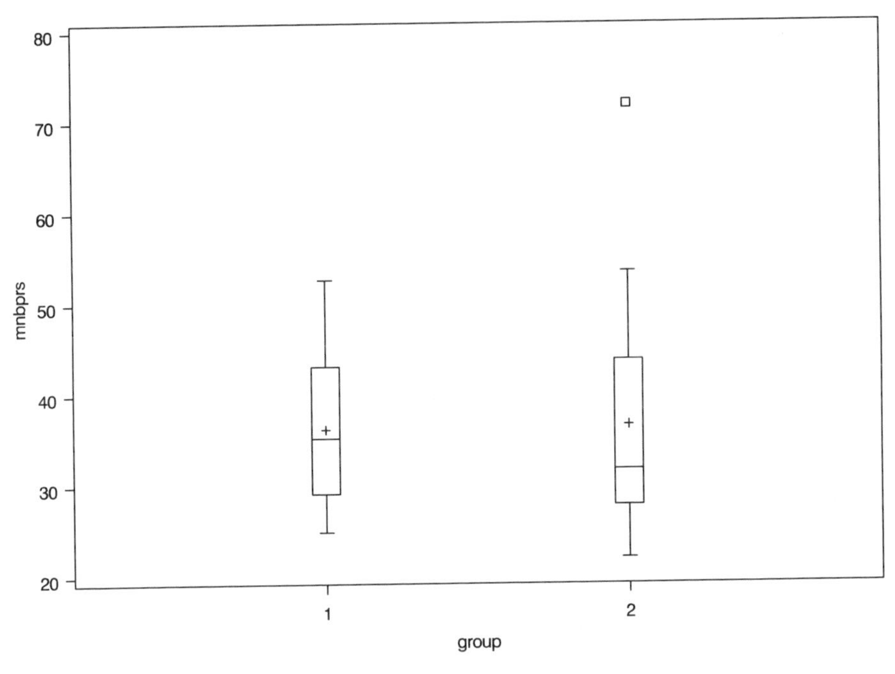

FIGURE 11.5
Boxplots of mean summary measures for the two treatment groups in the BPRS data.

The resulting plot is shown in Figure 11.5. The diagram indicates that the mean summary measure is more variable in the second treatment group and its distribution in this group is somewhat skew. There is little evidence of a difference in location of the summary measure distributions in each group.

Although the informal graphical material presented up to now has all indicated a lack of difference in the two treatment groups, most investigators would still require a formal test for a difference. Consequently we shall now apply a *t*-test to assess any difference between the treatment groups, and also calculate a confidence interval for this difference.

```
proc ttest data=bprs;
  class group;
  var mnbprs;
run;
```

The results are shown in Table 11.3. The *t*-test confirms the lack of any evidence for a group difference.

11.3.3 Incorporating Pretreatment Outcome Values into the Summary Measure Approach

Baseline measurements of the outcome variable in a longitudinal study are often correlated with the chosen summary measure, and using such measures

TABLE 11.3

Results from a *t*-Test on the Mean Summary Measure

The *t*-TEST Procedure

Statistics

Variable	group	N	Lower CL Mean	Mean	Upper CL Mean	Lower CL Std Dev	Std Dev
mnbprs	1	20	32.252	36.169	40.086	6.3646	8.3691
mnbprs	2	20	30.849	36.563	42.276	9.2848	12.209
mnbprs	Diff (1-2)		-7.094	-0.394	6.3067	8.5538	10.467

Statistics

Variable	group	Upper CL Std Dev	Std Err	Minimum	Maximum
mnbprs	1	12.224	1.8714	24.875	52.625
mnbprs	2	17.832	2.73	22	71.875
mnbprs	Diff (1-2)	13.489	3.3098		

T-Tests

Variable	Method	Variances	DF	t Value	Pr > |t|
mnbprs	Pooled	Equal	38	-0.12	0.9059
mnbprs	Satterthwaite	Unequal	33.6	-0.12	0.9060

Equality of Variances

Variable	Method	Num DF	Den DF	F Value	Pr > F
mnbprs	Folded F	19	19	2.13	0.1083

in the analysis can often lead to substantial gains in precision, but only when used appropriately, and that is as a covariate in an analysis of covariance (see Everitt and Pickles, 2004). We can illustrate the analysis using the data in Table 11.1 since the BPRS value corresponding to time zero is taken prior to the start of treatment. The SAS code needed for the analysis of covariance of the mean summary measure with treatment group and week 0 value as covariates is

```
proc glm data=bprs;
  class group;
  model mnbprs=x0 group;
run;
```

The results are shown in Table 11.4. We see that the baseline BPRS is strongly related to the BPRS values taken after treatment has begun, but there is still no evidence of a treatment difference even after conditioning on the baseline value.

11.3.4 Dealing with Missing Values When Using the Summary Measure Approach

One of the problems that often occurs in the collection of longitudinal data is that a patient may not have values of the outcome measure recorded on

TABLE 11.4

Results from an Analysis of Covariance of the BPRS Data with Baseline BPRS as Covariate

```
                         The GLM Procedure

                      Class Level Information

                   Class          Levels    Values

                   group               2    1 2


               Number of Observations Read           40
               Number of Observations Used           40

                         The GLM Procedure

Dependent Variable: mnbprs

                                     Sum of
Source                     DF       Squares    Mean Square   F Value   Pr > F

Model                       2   1871.515626     935.757813     15.10   <.0001

Error                      37   2292.965234      61.972033

Corrected Total            39   4164.480859


            R-Square     Coeff Var      Root MSE     mnbprs Mean

            0.449400      21.64745      7.872232        36.36563


Source                     DF     Type I SS    Mean Square   F Value   Pr > F

x0                          1   1868.066649    1868.066649     30.14   <.0001
group                       1      3.448977       3.448977      0.06   0.8148


Source                     DF   Type III SS    Mean Square   F Value   Pr > F

x0                          1   1869.965235    1869.965235     30.17   <.0001
group                       1      3.448977       3.448977      0.06   0.8148
```

all the occasions intended. This problem will be considered in detail in the next chapter, but as an example of where it has arisen we can examine the data shown in Table 11.5 (taken from Davis, 2002). The data come from a clinical trial comparing two treatments for maternal pain relief during labour. In this study 83 women in labour were randomized to receive an experimental pain medication (43 subjects) or placebo (40 subjects). Treatment was initiated when the cervical dilation was 8 cm. At 30-minute intervals, the amount of pain was self-reported by placing a mark on a 100-mm line (0 = no pain, 100 = very much pain). Table 11.5 gives the data for the first 20 subjects in each group.

If we use the mean as a summary measure for these data, the missing values can be dealt with simply by calculating, for each subject, the mean of their *available* values. So, for example, for subject 1 this would be the mean of four values, and for subject 2, the mean of three values. This is clearly very straightforward but Matthews (1993) points out a number of possible problems:

TABLE 11.5

Pain Scores from 83 Women in Labour: First 20 Subjects in Each Group

		Self-Reported Pain Scores at 30-Minute Intervals						
Group	**Patient**	**0**	**30**	**60**	**90**	**120**	**150**	**180**
1	1	0.0	0.0	0.0	0.0			
	2	0.0	0.0	0.0	0.0	2.5	2.3	14.0
	3	38.0	5.0	1.0	1.0	0.0	5.0	
	4	6.0	48.0	85.0	0.0	0.0		
	5	19.0	5.0					
	6	7.0	0.0	0.0	0.0			
	7	44.0	42.0	42.0	45.0			
	8	1.0	0.0	0.0	0.0	0.0	6.0	24.0
	9	24.5	35.0	13.0				
	10	1.0	30.5	81.5	67.5	98.5	97.0	
	11	35.5	44.5	55.0	69.0	72.5	39.5	26.0
	12	0.0	0.0	0.0	0.0	0.0	0.0	0.0
	13	8.0	30.5	26.0	24.0	29.0	45.0	91.0
	14	7.0	6.5	7.0	4.0	10.0		
	15	6.0	8.5	19.5	16.5	42.5	45.5	48.5
	16	32.5	9.5	7.5	5.5	4.5	0.0	7.0
	17	10.5	10.0	18.0	32.5	0.0	0.0	0.0
	18	11.5	20.5	32.5	37.0	39.0		
	19	72.0	91.5	4.5	32.0	10.5	10.5	10.5
	20	0.0	0.0	0.0	0.0	13.54	7.0	
2	1	4.0	9.0	30.0	75.0	49.0	97.0	
	2	0.0	0.0	1.0	27.5	95.0	100.0	
	3	9.0	6.0	25.0				
	4	52.5	18.0	12.5				
	5	90.5	99.0	100.0	100.0	100.0	100.0	100.0
	6	74.0	70.0	81.5	94.5	97.0		
	7	0.0	0.0	0.0	1.5	0.0	18.0	71.0
	8	0.0	51.5	56.0				
	9	6.5	7.0	7.0	9.0	25.0	36.0	20.0
	10	19.0	31.0	41.0	58.0			
	11	6.0	23.0	45.0	67.0	90.5		
	12	42.0	64.0	6.0				
	13	86.5	53.0	88.0	100.0	100.0		
	14	50.0	100.0	100.0	100.0	100.0		
	15	27.5	36.5	74.0	97.0	100.0	100.0	95.0
	16	0.0	0.0	6.0	6.0			
	17	62.0	79.0	80.5	85.0	90.0	97.5	97.0
	18	17.5	27.5	21.0	60.0	80.0	97.0	
	19	6.5	5.5	18.5	20.0	36.5	63.5	81.5
	20	8.0	9.0	35.5	39.0	70.0	92.0	98.0

Source: Davis, C.S., 2002, *Statistical Methods for the Analysis of Repeated Measurements*, Springer. With permission.

- If the summary measures are based on observations that have widely differing structures then, even within apparently homogeneous groups, they will not share a common distribution, contrary to the assumptions of most of the methods of analysis that are likely to be applied.
- The reason that observations are missing needs to be considered. (This problem is discussed in the next chapter.)

Here we shall ignore these possible difficulties and carry out the summary measure analysis using the following SAS code.

```
data labour;
  infile cards missover;
  input id x0-x6;
  group=1;
  if _n_>20 then group=2;
  mnpain=mean(of x0-x6);
cards;
 1   0.0   0.0   0.0   0.0
 2   0.0   0.0   0.0   0.0   2.5   2.3  14.0
 3  38.0   5.0   1.0   1.0   0.0   5.0
....
19   6.5   5.5  18.5  20.0  36.5  63.5  81.5
20   8.0   9.0  35.5  39.0  70.0  92.0  98.0
;
proc ttest data=labour;
  class group;
  var mnpain;
run;
```

The `infile` statement is not usually needed when the data are instream, i.e., included at the end of the data step after a `cards` or `datalines` statement. Including it allows options to be used to modify the way the data are read. In this case the `missover` option prevents SAS from going to a new line when there are fewer data values than variables. Instead, the remaining variables are set to missing values. The results are shown in Table 11.6. There is strong evidence of a treatment difference for these data. The 95% confidence interval for the difference is [–44.03, –13.18]. The experimental treatment appears to have lowered the average pain score by between 13 and 44 points on the visual analogue scale.

11.4 Summary Measure Approach for Binary Responses

Table 11.7 shows the data collected in a clinical trial comparing two treatments for a respiratory illness (Davis, 1991). In each of the two centres, eligible patients were randomly assigned to active treatment or placebo.

TABLE 11.6

Results from a t-Test for the Mean Summary Measure Applied to the Data in Table 11.5

The TTEST Procedure

Statistics

Variable	group		N	Lower CL Mean	Mean	Upper CL Mean	Lower CL Std Dev	Std Dev
mnpain		1	20	10.951	19.5	28.05	13.893	18.268
mnpain		2	20	34.642	48.104	61.566	21.875	28.764
mnpain	Diff (1-2)			-44.03	-28.6	-13.18	19.691	24.095

Statistics

Variable	group		Upper CL Std Dev	Std Err	Minimum	Maximum
mnpain		1	26.682	4.0848	0	62.667
mnpain		2	42.012	6.4319	3	98.5
mnpain	Diff (1-2)		31.053	7.6194		

T-Tests

Variable	Method	Variances	DF	t Value	Pr > |t|
mnpain	Pooled	Equal	38	-3.75	0.0006
mnpain	Satterthwaite	Unequal	32.2	-3.75	0.0007

Equality of Variances

Variable	Method	Num DF	Den DF	F Value	Pr > F
mnpain	Folded F	19	19	2.48	0.0547

During treatment, the respiratory status (categorized as 0 = poor, 1 = good) was determined at four visits. There were 111 patients (54 active, 57 placebo) with no missing data for responses or covariates. Here we shall consider how the response feature approach can be applied to this binary response, with the initial analysis ignoring all covariates except treatment group. We might, of course, simply ignore the binary nature of the response variable and compare the 'mean' responses over time in the two treatment groups by a t-test. Since the mean in this case is the proportion (p) of visits at which a patient's respiratory status was good, we could consider performing the test after taking some appropriate transformation, for example, arcsin (p) or arcsin ($\sqrt{p}$).

```
data resptrial;
  input id centre treat sex age bl v1-v4;
  ngood=sum(of v1-v4);
  visits=4;
  mnstatus=mean(of v1-v4);
  arcsin=arsin(mnstatus);
  arcroot=arsin(sqrt(mnstatus));
```

```
cards;
11  1   1   46  0   0   0   0   0
21  1   1   28  0   0   0   0   0
31  2   1   23  1   1   1   1   1
....
11022   2   63  1   1   1   1   1
11122   1   31  1   1   1   1   1
;
proc ttest data=resptrial;
  class treat;
  var mnstatus arcsin arcroot;
run;
```

TABLE 11.7

Respiratory Disorder Data

Patient	Center	Treatment	Sex	Age	BL	V1	V2	V3	V4
1	1	1	1	46	0	0	0	0	0
2	1	1	1	28	0	0	0	0	0
3	1	2	1	23	1	1	1	1	1
4	1	1	1	44	1	1	1	1	0
5	1	1	2	13	1	1	1	1	1
6	1	2	1	34	0	0	0	0	0
7	1	1	1	43	0	1	0	1	1
8	1	2	1	28	0	0	0	0	0
9	1	2	1	31	1	1	1	1	1
10	1	1	1	37	1	0	1	1	0
11	1	2	1	30	1	1	1	1	1
12	1	2	1	14	0	1	1	1	0
13	1	1	1	23	1	1	0	0	0
14	1	1	1	30	0	0	0	0	0
15	1	1	1	20	1	1	1	1	1
16	1	2	1	22	0	0	0	0	1
17	1	1	1	25	0	0	0	0	0
18	1	2	2	47	0	0	1	1	1
19	1	1	2	31	0	0	0	0	0
20	1	2	1	20	1	1	0	1	0
21	1	2	1	26	0	1	0	1	0
22	1	2	1	46	1	1	1	1	1
23	1	2	1	32	1	1	1	1	1
24	1	2	1	48	0	1	0	0	0
25	1	1	2	35	0	0	0	0	0
26	1	2	1	26	0	0	0	0	0
27	1	1	1	23	1	1	0	1	1
28	1	1	2	36	0	1	1	0	0
29	1	1	1	19	0	1	1	0	0
30	1	2	1	28	0	0	0	0	0

TABLE 11.7 (continued)

Respiratory Disorder Data

Patient	Center	Treatment	Sex	Age	BL	V1	V2	V3	V4
31	1	1	1	37	0	0	0	0	0
32	1	2	1	23	0	1	1	1	1
33	1	2	1	30	1	1	1	1	0
34	1	1	1	15	0	0	1	1	0
35	1	2	1	26	0	0	0	1	0
36	1	1	2	45	0	0	0	0	0
37	1	2	1	31	0	0	1	0	0
38	1	2	1	50	0	0	0	0	0
39	1	1	1	28	0	0	0	0	0
40	1	1	1	26	0	0	0	0	0
41	1	1	1	14	0	0	0	0	1
42	1	2	1	31	0	0	1	0	0
43	1	1	1	13	1	1	1	1	1
44	1	1	1	27	0	0	0	0	0
45	1	1	1	26	0	1	0	1	1
46	1	1	1	49	0	0	0	0	0
47	1	1	1	63	0	0	0	0	0
48	1	2	1	57	1	1	1	1	1
49	1	1	1	27	1	1	1	1	1
50	1	2	1	22	0	0	1	1	1
51	1	2	1	15	0	0	1	1	1
52	1	1	1	43	0	0	0	1	0
53	1	2	2	32	0	0	0	1	0
54	1	2	1	11	1	1	1	1	0
55	1	1	1	24	1	1	1	1	1
56	1	2	1	25	0	1	1	0	1
57	2	1	2	39	0	0	0	0	0
58	2	2	1	25	0	0	1	1	1
59	2	2	1	58	1	1	1	1	1
60	2	1	2	51	1	1	0	1	1
61	2	1	2	32	1	0	0	1	1
62	2	1	1	45	1	1	0	0	0
63	2	1	2	44	1	1	1	1	1
64	2	1	2	48	0	0	0	0	0
65	2	2	1	26	0	1	1	1	1
66	2	2	1	14	0	1	1	1	1
67	2	1	2	48	0	0	0	0	0
68	2	2	1	13	1	1	1	1	1
69	2	1	1	20	0	1	1	1	1
70	2	2	1	37	1	1	0	0	1
71	2	2	1	25	1	1	1	1	1
72	2	2	1	20	0	0	0	0	0
73	2	1	2	58	0	1	0	0	0
74	2	1	1	38	1	1	0	0	0
75	2	2	1	55	1	1	1	1	1
76	2	2	1	24	1	1	1	1	1
77	2	1	2	36	1	1	0	0	1
78	2	1	1	36	0	1	1	1	1
79	2	2	2	60	1	1	1	1	1
80	2	1	1	15	1	0	0	1	1

TABLE 11.7 (continued)

Respiratory Disorder Data

Patient	Center	Treatment	Sex	Age	BL	V1	V2	V3	V4
81	2	2	1	25	1	1	1	1	0
82	2	2	1	35	1	1	1	1	1
83	2	2	1	19	1	1	0	1	1
84	2	1	2	31	1	1	1	1	1
85	2	2	1	21	1	1	1	1	1
86	2	2	2	37	0	1	1	1	1
87	2	1	1	52	0	1	1	1	1
88	2	2	1	55	0	0	1	1	0
89	2	1	1	19	1	0	0	1	1
90	2	1	1	20	1	0	1	1	1
91	2	1	1	42	1	0	0	0	0
92	2	2	1	41	1	1	1	1	1
93	2	2	1	52	0	0	0	0	0
94	2	1	2	47	0	1	1	0	1
95	2	1	1	11	1	1	1	1	1
96	2	1	1	14	0	0	0	1	0
97	2	1	1	15	1	1	1	1	1
98	2	1	1	66	1	1	1	1	1
99	2	2	1	34	0	1	1	0	1
100	2	1	1	43	0	0	0	0	0
101	2	1	1	33	1	1	1	0	1
102	2	1	1	48	1	1	0	0	0
103	2	2	1	20	0	1	1	1	1
104	2	1	2	39	1	0	1	0	0
105	2	2	1	28	0	1	0	0	0
106	2	1	2	38	0	0	0	0	0
107	2	2	1	43	1	1	1	1	1
108	2	2	2	39	0	1	1	1	1
109	2	2	1	68	0	1	1	1	1
110	2	2	2	63	1	1	1	1	1
111	2	2	1	31	1	1	1	1	1

Note: Treatment: 1 = placebo, 2 = active; Sex: 1= male, 2 = female.
Source: Davis, C.S., 2002, *Statistical Methods for the Analysis of Repeated Measurements*, Springer. .

The results are shown in Table 11.8. There is clear evidence of a treatment difference whether the untransformed or transformed summary measure is analyzed. There is, on average, a higher proportion of "good" responses in the active treatment group.

A linear regression of the arcsin-transformed proportion of positive responses over the four post-baseline measurement occasions might be used to assess the effects of the baseline measurement, age, sex, and center.

```
proc glm data=resptrial;
  class centre treat sex;
  model arcroot=centre age sex bl treat;
run;
```

TABLE 11.8

Results of Summary Measure Analysis Applied to Respiratory Data in Table 11.7

The TTEST Procedure

Statistics

Variable	treat	N	Lower CL Mean	Mean	Upper CL Mean	Lower CL Std Dev	Std Dev
mnstatus	1	57	0.3373	0.443	0.5486	0.3361	0.3981
mnstatus	2	54	0.5841	0.6852	0.7863	0.3114	0.3704
mnstatus	Diff (1-2)		-0.387	-0.242	-0.097	0.3399	0.3849
arcsin	1	57	0.4293	0.5907	0.752	0.5134	0.6082
arcsin	2	54	0.8031	0.9715	1.1399	0.5186	0.6169
arcsin	Diff (1-2)		-0.611	-0.381	-0.15	0.5408	0.6124
arcroot	1	57	0.5377	0.6981	0.8586	0.5104	0.6046
arcroot	2	54	0.9134	1.0666	1.2198	0.4719	0.5614
arcroot	Diff (1-2)		-0.588	-0.368	-0.149	0.5157	0.584

Statistics

Variable	treat	Upper CL Std Dev	Std Err	Minimum	Maximum
mnstatus	1	0.4884	0.0527	0	1
mnstatus	2	0.4573	0.0504	0	1
mnstatus	Diff (1-2)	0.4438	0.0731		
arcsin	1	0.746	0.0806	0	1.5708
arcsin	2	0.7616	0.084	0	1.5708
arcsin	Diff (1-2)	0.7061	0.1163		
arcroot	1	0.7417	0.0801	0	1.5708
arcroot	2	0.693	0.0764	0	1.5708
arcroot	Diff (1-2)	0.6733	0.1109		

T-Tests

Variable	Method	Variances	DF	t Value	Pr > |t|
mnstatus	Pooled	Equal	109	-3.31	0.0013
mnstatus	Satterthwaite	Unequal	109	-3.32	0.0012
arcsin	Pooled	Equal	109	-3.27	0.0014
arcsin	Satterthwaite	Unequal	108	-3.27	0.0014
arcroot	Pooled	Equal	109	-3.32	0.0012
arcroot	Satterthwaite	Unequal	109	-3.33	0.0012

Equality of Variances

Variable	Method	Num DF	Den DF	F Value	Pr > F
mnstatus	Folded F	56	53	1.16	0.5984
arcsin	Folded F	53	56	1.03	0.9141
arcroot	Folded F	56	53	1.16	0.5881

The results are shown in Table 11.9. Only the regression coefficients for baseline response and treatment group are statistically significant.

A more satisfactory analysis can be achieved by using the generalized linear modelling approach described in Chapter 8. A standard logistic regression model might be applied, but because the number of occasions on which the response was good out of the four visits made by each participant is unlikely to be binomially distributed (the observations are likely to be correlated rather than independent), we need to allow for possible overdispersion. Fitting a model with logistic link and with treatment, sex, age, and baseline respiratory status as the main effects

TABLE 11.9

Results from the Linear Regression on the Arcsin-Transformed Proportion of Positive Responses for the Respiratory Data

```
                         The GLM Procedure

                      Class Level Information

                   Class         Levels    Values

                   centre             2    1 2

                   treat              2    1 2

                   sex                2    1 2


              Number of Observations Read          111
              Number of Observations Used          111

                         The GLM Procedure

Dependent Variable: arcroot

                                        Sum of
Source                      DF         Squares     Mean Square    F Value    Pr > F

Model                        5     16.51257785      3.30251557      14.20    <.0001

Error                      105     24.42553350      0.23262413

Corrected Total            110     40.93811135


             R-Square     Coeff Var      Root MSE     arcroot Mean

             0.403355      54.97165      0.482311         0.877382

Source                      DF       Type I SS     Mean Square    F Value    Pr > F

centre                       1      3.14379291      3.14379291      13.51    0.0004
age                          1      1.00083354      1.00083354       4.30    0.0405
sex                          1      0.40002818      0.40002818       1.72    0.1926
bl                           1      8.27903368      8.27903368      35.59    <.0001
treat                        1      3.68888954      3.68888954      15.86    0.0001


Source                      DF     Type III SS     Mean Square    F Value    Pr > F

centre                       1      0.97656959      0.97656959       4.20    0.0430
age                          1      0.43858914      0.43858914       1.89    0.1726
sex                          1      0.01684248      0.01684248       0.07    0.7884
bl                           1      8.74201567      8.74201567      37.58    <.0001
treat                        1      3.68888954      3.68888954      15.86    0.0001
```

```
proc logistic data=resptrial;
  class centre treat sex /param=ref ref=first;
  model ngood/visits=centre age sex bl treat /scale=d;
run;
```

The events/trials syntax is used on the `model` statement, and `scale=d` sets the dispersion parameter to be the deviance divided by its degrees of freedom. The results are shown in Table 11.10. The estimated value of the scale parameter, 2.47, is substantially above unity, confirming the presence of overdispersion. The estimated odds ratio for the effect of treatment is 3.67 with a 95% confidence interval of (1.77, 7.60). The *p*-values from the linear regression in Table 11.9 and the logistic regression in Table 11.10 are comparable,

TABLE 11.10

Results from Overdispersed Logistic Regression Model Fitted to Proportion of Positive Responses in the Respiratory Data

```
                    The LOGISTIC Procedure

                       Model Information

        Data Set                        WORK.RESPTRIAL
        Response Variable (Events)      ngood
        Response Variable (Trials)      visits
        Number of Observations          111
        Model                           binary logit
        Optimization Technique          Fisher's scoring


                        Response Profile

               Ordered      Binary           Total
                 Value      Outcome      Frequency

                     1      Event              249
                     2      Nonevent           195

                    Class Level Information

                                        Design
                                      Variables

                 Class       Value            1

                 centre      1                0
                             2                1

                 treat       1                0
                             2                1

                 sex         1                0
                             2                1


                    Model Convergence Status

        Convergence criterion (GCONV=1E-8) satisfied.


        Deviance and Pearson Goodness-of-Fit Statistics

 Criterion        DF          Value      Value/DF      Pr > ChiSq

 Deviance        105       259.2222        2.4688          <.0001
 Pearson         105       222.9025        2.1229          <.0001

            Number of events/trials observations: 111

NOTE: The covariance matrix has been multiplied by the heterogeneity factor
      (Deviance / DF) 2.46878.


                    The LOGISTIC Procedure

                     Model Fit Statistics

                                          Intercept
                            Intercept           and
             Criterion           Only    Covariates

             AIC              248.652       207.731
             SC               252.748       232.306
             -2 Log L         246.652       195.731
```

TABLE 11.10 (continued)

Results from Overdispersed Logistic Regression Model Fitted to Proportion of Positive Responses in the Respiratory Data

Testing Global Null Hypothesis: BETA=0

Test	Chi-Square	DF	Pr > ChiSq
Likelihood Ratio	50.9209	5	<.0001
Score	46.0339	5	<.0001
Wald	37.0374	5	<.0001

Type III Analysis of Effects

Effect	DF	Wald Chi-Square	Pr > ChiSq
centre	1	3.1834	0.0744
age	1	1.7011	0.1921
sex	1	0.0663	0.7968
bl	1	24.6428	<.0001
treat	1	12.1889	0.0005

Analysis of Maximum Likelihood Estimates

Parameter		DF	Estimate	Standard Error	Wald Chi-Square	Pr > ChiSq
Intercept		1	-0.9002	0.5305	2.8789	0.0897
centre	2	1	0.6716	0.3764	3.1834	0.0744
age		1	-0.0182	0.0139	1.7011	0.1921
sex	2	1	0.1192	0.4630	0.0663	0.7968
bl		1	1.8820	0.3791	24.6428	<.0001
treat	2	1	1.2992	0.3721	12.1889	0.0005

Odds Ratio Estimates

Effect	Point Estimate	95% Wald Confidence Limits	
centre 2 vs 1	1.957	0.936	4.093
age	0.982	0.956	1.009
sex 2 vs 1	1.127	0.455	2.792
bl	6.567	3.124	13.806
treat 2 vs 1	3.666	1.768	7.603

The LOGISTIC Procedure

Association of Predicted Probabilities and Observed Responses

Percent Concordant	79.1	Somers' D	0.590
Percent Discordant	20.2	Gamma	0.594
Percent Tied	0.7	Tau-a	0.291
Pairs	48555	c	0.795

but the estimates from the logit model are on a more natural scale. There is no relatively straightforward interpretation of the estimates from the model fitted to the arcsin-transformed responses, although calculation of an odds ratio at the mean value of the sample covariates could be attempted.

11.5 Summary

The methods described in this chapter provide for the exploration and simple analysis of longitudinal data collected in the course of a clinical trial. The graphical methods can provide insights into both potentially interesting patterns of response over time and the structure of any treatment differences. In addition, they can indicate possible outlying observations that may need special attention. The response feature approach to analysis has the distinct advantage that it is straightforward, can be tailored to consider aspects of the data thought to be particularly relevant, and produces results that are relatively simple to understand. The method can accommodate data containing missing values without difficulty, although it might be misleading if the observations are anything other than missing completely at random (see next chapter).

12

The Analysis of Longitudinal Data II: Models for Normal Response Variables

12.1 Introduction

The summary measure approach to the analysis of longitudinal data described in the previous chapter provides a useful first step in making inferences about the data but will only rarely give the complete picture. A more complete analysis will need to involve fitting a suitable model to the data and estimating parameters that link the explanatory variables of interest to the repeated measures of the response variable. The main objective in longitudinal studies is to characterize change in the repeated values of the response variable and to determine the explanatory variables most associated with any change.

Because several observations of the response variable are made on the same individual, it is likely that the measurements will be correlated rather than independent, even after conditioning on the explanatory variables. Consequently, models for repeated measures data need to include parameters relating the explanatory variables to the repeated measurements — parameters analogous to those in the usual multiple regression model (see Chapter 6), and, in addition, parameters that account adequately for the correlational structure of the repeated measurements. It is the former parameters that are generally of most interest, with the latter often being regarded as *nuisance parameters*. But providing an adequate model for the correlational structure of the repeated measures is necessary to avoid misleading inferences about those parameters that are of most importance to the researcher.

Over the last decade, methodology for the analysis of repeated measures data has been the subject of much research and development, and there are now a variety of powerful techniques available. Comprehensive accounts of these methods are given in Diggle et al. (1994) and Davis (2002). In this chapter we will concentrate on a single class of methods, *linear mixed effects models*, suitable for responses that can be assumed to be approximately normally distributed. Non-normal responses will be the subject of Chapter 13.

12.2 Linear Mixed Effects Models for Repeated Measures Data

Linear mixed effects models for repeated measures data formalize the sensible idea that an individual's pattern of responses is likely to depend on many characteristics of that individual, including some that are unobserved. These unobserved variables are then included in the model as random variables, that is, *random effects*. The essential feature of the model is that correlation amongst the repeated measurements on the same unit arises from shared, unobserved variables. Conditional on the values of the random effects, the repeated measurements are assumed to be independent, the so-called *local independence* assumption.

Linear mixed effects models are introduced in Display 12.1, where two commonly used approaches, the *random intercept* and *random intercept and slope* models, are described.

We will use the data in Table 12.1 reported in Zerbe (1979) and also given in Davis (2002), to illustrate the application of linear mixed effects models, in particular the two models described in Display 12.1. These data consist of plasma inorganic phosphate measurements obtained from 13 control and 20 obese patients 0, 0.5, 1, 1.5, 2, and 3 hours after an oral glucose challenge. The data are read in as follows:

```
data pip;
 input id x1-x8;
 if id>13 then group=2;
 else group=1;
cards;
 1   4.3   3.3   3.0   2.6   2.2   2.5   3.4   4.4
 2   3.7   2.6   2.6   1.9   2.9   3.2   3.1   3.9
 3   4.0   4.1   3.1   2.3   2.9   3.1   3.9   4.0
....
32   4.5   4.0   3.7   3.3   2.4   2.3   3.1   3.3
33   4.6   4.4   3.8   3.8   3.8   3.6   3.8   3.8
;
data pipl;
   set pip;
   array xs {*} x1-x8;
   array t{8} t1-t8 (0 .5 1 1.5 2 3 4 5);
   do i=1 to 8;
     time=t{i};
```

DISPLAY 12.1

Two Simple Linear Mixed Effects Models

- Consider a simple set of longitudinal data in which a number of individuals each have values of a response variable recorded at times $t_1, t_2, \ldots, t_r$. (We assume the same set of time points for each individual to make the subsequent description simpler, but it is as simple to model data in which each individual is observed at a different set of time points.)
- Let y_{ij} represent the value of the response for individual i at time t_j. A possible model for the y_{ij} might be

$$y_{ij} = \beta_0 + \beta_1 t_j + u_i + \varepsilon_{ij} \qquad \text{(A)}$$

- Here the total residual that would be present in the usual linear regression model has been partitioned into a subject-specific random component u_i, which is constant over time, plus a residual ε_{ij}, which varies randomly over time. The u_i are assumed to be normally distributed with zero mean and variance σ_u^2. Similarly, the ε_{ij} are assumed normally distributed with zero mean and variance σ^2. The u_i and the ε_{ij} are assumed to be independent of each other and of the t_j.
- The model in (A) is known as a *random intercept model*; the u_i are the random intercepts. The repeated measurements for a specimen vary about that specimen's own regression line, which can differ in intercept but not in slope from the regression lines of other specimens. The random effects model possible heterogeneity in the intercepts of the individuals.
- In this model time has a fixed effect.
- The random intercept model implies that the total variance of each repeated measurement is

$$\mathrm{Var}\left(u_i + \varepsilon_{ij}\right) = \sigma_u^2 + \sigma^2$$

- Due to this decomposition of the total residual variance into a between-subject component, σ_u^2, and a within-subject component, σ^2, the model is sometimes referred to as a *variance component model*.
- The covariance between the total residuals at two time points t_j and $t_{j'}$, in the same specimen i is

$$\mathrm{Cov}\left(u_i + \varepsilon_{ij}, u_i + \varepsilon_{ij'}\right) = \sigma_u^2$$

DISPLAY 12.1 (continued)

Two Simple Linear Mixed Effects Models

- Note that these covariances are induced by the shared random intercept; for specimens with $u_i > 0$, the total residuals will tend to be greater than the mean, for specimens with $u_i < 0$, they will tend to be less than the mean.
- It follows from the two relations above that the residual correlations are given by

$$Cor\left(u_i + \varepsilon_{ij}, u_i + \varepsilon_{ij'}\right) = \frac{\sigma_u^2}{\sigma_u^2 + \sigma^2}$$

- This is an *intraclass correlation,* interpreted as the proportion of the total residual variance that is due to residual variability between subjects.
- A random intercept model constrains the variance of each repeated measure to be the same and the covariance between any pair of measurements to be equal. This is usually called the *compound symmetry* structure.
- These constraints are often not realistic for repeated measures data. For example, for longitudinal data it is more common for measures taken closer to each other in time to be more highly correlated than those taken further apart. In addition, the variances of the later repeated measures are often greater than those of measures taken earlier.
- Consequently, for many such data sets the random intercept model will not do justice to the observed pattern of covariances between the repeated measures. A model that allows a more realistic structure for the covariances is one that allows heterogeneity in both slopes and intercepts, the *random slope and intercept model.*
- It should also be noted that reestimating the model after adding or subtracting a constant from t_j, e.g., its mean, will lead to different variance and composure estimates but will not affect fixed effects.
- In this model there are two types of random effects, the first modelling heterogeneity in intercepts, u_{i1}, and the second modelling heterogeneity in slopes, u_{i2}.
- Explicitly the model is

$$y_{ij} = \beta_0 + \beta_1 t_j + u_{i1} + u_{i2} t_j + \varepsilon_{ij} \qquad \text{(B)}$$

where the parameters are not, of course, the same as in (A).

DISPLAY 12.1 (continued)

Two Simple Linear Mixed Effects Models

- The two random effects are assumed to have a bivariate normal distribution with zero means for both variables, variances $\sigma^2_{u_1}, \sigma^2_{u_2}$, and covariance $\sigma_{u_1u_2}$.
- With this model the total residual is $u_{i1} + u_{i2}t_j + \varepsilon_{ij}$ with variance

$$Var\left(u_{i1} + u_{i2}t_j + \varepsilon_{ij}\right) = \sigma^2_{u_1} + 2\sigma_{u_1u_2}t_j + \sigma^2_{u_2}x_j^2 + \sigma^2$$

  which is no longer constant for different values of t_j.
- Similarly the covariance between two total residuals of the same individual

$$Cov\left(u_{i1} + u_{i2}t_j + \varepsilon_{ij}, u_{i1} + u_{i2}t_{j'} + \varepsilon_{ij'}\right) = \sigma^2_{u_1} + \sigma_{u_1u_2}\left(t_j + t_{j'}\right) + \sigma^2_{u_2}t_jt_{j'}$$

  is not constrained to be the same for all pairs j and j'.
- Linear mixed-effects models can be estimated by maximum likelihood. However, this method tends to produce biased estimates of the variance components. A modified version of maximum likelihood, known as *restricted maximum likelihood,* is therefore often recommended; this provides consistent estimates of the variance components. Details are given in Diggle et al. (1994) and Longford (1993). Often the two estimation methods will give similar results.
- Competing linear mixed-effects models can be compared using a likelihood ratio test. If, however, the models have been estimated by restricted maximum likelihood, this test can only be used if both models have the same set of fixed effects (see Longford, 1993).

```
      pip=xs{i};
      output;
    end;
    label time='hours after glucose';
run;
proc format;
    value group 1='Control' 2='Obese';
run;
```

TABLE 12.1

Plasma Inorganic Phosphate Levels from 33 Subjects

		Hours after Glucose Challenge							
Group	ID	0	0.5	1	1.5	2	3	4	5
Control	1	4.3	3.3	3.0	2.6	2.2	2.5	3.4	4.4
	2	3.7	2.6	2.6	1.9	2.9	3.2	3.1	3.9
	3	4.0	4.1	3.1	2.3	2.9	3.1	3.9	4.0
	4	3.6	3.0	2.2	2.8	2.9	3.9	3.8	4.0
	5	4.1	3.8	2.1	3.0	3.6	3.4	3.6	3.7
	6	3.8	2.2	2.0	2.6	3.8	3.6	3.0	3.5
	7	3.8	3.0	2.4	2.5	3.1	3.4	3.5	3.7
	8	4.4	3.9	2.8	2.1	3.6	3.8	4.0	3.9
	9	5.0	4.0	3.4	3.4	3.3	3.6	4.0	4.3
	10	3.7	3.1	2.9	2.2	1.5	2.3	2.7	2.8
	11	3.7	2.6	2.6	2.3	2.9	2.2	3.1	3.9
	12	4.4	3.7	3.1	3.2	3.7	4.3	3.9	4.8
	13	4.7	3.1	3.2	3.3	3.2	4.2	3.7	4.3
Obese	14	4.3	3.3	3.0	2.6	2.2	2.5	2.4	3.4
	15	5.0	4.9	4.1	3.7	3.7	4.1	4.7	4.9
	16	4.6	4.4	3.9	3.9	3.7	4.2	4.8	5.0
	17	4.3	3.9	3.1	3.1	3.1	3.1	3.6	4.0
	18	3.1	3.1	3.3	2.6	2.6	1.9	2.3	2.7
	19	4.8	5.0	2.9	2.8	2.2	3.1	3.5	3.6
	20	3.7	3.1	3.3	2.8	2.9	3.6	4.3	4.4
	21	5.4	4.7	3.9	4.1	2.8	3.7	3.5	3.7
	22	3.0	2.5	2.3	2.2	2.1	2.6	3.2	3.5
	23	4.9	5.0	4.1	3.7	3.7	4.1	4.7	4.9
	24	4.8	4.3	4.7	4.6	4.7	3.7	3.6	3.9
	25	4.4	4.2	4.2	3.4	3.5	3.4	3.8	4.0
	26	4.9	4.3	4.0	4.0	3.3	4.1	4.2	4.3
	27	5.1	4.1	4.6	4.1	3.4	4.2	4.4	4.9
	28	4.8	4.6	4.6	4.4	4.1	4.0	3.8	3.8
	29	4.2	3.5	3.8	3.6	3.3	3.1	3.5	3.9
	30	6.6	6.1	5.2	4.1	4.3	3.8	4.2	4.8
	31	3.6	3.4	3.1	2.8	2.1	2.4	2.5	3.5
	32	4.5	4.0	3.7	3.3	2.4	2.3	3.1	3.3
	33	4.6	4.4	3.8	3.8	3.8	3.6	3.8	3.8

Source: Davis, C.S., 2002, *Statistical Methods for the Analysis of Repeated Measurements*, Springer. With permission.

Both wide and long forms of the data set are created as described in the previous chapter. One difference in this example arises because the measurement times are not evenly spaced, so the index to the array cannot be used as the 'time' variable. Instead, a separate array of measurement times is set up. We also create a format for later labelling of the two groups. The fact that the format bears the same name, `group`, as the variable to which it is to be applied is not a problem. Indeed, it can be useful when formats are defined for a large number of variables.

Here we will begin by plotting the data to gain some idea of what form of linear mixed-effects model might be appropriate. First we plot the raw

TABLE 12.2

Part of Glucose Challenge Data in "Long" Form

	Subject	Time	Group	Plasma
1	1	0.0	Control	4.3
2	1	0.5	Control	3.3
3	1	1.0	Control	3.0
4	1	1.5	Control	2.6
5	1	2.0	Control	2.2
6	1	3.0	Control	2.5
7	1	4.0	Control	3.4
8	1	5.0	Control	4.4
9	2	0.0	Control	3.7
10	2	0.5	Control	2.6
11	2	1.0	Control	2.6
12	2	1.5	Control	1.9
13	2	2.0	Control	2.9
14	2	3.0	Control	3.2
15	2	4.0	Control	3.1
16	2	5.0	Control	3.9
17	3	0.0	Control	4.0
18	3	0.5	Control	4.1
19	3	1.0	Control	3.1
20	3	1.5	Control	2.3

data separately for the control and the obese groups. In these and subsequent plots we are going to make use of some of the plotting macros, so these are included first.

```
%inc 'c:\sasbook\macros\panelplot.sas';
%inc 'c:\sasbook\macros\template.sas';
%inc 'c:\sasbook\macros\plotmat.sas';
proc sort data=pipl; by group id; run;
proc gplot data=pipl gout=fig12_1 uniform;
 plot pip*time=id /nolegend hminor=0;
 by group;
 symbol1 i=join v=none r=50;
 format group group.;
run;
%panelplot(igout=fig12_1,ncols=2);
```

The data are sorted by `group` and `id` within `group`, so that the `gplot` step can produce separate plots for each group via the `by group;` statement. The `uniform` option on the `proc` statement ensures that the separate plots share the same scale for their axes, which aids comparison. The `format` statement applies the format `group` to the variable of the same name. To identify it as a format the name must be suffixed with a dot. Although the separate plots are produced, the panelplot macro combines them into the single plot shown in Figure 12.1.

The profiles in both groups show some curvature, suggesting that a quadratic effect of time may be needed in any model. There also appears to be some suspicion of a difference in the shape of the curves in the two groups, suggesting perhaps the need to consider a group × time interaction.

Next we plot the scatterplot matrices of the repeated measurements for the two groups using

```
data group1 group2;
  set pip;
  if group=1 then output group1;
  else output group2;
run;
goptions reset=symbol;
%plotmat(group1,x1-x8);
%plotmat(group2,x1-x8);
```

The short data step splits the data set into two, one for each group. This is a simple example of how a data step can create more than one data set. The plots are shown in Figure 12.2 and Figure 12.3. Both plots indicate that the correlations of pairs of measurements made at different times differ, so the compound symmetry structure for these correlations (see Display 12.1) is unlikely to be appropriate.

On the basis of the plots in Figure 12.1 to Figure 12.3, a suitable model for the glucose challenge data will need to include a quadratic effect for time and allow the correlations structure to depart from the compound symmetry assumption outlined in Display 12.1. We will begin by fitting the following random intercept and slope model:

$$y_{ij} = \beta_0 + \beta_1\text{group} + \beta_2\text{time} + \beta_3\text{time}^2 + u_{i1} + u_{i2}\text{time} + \varepsilon_{ij}$$

We can fit this model using proc mixed as follows

```
proc sort data=pipl; by id time; run;
proc mixed data=pipl covtest noclprint;
  class group id;
  model pip=group time|time /s ddfm=bw;
  random int time /subject=id type=un;
run;
```

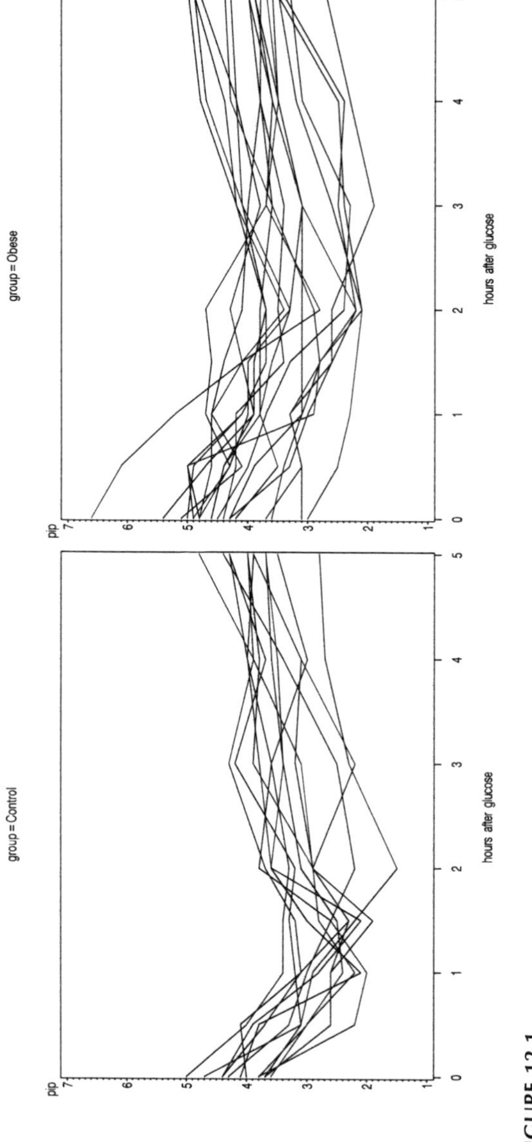

FIGURE 12.1
Glucose challenge data for control and obese groups.

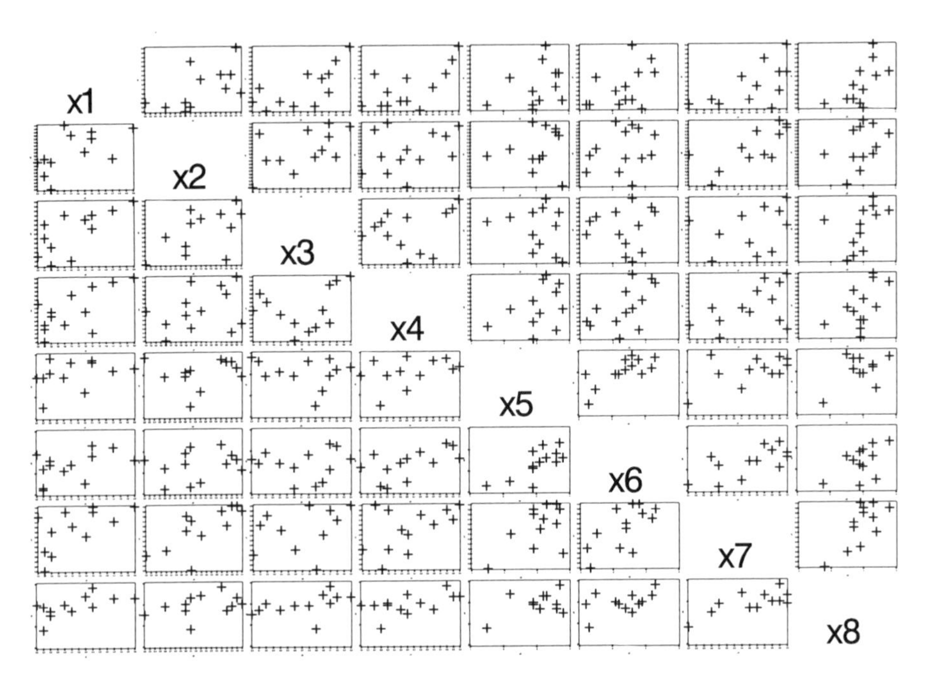

FIGURE 12.2
Scatterplot matrix for control group in Table 12.1.

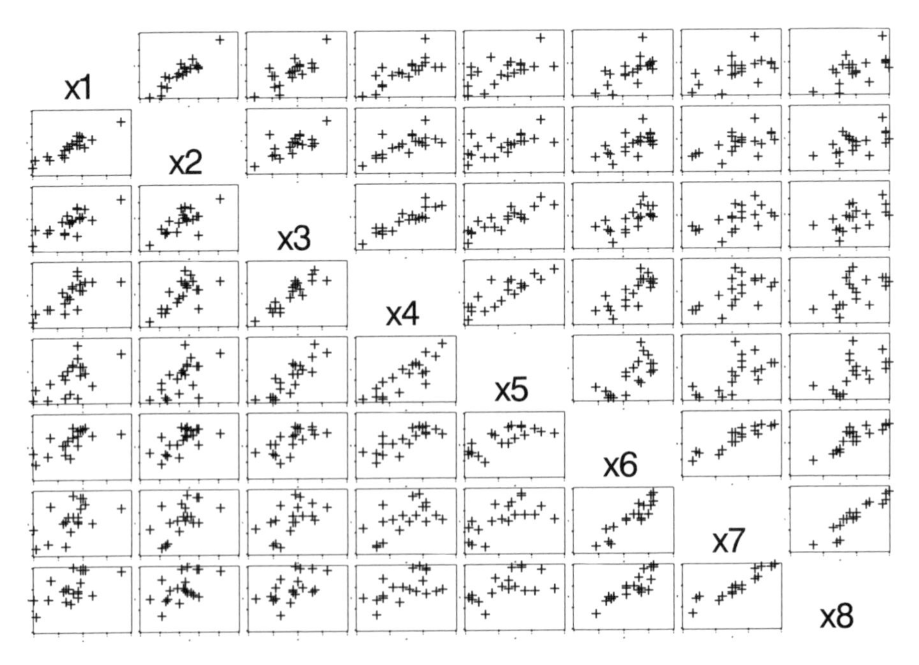

FIGURE 12.3
Scatterplot matrix for obese group in Table 12.1.

Proc mixed is the SAS procedure for linear mixed models with normal responses. Its syntax is similar to that of proc glm, with additional statements and options to deal with the random effects. The first point to note is that it takes as input the long form of the data set. With large data sets it is advisable to sort the data by subject and measurement occasion within subject. The `class` statement performs its usual function of identifying categorical variables. If the subject identifier is not a numeric variable, or the data have not been sorted, it should be included on the `class` statement. The `noclprint` option on the `proc` statement stops the listing of the levels of the categorical variables in the output, which is useful when the data contain observations on a large number of subjects. In that case, `noclprint=`*n* could be used to suppress the class level listing for variables with more than *n* levels. The `model` statement specifies the fixed effects in the model in the same way as for `proc glm`. Here we use the bar operator (|) as the shorthand for time time*time and, as this implies, interactions and polynomial terms can be specified with the asterisk. The `s` (`solution`) option requests that the fixed effects parameter estimates be included in the output. In mixed models the denominator degrees of freedom for the *F* and *t* tests of the fixed effects need to be estimated from the data. Proc mixed offers five methods of estimation. In general these will lead to different results, but for longitudinal analyses with reasonably sized samples any method is likely to yield degrees of freedom large enough to lead to very similar *p*-values. We have selected the `bw` (`betwithin`) method as suitable for longitudinal analysis, although the Satterthwaite or Kenward–Roger methods could also have been chosen.

The `random` statement specifies the random effects and their related options. A random intercept is not included in the model by default and needs to be specified as `int` or `intercept` on the `random` statement. Including `time` as a random effect specifies random slopes in `time`, i.e., the u_{i2}time term in the model. The `subject=` option specifies the subject identifier. The `type=` option specifies the covariance structure of the random effects. In the terminology adopted by SAS the random parameters are referred to as 'covariance parameters' and are represented in the model as a covariance matrix which has a structure specified by the `type` option. `Type=vc` (variance components) is the default and estimates the variance for each random effect whilst constraining any covariance between them to zero. `Type=un` (unstructured) allows the random intercepts and slopes to covary and estimates the covariance between them. The `covtest` option on the `proc mixed` statement produces asymptotic standard errors and Wald tests for the covariance parameters.

The results are shown in Table 12.3. The regression coefficients for linear and quadratic time are both highly significant. The group effect just fails to reach significance at the 5% level. When an unstructured covariance matrix is specified for the random effects, their estimates are labelled in the output with the row and column number of the matrix. UN(1,1) is the variance of the random intercept term, u_{i1} above, and is estimated to be 0.3943. UN(2,2)

TABLE 12.3

Results from Random Slope and Intercept Model with Fixed Quadratic Time Effect Fitted to Glucose Challenge Data

```
                         The Mixed Procedure

                          Model Information

          Data Set                     WORK.PIPL
          Dependent Variable           pip
          Covariance Structure         Unstructured
          Subject Effect               id
          Estimation Method            REML
          Residual Variance Method     Profile
          Fixed Effects SE Method      Model-Based
          Degrees of Freedom Method    Between-Within


                             Dimensions

               Covariance Parameters                 4
               Columns in X                          5
               Columns in Z Per Subject              2
               Subjects                             33
               Max Obs Per Subject                   8
               Observations Used                   264
               Observations Not Used                 0
               Total Observations                  264


                          Iteration History

     Iteration    Evaluations    -2 Res Log Like       Criterion

             0              1       570.33709221
             1              2       424.01656924      0.00000368
             2              1       424.01647003      0.00000000


                      Convergence criteria met.


                    Covariance Parameter Estimates

                                              Standard         Z
   Cov Parm      Subject      Estimate           Error     Value        Pr Z

   UN(1,1)       id             0.3943          0.1237      3.19      0.0007
   UN(2,1)       id           -0.04477         0.02346     -1.91      0.0564
   UN(2,2)       id            0.01592        0.006092      2.61      0.0045
   Residual                     0.1757         0.01770      9.92      <.0001

                           Fit Statistics

               -2 Res Log Likelihood            424.0
               AIC (smaller is better)          432.0
               AICC (smaller is better)         432.2
               BIC (smaller is better)          438.0

                         The Mixed Procedure

                   Null Model Likelihood Ratio Test

                     DF     Chi-Square      Pr > ChiSq

                      3         146.32          <.0001
```

TABLE 12.3 (continued)

Results from Random Slope and Intercept Model with Fixed Quadratic Time Effect Fitted to Glucose Challenge Data

Solution for Fixed Effects

Effect	Group	Estimate	Standard Error	DF	t Value	Pr > |t|
Intercept		4.3372	0.1448	31	29.96	<.0001
group	1	-0.3826	0.1928	31	-1.98	0.0562
group	2	0	.	.	.	.
time		-0.8311	0.06214	229	-13.38	<.0001
time*time		0.1636	0.01125	229	14.55	<.0001

Type 3 Tests of Fixed Effects

Effect	Num DF	Den DF	F Value	Pr > F
group	1	31	3.94	0.0562
time	1	229	178.89	<.0001
time*time	1	229	211.56	<.0001

is the variance of the random slopes in time, u_{i2}, estimated as 0.01592 and UN(2,1) is the intercept–slope covariance term estimated as –0.04477.

Here to demonstrate what happens if we make a very misleading assumption about the correlational structure of the repeated measurements, we will compare the results in Table 12.3 with those obtained if we assume that the repeated measurements are independent. The independence model can be fitted in the usual way using `proc glm` as follows:

```
proc glm data=pipl;
  class group;
  model pip=group time|time /solution;
run;
```

The results are shown in Table 12.4. We see that under the independence assumption the standard error for the group effect is about half of that given in Table 12.3 and if used would lead to the claim of strong evidence of a difference between control and obese patients.

To informally assess how the fitted linear mixed effects model describes the glucose challenge data, we will now plot the predicted values from the model separately for each group. To do this we use the same `proc mixed` step as before, changing the model statement to

```
model pip=group time|time /s ddfm=bw outp=mixout;
```

The `outp=mixout` option saves the predicted values to the `mixout` data set. These are then plotted in the same way as the observed values were for Figure 12.1. The result is shown in Figure 12.4. We can see that the model has captured the profiles of the control group relatively well but not perhaps

TABLE 12.4

Results from Independence Model Fitted to Glucose Challenge Data

```
                              The GLM Procedure

                           Class Level Information

                         Class          Levels    Values

                         group               2    1 2

                          Number of observations    264

                              The GLM Procedure

Dependent Variable: pip

                                            Sum of
 Source                          DF        Squares    Mean Square   F Value   Pr > F

 Model                            3     50.5489659     16.8496553     35.13   <.0001

 Error                          260    124.7072462      0.4796433

 Corrected Total                263    175.2562121


              R-Square     Coeff Var      Root MSE      pip Mean

              0.288429      19.25812      0.692563      3.596212


 Source                          DF      Type I SS    Mean Square   F Value   Pr > F

 group                            1    13.16492366    13.16492366     27.45   <.0001
 time                             1     0.21361067     0.21361067      0.45   0.5051
 time*time                        1    37.17043160    37.17043160     77.50   <.0001


 Source                          DF    Type III SS    Mean Square   F Value   Pr > F

 group                            1    13.16492366    13.16492366     27.45   <.0001
 time                             1    35.91881784    35.91881784     74.89   <.0001
 time*time                        1    37.17043160    37.17043160     77.50   <.0001


                                                 Standard
      Parameter             Estimate                Error    t Value    Pr > |t|

      Intercept          4.366489007 B         0.10009072      43.63      <.0001
      group      1      -0.457019231 B         0.08723374      -5.24      <.0001
      group      2       0.000000000 B          .                .         .
      time              -0.831145729           0.09604513      -8.65      <.0001
      time*time          0.163609832           0.01858531       8.80      <.0001

NOTE: The X'X matrix has been found to be singular, and a generalized inverse
      was used to solve the normal equations.  Terms whose estimates are
      followed by the letter 'B' are not uniquely estimable.
```

those of the obese group. We need to consider a further model that contains a group × time interaction by amending the model statement to

```
model pip=group time|time group*time/s ddfm=bw
outp=mixout;
```

The results for this model are given in Table 12.5. The interaction effect is highly significant. The fitted values from this model are shown in Figure 12.5. (The code is very similar to that given for producing Figure 12.4.) The

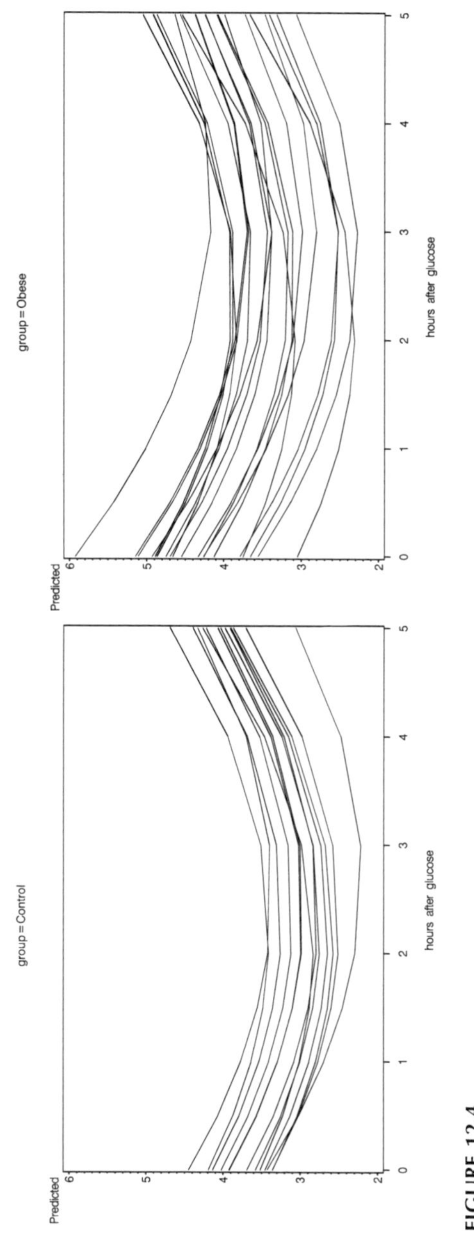

FIGURE 12.4
Fitted values from random intercept and slope model with fixed quadratic effect for glucose challenge data.

TABLE 12.5

Results from Random Intercept Slope and Model with Quadratic Time Effect and Group × Time Interaction Fitted to Glucose Challenge Data

```
                          The Mixed Procedure

                           Model Information

          Data Set                       WORK.PIPL
          Dependent Variable             pip
          Covariance Structure           Unstructured
          Subject Effect                 id
          Estimation Method              REML
          Residual Variance Method       Profile
          Fixed Effects SE Method        Model-Based
          Degrees of Freedom Method      Between-Within


                              Dimensions

               Covariance Parameters                4
               Columns in X                         7
               Columns in Z Per Subject             2
               Subjects                            33
               Max Obs Per Subject                  8


                         Number of Observations

             Number of Observations Read             264
             Number of Observations Used             264
             Number of Observations Not Used           0


                           Iteration History

         Iteration    Evaluations    -2 Res Log Like       Criterion

                 0              1       564.72900461
                 1              1       417.95581545      0.00000000


                        Convergence criteria met.


                     Covariance Parameter Estimates

                                                 Standard         Z
      Cov Parm      Subject       Estimate         Error      Value         Pr Z

      UN(1,1)       id              0.3539        0.1051       3.37       0.0004
      UN(2,1)       id            -0.02907       0.01770      -1.64       0.1006
      UN(2,2)       id            0.009834      0.004660       2.11       0.0174
      Residual                      0.1757       0.01770       9.92       <.0001


                             Fit Statistics

              -2 Res Log Likelihood               418.0
              AIC (smaller is better)             426.0
              AICC (smaller is better)            426.1
              BIC (smaller is better)             431.9

                          The Mixed Procedure

                    Null Model Likelihood Ratio Test

                      DF    Chi-Square       Pr > ChiSq

                       3        146.77           <.0001
```

TABLE 12.5 (continued)

Results from Random Intercept Slope and Model with Quadratic Time Effect and Group × Time Interaction Fitted to Glucose Challenge Data

Solution for Fixed Effects

Effect	Group	Estimate	Standard Error	DF	t Value	Pr > |t|
Intercept		4.5041	0.1486	31	30.30	<.0001
group	1	-0.8064	0.2289	31	-3.52	0.0014
group	2	0	.	.	.	.
time		-0.8959	0.06350	228	-14.11	<.0001
time*time		0.1636	0.01125	228	14.55	<.0001
time*group	1	0.1644	0.04787	228	3.43	0.0007
time*group	2	0	.	.	.	.

Type 3 Tests of Fixed Effects

Effect	Num DF	Den DF	F Value	Pr > F
group	1	31	12.41	0.0014
time	1	228	178.82	<.0001
time*time	1	228	211.56	<.0001
time*group	1	228	11.79	0.0007

plot shows that the new model has produced predicted values that more accurately reflect the raw data plotted in Figure 12.1. The predicted profiles for the obese group are "flatter" as required.

We now check the assumptions of the final model fitted to the glucose challenge data, i.e., that the random effect terms and residuals are normally distributed. The residuals are in the same data set as the predicted values, created with the outp option on the model statement shown earlier. How the random effects are predicted is explained briefly in Display 12.2. They are produced and saved as follows:

```
proc mixed data=pipl covtest noclprint;
  class group id;
  model pip=group time|time group*time/
s ddfm=bw outp=mixout;
  random int time /subject=id type=un s;
  ods output solutionr=reffs;
  ods listing exclude solutionr;
run;
```

Three elements have been added to the proc mixed step. The s (solution) option has been added to the random statement. This requests that the random effects be calculated and, by default, they are printed in the output. The ods output statement is used to store them in a data set. Solutionr is the ods table name and reffs is the name we have chosen for the data set being created. Finally, the ods listing statement excludes the random effects table from the output listing. With a large number of

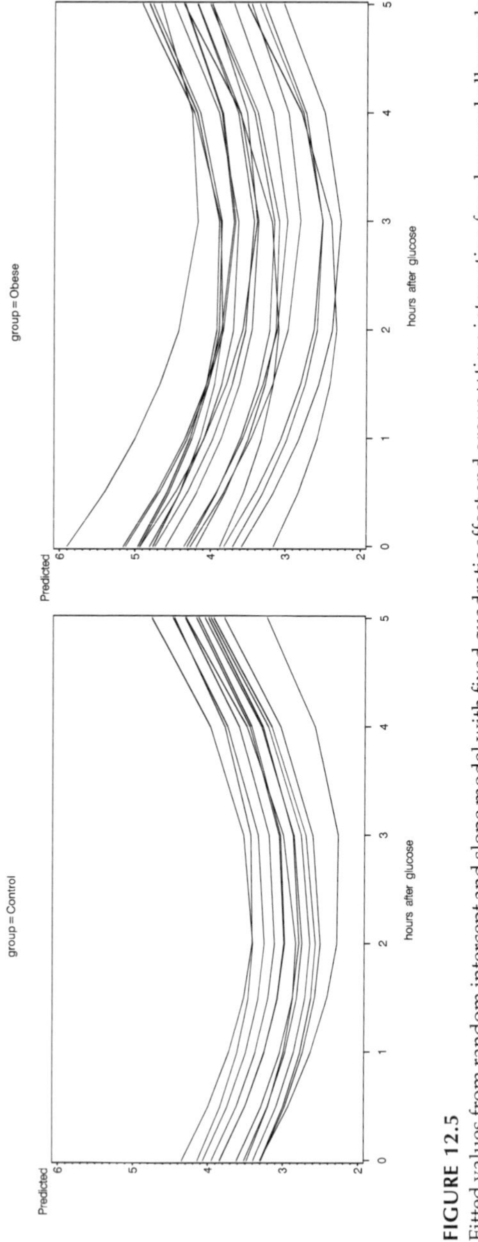

FIGURE 12.5
Fitted values from random intercept and slope model with fixed quadratic effect and group × time interaction for glucose challenge data.

DISPLAY 12.2

Prediction of Random Effects

- The random effects are not estimated as part of the model. However, having estimated the model, we can *predict* the values of the random effects.
- According to Bayes' Theorem, the *posterior probability* of the random effects is given by

$$\Pr\left(\mathbf{u}\middle|\mathbf{y},\mathbf{x}\right)=f\left(\mathbf{y}\middle|\mathbf{u},\mathbf{x}\right)g\left(\mathbf{u}\right)$$

  where $f\left(\mathbf{y}\middle|\mathbf{u},\mathbf{x}\right)$ is the conditional density of the responses given the random effects and covariates (a product of normal densities) and $g\left(\mathbf{u}\right)$ is the *prior* density of the random effects (multivariate normal). The means of this posterior distribution can be used as estimates of the random effects and are known as *empirical Bayes* estimates.
- The empirical Bayes estimator is also known as a shrinkage estimator because the predicted random effects are smaller in absolute value than are their fixed effect counterparts.
- *Best linear unbiased predictions* (BLUP) are linear combinations of the responses that are unbiased estimators of the random effects and mimimize the mean square error.

subjects the random effects table will run to several pages of output, so it is useful to be able to suppress it when it is not required.

`Proc univariate` is used to produce normal probability plots, which are combined using the `panelplot` macro as follows:

```
proc sort data=reffs; by effect; run;
goptions reset=symbol;
proc univariate data=reffs gout=fig12_6 noprint;
  var estimate;
  probplot estimate /normal;
  by effect;
run;
title h=1 "Residuals";
proc univariate data=mixout gout=fig12_6 noprint;
  var resid;
  probplot resid /normal;
```

```
run;
title;
%panelplot(igout=fig12_6,ncols=3);
```

The resulting plot is shown in Figure 12.6. The plot of the residuals is linear as required, but there is some slight deviation form linearity for each of the predicted random effects.

12.3 Dropouts in Longitudinal Data

A problem that frequently occurs when collecting longitudinal data is that some of the intended measurements are, for one reason or another, not made. In clinical trials, for example, some patients may miss one or more protocol scheduled visits after treatment has begun and so fail to have the required outcome measure taken. Other patients do not complete the intended follow-up for some reason and drop out of the study before the end date specified in the protocol. Both situations result in missing values of the outcome measure; in the first case these are intermittent, but dropping out of the study implies that once an observation at a particular time point is missing so are all the remaining planned observations. Many studies will contain missing values of both types, although in practice it is dropouts that cause most problems when analysing the resulting data set.

An example of a set of longitudinal data in which a number of patients have dropped out is given in Table 12.6. These data are essentially a subset of those collected in a clinical trial that is described in detail in Proudfoot et al. (2003). The trial was designed to assess the effectiveness of interactive program using multimedia techniques for the delivery of cognitive behavioural therapy for depressed patients and known as Beating the Blues (BtB). In a randomized controlled trial of the program, patients with depression recruited in primary care were randomized to either the BtB program, or to Treatment as Usual (TAU). The outcome measure used in the trial was the Beck Depression Inventory II (BDI; Beck et al., 1996), with higher values indicating more depression. Measurements of this variable were made on five occasions, one prior to the start of treatment and at two-month intervals after treatment began. In addition, whether or not a participant in the trial was already taking antidepressant medication was noted along with the length of time participants had been depressed.

We can read the data in creating both the wide and long formats in the same data step.

```
data btb  (keep=sub--treatment BDIpre--BDI8m)
     btbl (keep=sub--treatment bdi time);
```

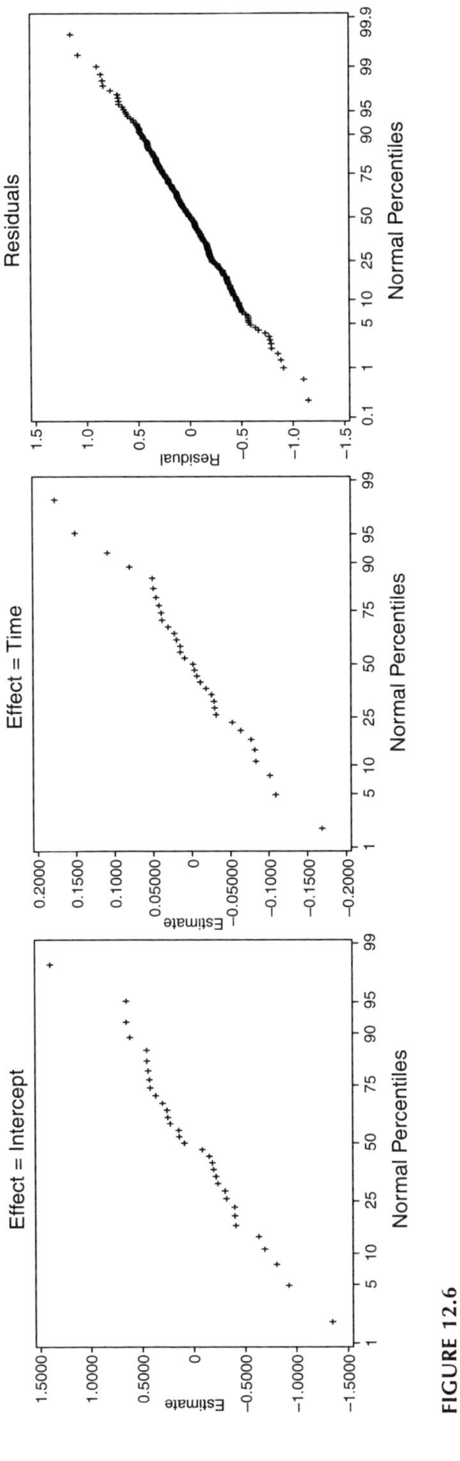

FIGURE 12.6
Probability plots of predicted random intercepts, random slopes, and residuals for final model fitted to glucose challenge data.

TABLE 12.6

Subset of Data from the Original BtB Trial

Sub	Drug	Duration (months)	Treatment	BDIpre	BDI2m	BDI3m	BDI5m	BDI8m
1	n	>6	TAU	29	2	2	NA	NA
2	y	>6	BtB	32	16	24	17	20
3	y	<6	TAU	25	20	NA	NA	NA
4	n	>6	BtB	21	17	16	10	9
5	y	>6	BtB	26	23	NA	NA	NA
6	y	<6	BtB	7	0	0	0	0
7	y	<6	TAU	17	7	7	3	7
8	n	>6	TAU	20	20	21	19	13
9	y	<6	BtB	18	13	14	20	11
10	y	>6	BtB	20	5	5	8	12
11	n	>6	TAU	30	32	24	12	2
12	y	<6	BtB	49	35	NA	NA	NA
13	n	>6	TAU	26	27	23	NA	NA
14	y	>6	TAU	30	26	36	27	22
15	y	>6	BtB	23	13	13	12	23
16	n	<6	TAU	16	13	3	2	0
17	n	>6	BtB	30	30	29	NA	NA
18	n	<6	BtB	13	8	8	7	6
19	n	>6	TAU	37	30	33	31	22
20	y	<6	BtB	35	12	10	8	10
21	n	>6	BtB	21	6	NA	NA	NA
22	n	<6	TAU	26	17	17	20	12
23	n	>6	TAU	29	22	10	NA	NA
24	n	>6	TAU	20	21	NA	NA	NA
25	n	>6	TAU	33	23	NA	NA	NA
26	n	>6	BtB	19	12	13	NA	NA
27	y	<6	TAU	12	15	NA	NA	NA
28	y	>6	TAU	47	36	49	34	NA
29	y	>6	BtB	36	6	0	0	2
30	n	<6	BtB	10	8	6	3	3
31	n	<6	TAU	27	7	15	16	0
32	n	<6	BtB	18	10	10	6	8
33	y	<6	BtB	11	8	3	2	15
34	y	<6	BtB	6	7	NA	NA	NA
35	y	>6	BtB	44	24	20	29	14
36	n	<6	TAU	38	38	NA	NA	NA
37	n	<6	TAU	21	14	20	1	8
38	y	>6	TAU	34	17	8	9	13
39	y	<6	BtB	9	7	1	NA	NA
40	y	>6	TAU	38	27	19	20	30
41	y	<6	BtB	46	40	NA	NA	NA
42	n	<6	TAU	20	19	18	19	18
43	y	>6	TAU	17	29	2	0	0
44	n	>6	BtB	18	20	NA	NA	NA
45	y	>6	BtB	42	1	8	10	6
46	n	<6	BtB	30	30	NA	NA	NA
47	y	<6	BtB	33	27	16	30	15
48	n	<6	BtB	12	1	0	0	NA

TABLE 12.6 (continued)

Subset of Data from the Original BtB Trial

Sub	Drug	Duration (months)	Treatment	BDIpre	BDI2m	BDI3m	BDI5m	BDI8m
49	y	<6	BtB	2	5	NA	NA	NA
50	n	>6	TAU	36	42	49	47	40
51	n	<6	TAU	35	30	NA	NA	NA
52	n	<6	BtB	23	20	NA	NA	NA
53	n	>6	TAU	31	48	38	38	37
54	y	<6	BtB	8	5	7	NA	NA
55	y	<6	TAU	23	21	26	NA	NA
56	y	<6	BtB	7	7	5	4	0
57	n	<6	TAU	14	13	14	NA	NA
58	n	<6	TAU	40	36	33	NA	NA
59	y	<6	BtB	23	30	NA	NA	NA
60	n	>6	BtB	14	3	NA	NA	NA
61	n	>6	TAU	22	20	16	24	16
62	n	>6	TAU	23	23	15	25	17
63	n	<6	TAU	15	7	13	13	NA
64	n	>6	TAU	8	12	11	26	NA
65	n	>6	BtB	12	18	NA	NA	NA
66	n	>6	TAU	7	6	2	1	NA
67	y	<6	TAU	17	9	3	1	0
68	y	<6	BtB	33	18	16	NA	NA
69	n	<6	TAU	27	20	NA	NA	NA
70	n	<6	BtB	27	30	NA	NA	NA
71	n	<6	BtB	9	6	10	1	0
72	n	>6	BtB	40	30	12	NA	NA
73	n	>6	TAU	11	8	7	NA	NA
74	n	<6	TAU	9	8	NA	NA	NA
75	n	>6	TAU	14	22	21	24	19
76	y	>6	BtB	28	9	20	18	13
77	n	>6	BtB	15	9	13	14	10
78	y	>6	BtB	22	10	5	5	12
79	n	<6	TAU	23	9	NA	NA	NA
80	n	>6	TAU	21	22	24	23	22
81	n	>6	TAU	27	31	28	22	14
82	y	>6	BtB	14	15	NA	NA	NA
83	n	>6	TAU	10	13	12	8	20
84	y	<6	TAU	21	9	6	7	1
85	y	>6	BtB	46	36	53	NA	NA
86	n	>6	BtB	36	14	7	15	15
87	y	>6	BtB	23	17	NA	NA	NA
88	y	>6	TAU	35	0	6	0	1
89	y	<6	BtB	33	13	13	10	8
90	n	<6	BtB	19	4	27	1	2
91	n	<6	TAU	16	NA	NA	NA	NA
92	y	<6	BtB	30	26	28	NA	NA
93	y	<6	BtB	17	8	7	12	NA
94	n	>6	BtB	19	4	3	3	3
95	n	>6	BtB	16	11	4	2	3
96	y	>6	BtB	16	16	10	10	8

TABLE 12.6 (continued)

Subset of Data from the Original BtB Trial

Sub	Drug	Duration (months)	Treatment	BDIpre	BDI2m	BDI3m	BDI5m	BDI8m
97	y	<6	TAU	28	NA	NA	NA	NA
98	n	>6	BtB	11	22	9	11	11
99	n	<6	TAU	13	5	5	0	6
100	y	<6	TAU	43	NA	NA	NA	NA

```
  array bdis {*} BDIpre BDI2m BDI3m BDI5m BDI8m;
  array t {*} t1-t5 (0 2 3 5 8);
  input sub drug$ Duration$ Treatment$ @;
  do i=1 to 5;
    input bdi @;
    bdis{i}=bdi;
    time=t{i};
    output btbl;
  end;
  output btb;
cards;
  1   n   >6m   TAU     29   2   2   .   .
  2   y   >6m   BtheB   32   16  24  17  20
  3   y   <6m   TAU     25   20  .   .   .
 . . . .
 99   n   <6m   TAU     13   5   5   0   6
100   y   <6m   TAU     43   .   .   .   .
;
```

We have already seen how to use the `array`, iterative `do`, and `output` statements to restructure a data set. This example shows the use of two `output` statements, each naming the data set that the observation is to be written to. The `data` statement also names two data sets, and the `keep` option specifies the variables they are to contain.

To begin, we shall graph the data by plotting the boxplots of each of the five repeated measures separately for each treatment group.

```
proc sort data=btbl;
  by treatment time;
run;
proc boxplot data=btbl gout=fig12_7;
```

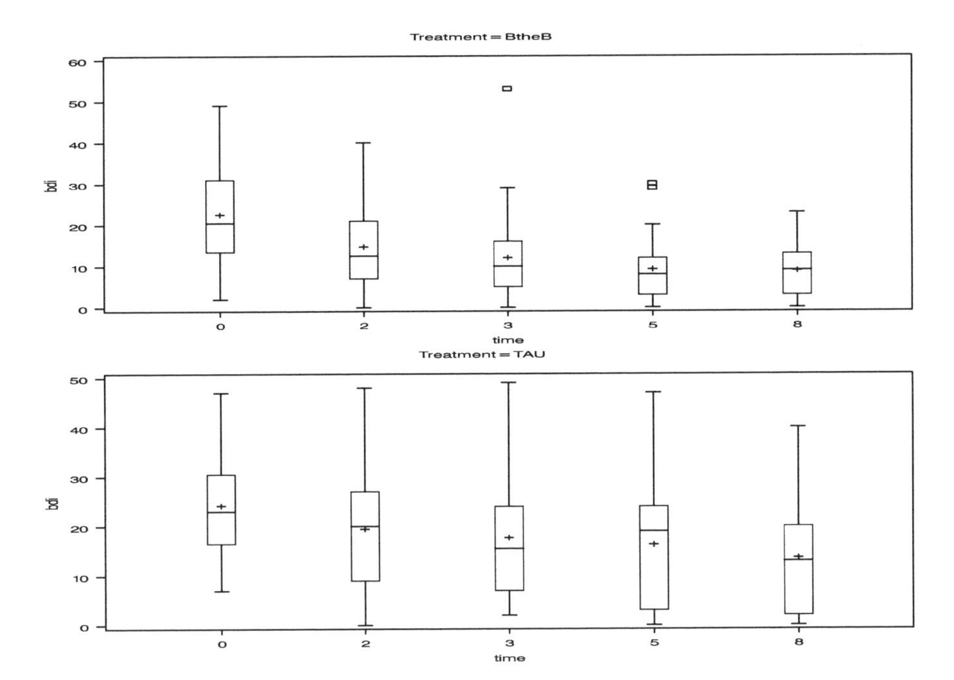

FIGURE 12.7
Boxplots for the repeated measures by treatment group for the BtB data.

```
    plot bdi*time / boxstyle=schematic;
    by treatment;
  run;
  %panelplot(igout=fig12_7,nrows=2);
```

The resulting diagram is shown in Figure 12.7.

Figure 12.7 shows that there is decline in BDI values in both groups with perhaps the values in the BtB group being lower at each postrandomization visit. We shall fit both random intercept and random intercept and slope models to the data, including the pre-BDI values, treatment group, drugs, and duration as fixed effect covariates.

The data contain a number of missing values, and in applying `proc mixed` to the long form of the data set these will be dropped from the analysis. But notice it is only the missing values that are removed, *not* participants who have at least one missing value. *All* the available data are used in the model fitting process.

We begin by fitting the random intercept and slope model:

```
proc mixed data=btbl covtest noclprint=3;
 class drug duration treatment sub;
```

```
  model bdi=drug duration treatment time /
    s cl ddfm=bw;
  random int time /subject=sub type=un;
run;
```

The random effects (covariance parameters) estimates and associated Wald tests for this model are

Covariance Parameter Estimates

Cov Parm	Subject	Estimate	Standard Error	Z Value	Pr Z
UN(1,1)	sub	78.8941	15.1932	5.19	<.0001
UN(2,1)	sub	0.08138	1.9103	0.04	0.9660
UN(2,2)	sub	0.2573	0.2823	0.91	0.1811
Residual		38.1343	3.6849	10.35	<.0001

Clearly, a simpler model with only a random intercept is adequate for these data. This model can be fitted by amending the `random` statement to

```
random int /subject=sub;
```

The results from fitting this model are given in Table 12.7. The treatment and time effects are significant, but those for drugs and duration are not. The confidence interval for the treatment effect implies that treatment with BtB reduces the depression score on average by between about one fifth of a point and eight points, conditional on the values of the other covariates. Clearly, the lower end of the interval would not represent a decrease that was of any clinical use, but the value at the upper end represents a considerable decrease in a patient's depression.

We now need to consider briefly how the dropouts may affect the analyses reported above. To understand the problems that patients dropping out can cause for the analysis of data from a longitudinal trial, we need to consider a classification of dropout mechanisms first introduced by Rubin (1976). The type of mechanism involved has implications for which approaches to analysis are suitable and which are not. Rubin's suggested classification involves three types of dropout mechanism:

- *Dropout completely at random* (DCAR). Here, the probability that a patient drops out does not depend on either the observed or missing values of the response. Consequently the observed (nonmissing) values effectively constitute a simple random sample of the values for all subjects. Possible examples include missing laboratory measurements because of a dropped test tube (if it was not dropped

TABLE 12.7

Results from Random Intercept Model Fitted to the BtB Data

The Mixed Procedure

Model Information

Data Set	WORK.BTBL
Dependent Variable	bdi
Covariance Structure	Variance Components
Subject Effect	sub
Estimation Method	REML
Residual Variance Method	Profile
Fixed Effects SE Method	Model-Based
Degrees of Freedom Method	Between-Within

Class Level Information

Class	Levels	Values
drug	2	n y
Duration	2	<6m >6m
Treatment	2	BtheB TAU
sub	100	not printed

Dimensions

Covariance Parameters	2
Columns in X	8
Columns in Z Per Subject	1
Subjects	100
Max Obs Per Subject	5

Number of Observations

Number of Observations Read	500
Number of Observations Used	380
Number of Observations Not Used	120

Iteration History

Iteration	Evaluations	-2 Res Log Like	Criterion
0	1	2853.51771595	
1	2	2677.33928605	0.00091213
2	1	2676.30996724	0.00005384
3	1	2676.25424133	0.00000023
4	1	2676.25400888	0.00000000

Convergence criteria met.

The Mixed Procedure

Covariance Parameter Estimates

Cov Parm	Subject	Estimate	Standard Error	Z Value	Pr Z
Intercept	sub	80.5443	13.6702	5.89	<.0001
Residual		40.0945	3.4121	11.75	<.0001

Fit Statistics

-2 Res Log Likelihood	2676.3
AIC (smaller is better)	2680.3
AICC (smaller is better)	2680.3
BIC (smaller is better)	2685.5

TABLE 12.7 (continued)

Results from Random Intercept Model Fitted to the BtB Data

Solution for Fixed Effects

Effect	drug	Duration	Treatment	Estimate	Standard Error	DF	t Value	Pr > |t|	Alpha
Intercept				26.4177	2.3184	96	11.39	<.0001	0.05
drug	n			-2.0513	2.0474	96	-1.00	0.3189	0.05
drug	y			0	.	.	.	.	.
Duration		<6m		-3.4439	1.9473	96	-1.77	0.0801	0.05
Duration		>6m		0	.	.	.	.	.
Treatment			BtheB	-4.2928	2.0172	96	-2.13	0.0359	0.05
Treatment			TAU	0	.	.	.	.	.
time				-1.3882	0.1354	279	-10.26	<.0001	0.05

Solution for Fixed Effects

Effect	drug	Duration	Treatment	Lower	Upper
Intercept				21.8157	31.0197
drug	n			-6.1153	2.0127
drug	y			.	.
Duration		<6m		-7.3092	0.4215
Duration		>6m		.	.
Treatment			BtheB	-8.2969	-0.2888
Treatment			TAU	.	.
time				-1.6547	-1.1218

Type 3 Tests of Fixed Effects

Effect	Num DF	Den DF	F Value	Pr > F
drug	1	96	1.00	0.3189
Duration	1	96	3.13	0.0801
Treatment	1	96	4.53	0.0359
time	1	279	105.17	<.0001

because of the knowledge of any measurement), the accidental death of a participant in a study, or a participant moving to another area. Intermittent missing values in a longitudinal data set, whereby a patient misses a clinic visit for transitory reasons ("went shopping instead" or the like) can reasonably be assumed to be DCAR. Completely random dropout causes the least problem for data analysis, but it is a strong assumption.

- *Dropout at random* (DAR). The dropout at random mechanism occurs when the probability of dropping out depends on the outcome measures that have been observed in the past, but given this information is conditionally independent of all the future (unrecorded) values of the outcome variable following dropout. Here, 'missingness' depends only on the observed data with the distribution of future values for a subject who drops out at a particular time the same as the distribution of the future values of a subject who remains in at that time, if they have the same covariates and the same past history of outcome up to and including the specific time point. Murray and Findlay (1988) provide an example of this type of missing value from a study of hypertensive drugs in which the outcome measure was diastolic blood pressure. The protocol of the study specified that the participant was to be removed from the study when his/her blood pressure became too high. Here, blood pressure at the time of dropout was observed before the participant dropped out, so although the dropout mechanism is not DCAR since it depends on the values of blood pressure, it *is* DAR, because dropout depends only on the observed part of the data. A further example of a DAR mechanism is provided by Heitjan (1997) and involves a study in which the response measure is body mass index (BMI). Suppose that the measure is missing because subjects who had high body mass index values at earlier visits avoided being measured at later visits out of embarrassment, regardless of whether they had gained or lost weight in the intervening period. The missing values here are DAR but *not* DCAR; consequently, methods applied to the data that assumed the latter might give misleading results (see later discussion).

- *Nonignorable* (sometimes referred to as *informative*). The final type of dropout mechanism is one where the probability of dropping out depends on the unrecorded missing values: observations are likely to be missing when the outcome values that would have been observed had the patient not dropped out are systematically higher or lower than usual (corresponding perhaps to the patient's condition becoming worse or improving). A nonmedical example is when individuals with lower income levels or very high incomes are less likely to provide their personal income in an interview. In a medical setting, possible examples are a participant dropping out of a longitudinal study when his/her blood pressure became too high and this value was not observed, or when pain became intolerable and we did not record the associated pain value. For the BDI example introduced above, if subjects were more likely to avoid being measured if they had put on extra weight since the last visit, then the data are nonignorably missing. Dealing with data containing missing values that result from this type of dropout mechanism is difficult. The correct analyses for such data must estimate the dependence of the missingness probability on the missing values. Models and software that attempt this are available (see, for example, Diggle and Kenward, 1994) but their use is not routine and, in addition, it must be remembered that the associated parameter estimates can be unreliable.

Under what type of dropout mechanism are the mixed effects models considered in this chapter valid? The good news is that such models can be shown to give valid results under the relatively weak assumption that the dropout mechanism is DAR (see Carpenter et al., 2002). When the missing values are thought to be informative, any analysis is potentially problematical. But Diggle and Kenward (1994) have developed a modeling framework for longitudinal data with informative dropouts, in which random or completely random dropout mechanisms are also included as explicit models. The essential feature of the procedure is a logistic regression model for the probability of dropping out, in which the explanatory variables can include previous values of the response variable, and, in addition, the *unobserved* value at dropout as a *latent* variable (i.e., an unobserved variable). In other words, the dropout probability is allowed to depend on both the *observed* measurement history and the unobserved value at dropout. This allows both a formal assessment of the type of dropout mechanism in the data and the estimation of effects of interest, for example, treatment effects under different assumptions about the dropout mechanism. A full technical account of the model is given in Diggle and Kenward (1994), and a detailed example that uses the approach is described in Carpenter et al. (2002).

One of the problems for an investigator struggling to identify the dropout mechanism in a data set is that there are no routine methods to help, although a number of largely ad hoc graphical procedures can be used as described in Diggle (1998), Everitt (2002), and Carpenter et al. (2002).

12.4 Summary

Linear mixed effects models are extremely useful for modelling longitudinal data in particular and repeated measures data more generally. The models allow the correlations between the repeated measurements to be accounted for so that correct inferences can be drawn about the effects of covariates of interest on the repeated response values. In this chapter we have concentrated on responses that are continuous and conditional on the explanatory variables and random effects have a normal distribution. But random effects models can also be applied to non-normal responses, for example binary variables — see, for example, Everitt (2002) and the next chapter.

The lack of independence of repeated measures data is what makes the modelling of such data a challenge. But even when only a single measurement of a response is involved, correlation can, in some circumstances, occur between the response values of different individuals and cause similar problems. As an example, consider a randomized clinical trial in which subjects are recruited at multiple study centres. The multicentre design can help to provide adequate sample sizes and enhance the generalizability of the results. However, factors that vary by centre, including patient characteristics and medical practice patterns, may exert a sufficiently powerful effect to make inferences that ignore the "clustering" seriously misleading. Consequently, it may be necessary to incorporate random effects for centres into the analysis.

13

The Analysis of Longitudinal Data III: Non-Normal Responses

13.1 Introduction

In many longitudinal studies carried out in medicine, it will be clear that the assumption of normality for the response variable is simply not justified. Two examples are shown in Table 13.1 and Table 13.2. The first, in Table 13.1, results from a clinical trial comparing two treatments for a respiratory illness (Davis, 1991). In each of two centres, eligible patients were randomly assigned to active treatment or placebo. During treatment, the respiratory status (categorized as 0 = poor, 1 = good) was determined at each of four visits. A total of 111 patients were entered into the trial, 54 into the active group and 57 into the placebo group. The sex and age of each participant were also recorded, along with baseline respiratory status. Here the response variable is binary, making the models described in the previous chapter inappropriate for these data. (These data were used previously in Chapter 11.)

The data in Table 13.2 arise from a clinical trial reported in Thall and Vail (1990). Here 59 patients with epilepsy were randomized to receive either the antiepileptic drug progabide or a placebo in addition to standard chemotherapy. The number of seizures was counted over four 2-week periods. In addition, a baseline seizure rate was recorded for each patient, based on the 8-week pre-randomization seizure count.

Finally, the age of each patient was recorded. In this example the observations are counts that can take only positive values and so again making the normality assumption cannot be justified.

In the models for Gaussian responses described in Chapter 12, estimation of the regression parameters linking explanatory variables to the response variable and their standard errors needed to take account of the correlational structure of the data, but their interpretation could be undertaken independent of this structure. When modelling non-normal responses, this independence of estimation and interpretation no longer holds. Different assumptions about how the correlations are generated can lead to regression coefficients with different interpretations. The essential difference is between *marginal models* and *conditional models*.

TABLE 13.1

Respiratory Disorder Data

Patient	Centre	Treatment	Sex	Age	BL	V1	V2	V3	V4
1	1	1	1	46	0	0	0	0	0
2	1	1	1	28	0	0	0	0	0
3	1	2	1	23	1	1	1	1	1
4	1	1	1	44	1	1	1	1	0
5	1	1	2	13	1	1	1	1	1
6	1	2	1	34	0	0	0	0	0
7	1	1	1	43	0	1	0	1	1
8	1	2	1	28	0	0	0	0	0
9	1	2	1	31	1	1	1	1	1
10	1	1	1	37	1	0	1	1	0
11	1	2	1	30	1	1	1	1	1
12	1	2	1	14	0	1	1	1	0
13	1	1	1	23	1	1	0	0	0
14	1	1	1	30	0	0	0	0	0
15	1	1	1	20	1	1	1	1	1
16	1	2	1	22	0	0	0	0	1
17	1	1	1	25	0	0	0	0	0
18	1	2	2	47	0	0	1	1	1
19	1	1	2	31	0	0	0	0	0
20	1	2	1	20	1	1	0	1	0
21	1	2	1	26	0	1	0	1	0
22	1	2	1	46	1	1	1	1	1
23	1	2	1	32	1	1	1	1	1
24	1	2	1	48	0	1	0	0	0
25	1	1	2	35	0	0	0	0	0
26	1	2	1	26	0	0	0	0	0
27	1	1	1	23	1	1	0	1	1
28	1	1	2	36	0	1	1	0	0
29	1	1	1	19	0	1	1	0	0
30	1	2	1	28	0	0	0	0	0
31	1	1	1	37	0	0	0	0	0
32	1	2	1	23	0	1	1	1	1
33	1	2	1	30	1	1	1	1	0
34	1	1	1	15	0	0	1	1	0
35	1	2	1	26	0	0	0	1	0
36	1	1	2	45	0	0	0	0	0
37	1	2	1	31	0	0	1	0	0
38	1	2	1	50	0	0	0	0	0
39	1	1	1	28	0	0	0	0	0
40	1	1	1	26	0	0	0	0	0
41	1	1	1	14	0	0	0	0	1
42	1	2	1	31	0	0	1	0	0
43	1	1	1	13	1	1	1	1	1
44	1	1	1	27	0	0	0	0	0
45	1	1	1	26	0	1	0	1	1
46	1	1	1	49	0	0	0	0	0
47	1	1	1	63	0	0	0	0	0
48	1	2	1	57	1	1	1	1	1
49	1	1	1	27	1	1	1	1	1
50	1	2	1	22	0	0	1	1	1
51	1	2	1	15	0	0	1	1	1

TABLE 13.1 (continued)

Respiratory Disorder Data

Patient	Centre	Treatment	Sex	Age	BL	V1	V2	V3	V4
52	1	1	1	43	0	0	0	1	0
53	1	2	2	32	0	0	0	1	0
54	1	2	1	11	1	1	1	1	0
55	1	1	1	24	1	1	1	1	1
56	1	2	1	25	0	1	1	0	1
57	2	1	2	39	0	0	0	0	0
58	2	2	1	25	0	0	1	1	1
59	2	2	1	58	1	1	1	1	1
60	2	1	2	51	1	1	0	1	1
61	2	1	2	32	1	0	0	1	1
62	2	1	1	45	1	1	0	0	0
63	2	1	2	44	1	1	1	1	1
64	2	1	2	48	0	0	0	0	0
65	2	2	1	26	0	1	1	1	1
66	2	2	1	14	0	1	1	1	1
67	2	1	2	48	0	0	0	0	0
68	2	2	1	13	1	1	1	1	1
69	2	1	1	20	0	1	1	1	1
70	2	2	1	37	1	1	0	0	1
71	2	2	1	25	1	1	1	1	1
72	2	2	1	20	0	0	0	0	0
73	2	1	2	58	0	1	0	0	0
74	2	1	1	38	1	1	0	0	0
75	2	2	1	55	1	1	1	1	1
76	2	2	1	24	1	1	1	1	1
77	2	1	2	36	1	1	0	0	1
78	2	1	1	36	0	1	1	1	1
79	2	2	2	60	1	1	1	1	1
80	2	1	1	15	1	0	0	1	1
81	2	2	1	25	1	1	1	1	0
82	2	2	1	35	1	1	1	1	1
83	2	2	1	19	1	1	0	1	1
84	2	1	2	31	1	1	1	1	1
85	2	2	1	21	1	1	1	1	1
86	2	2	2	37	0	1	1	1	1
87	2	1	1	52	0	1	1	1	1
88	2	2	1	55	0	0	1	1	0
89	2	1	1	19	1	0	0	1	1
90	2	1	1	20	1	0	1	1	1
91	2	1	1	42	1	0	0	0	0
92	2	2	1	41	1	1	1	1	1
93	2	2	1	52	0	0	0	0	0
94	2	1	2	47	0	1	1	0	1
95	2	1	1	11	1	1	1	1	1
96	2	1	1	14	0	0	0	1	0
97	2	1	1	15	1	1	1	1	1
98	2	1	1	66	1	1	1	1	1
99	2	2	1	34	0	1	1	0	1
100	2	1	1	43	0	0	0	0	0
101	2	1	1	33	1	1	1	0	1
102	2	1	1	48	1	1	0	0	0

TABLE 13.1 (continued)

Respiratory Disorder Data

Patient	Centre	Treatment	Sex	Age	BL	V1	V2	V3	V4
103	2	2	1	20	0	1	1	1	1
104	2	1	2	39	1	0	1	0	0
105	2	2	1	28	0	1	0	0	0
106	2	1	2	38	0	0	0	0	0
107	2	2	1	43	1	1	1	1	1
108	2	2	2	39	0	1	1	1	1
109	2	2	1	68	0	1	1	1	1
110	2	2	2	63	1	1	1	1	1
111	2	2	1	31	1	1	1	1	1

Note: Treatment: 1 = placebo, 2 = active; Sex: 1= male, 2 = female.

TABLE 13.2

Data from a Clinical Trial of Patients Suffering from Epilepsy

Subject ID	Period 1	Period 2	Period 3	Period 4	Treatment	Baseline	Age
1	5	3	3	3	0	11	31
2	3	5	3	3	0	11	30
3	2	4	0	5	0	6	25
4	4	4	1	4	0	8	36
5	7	18	9	21	0	66	22
6	5	2	8	7	0	27	29
7	6	4	0	2	0	12	31
8	40	20	23	12	0	52	42
9	5	6	6	5	0	23	37
10	14	13	6	0	0	10	28
11	26	12	6	22	0	52	36
12	12	6	8	4	0	33	24
13	4	4	6	2	0	18	23
14	7	9	12	14	0	42	36
15	16	24	10	9	0	87	26
16	11	0	0	5	0	50	26
17	0	0	3	3	0	18	28
18	37	29	28	29	0	111	31
19	3	5	2	5	0	18	32
20	3	0	6	7	0	20	21
21	3	4	3	4	0	12	29
22	3	4	3	4	0	9	21
23	2	3	3	5	0	17	32
24	8	12	2	8	0	28	25
25	18	24	76	25	0	55	30
26	2	1	2	1	0	9	40
27	3	1	4	2	0	10	19
28	13	15	13	12	0	47	22
29	11	14	9	8	1	76	18
30	8	7	9	4	1	38	32
31	0	4	3	0	1	19	20
32	3	6	1	3	1	10	30
33	2	6	7	4	1	19	18

TABLE 13.2 (continued)

Data from a Clinical Trial of Patients Suffering from Epilepsy

Subject ID	Period 1	Period 2	Period 3	Period 4	Treatment	Baseline	Age
34	4	3	1	3	1	24	24
35	22	17	19	16	1	31	30
36	5	4	7	4	1	14	35
37	2	4	0	4	1	11	27
38	3	7	7	7	1	67	20
39	4	18	2	5	1	41	22
40	2	1	1	0	1	7	28
41	0	2	4	0	1	22	23
42	5	4	0	3	1	13	40
43	11	14	25	15	1	46	33
44	10	5	3	8	1	36	21
45	19	7	6	7	1	38	35
46	1	1	2	3	1	7	25
47	6	10	8	8	1	36	26
48	2	1	0	0	1	11	25
49	102	65	72	63	1	151	22
50	4	3	2	4	1	22	32
51	8	6	5	7	1	41	25
52	1	3	1	5	1	32	35
53	18	11	28	13	1	56	21
54	6	3	4	0	1	24	41
55	3	5	4	3	1	16	32
56	1	23	19	8	1	22	26
57	2	3	0	1	1	25	21
58	0	0	0	0	1	13	36
59	1	4	3	2	1	12	37

13.2 Marginal Models and Conditional Models

13.2.1 Marginal Models

Longitudinal data can be considered as a series of cross sections, and marginal models for such data use the generalized linear model (see Chapter 8) to fit each cross section. In this approach the relationship of the marginal mean and the explanatory variables is modelled separately from the within-subject correlation. The marginal regression coefficients have the same interpretation as coefficients from a cross-sectional analysis, and marginal models are natural analogues for correlated data of generalized linear models for independent data. Fitting marginal models to non-normal longitudinal data involves the use of a procedure known as *generalized estimating equations,* introduced by Liang and Zeger (1986). This approach may be viewed as a multivariate extension of the generalized linear model and the quasi-likelihood method. A brief account of generalized estimating equations is given in Display 13.1.

DISPLAY 13.1

Generalized Estimating Equations (GEE)

- The problem with applying a direct analogue of the generalized linear model to longitudinal data with non-normal responses is that there is usually no suitable likelihood function with the required combination of the appropriate link function, error distribution, and correlation structure.
- To overcome this problem, Liang and Zeger (1986) introduced a general method for incorporating within-subject correlation in GLMs, which is essentially an extension of the quasi-likelihood approach mentioned briefly in Chapter 8.
- As in conventional generalized linear models (GLMs), the variances of the responses given the covariates are assumed to be of the form $V(y) = \phi V(\mu)$, where the variance function is determined by the choice of distribution family (see Chapter 8).
- Since overdispersion is common in longitudinal data, the dispersion parameter ϕ is typically estimated even if the distribution requires $\phi = 1$.
- The feature of GEE that differs from the usual generalized linear model is that different responses on the same individual are allowed to be correlated given the covariates.
- These correlations are assumed to have a relatively simple structure parameterized by a small number of parameters. The following correlation structures are commonly used.
  a. An identity matrix leading to the independence working model in which the generalized estimating equation reduces to the univariate estimating equation given in Chapter 6, obtained by assuming that the repeated measurements are independent.
  b. An *exchangeable* correlation matrix with a single parameter similar to that described in Chapter 12. Here the correlation between each pair of repeated measurements is assumed to be the same, i.e., $\text{corr}(Y_{ij}, Y_{ik}) = \alpha$.
  c. An AR-1 *autoregressive* correlation matrix, also with a single parameter, but in which $\text{corr}(Y_{ij}, Y_{ik}) = \alpha^{|k-j|}, j \neq k$. This can allow the correlations of measurements taken further apart to be less than those taken closer to one another.
  e. An unstructured correlation matrix with $T(T-1)/2$ parameters in which $(Y_{ij}, Y_{ik}) = \alpha_{jk}$.
- For given values of the regression parameters $\beta_1, \ldots, \beta_q$, the α-parameters of the working correlation matrix can be estimated along with the dispersion parameter ϕ (see Zeger and Liang, 1986, for details).

DISPLAY 13.1 (continued)

Generalized Estimating Equations

- These estimates can then be used in the so-called generalized estimating equations to obtain estimates of the regression parameters.
- The GEE algorithm proceeds by iterating between (1) estimation of the regression parameters using the correlation and dispersion parameters from the previous iteration and (2) estimation of the correlation and dispersion parameters using the regression parameters from the previous iteration.
  The estimated regression coefficients are 'robust' in the sense that they are consistent from misspecified correlation structures, assuming that the mean structure is correctly specified.

13.2.2 Conditional Models

The random effects approach described in the previous chapter can be extended to non-normal responses, although the resulting models can be difficult to estimate because the likelihood involves integrals over the random effects distribution that generally do not have closed forms. As a consequence, it is often only possible to fit relatively simple models. In these models estimated regression coefficients have to be interpreted, *conditional* on the random effects. The regression parameters in the model are said to be *subject specific* and such effects will differ from the marginal or population averaged effects estimated using GEE, except when using an identity link function and a normal error distribution. Display 13.2 describes a random intercept model for repeated measurements of a binary response.

13.3 Analysis of the Respiratory Data

We shall apply both the generalized estimating equations approach (see Display 13.1) and the random effects model described in Display 13.2 to the respiratory data in Table 13.1. This will enable us to compare the population-averaged and subject-specific regression estimates. We shall include as covariates in each model treatment, time, sex, age, centre, and baseline respiratory status. As explained in the previous chapter, we begin by producing both 'wide' and 'long' forms of the data set.

```
data respw;
  input id centre treat sex age bl v1-v4;
cards;
```

DISPLAY 13.2

Random Intercept Model for Repeated Measurements of a Binary Response

- Consider a set of longitudinal data in which y_{ij} is the value of a binary response for individual i at say time t_j. The logistic regression model (see Chapter 7) for the response is now written as

$$\text{logit}\left[\Pr\left(y_{ij}=1 \mid u_i\right)\right]=\beta_0+\beta_1 t_j+u_i \qquad \text{(A)}$$

  where u_i is a random effect assumed to be normally distributed with zero mean and variance σ_u^2.
- Here the regression parameter β_1 again represents the change in the log odds per unit change in time, but this is now *conditional* on the random effect u_i.
- We can illustrate this difference graphically by simulating the model in (A); the result is shown below:

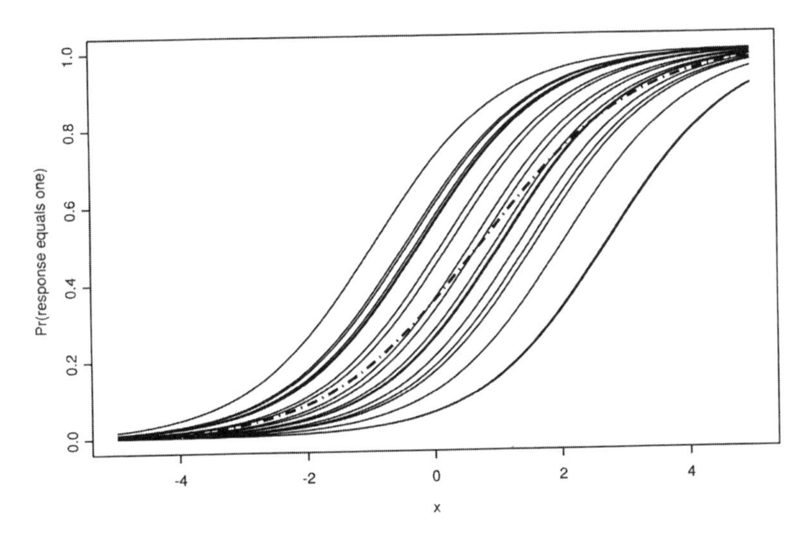

- Here the thin curves represent subject-specific relationships between the probability that the response equals one and a covariate x for model (A). The horizontal shifts are due to different values of the random intercept.
- The thick curve represents the population-averaged relationship, formed by averaging the thin curves for each value of x. It is, in effect, the thick curve that would be estimated in a marginal model.

DISPLAY 13.2 (continued)

- The population averaged regression parameters tend to be attenuated (closest to zero) relative to the subject-specific regression parameters. A marginal regression model does not address questions concerning heterogeneity between individuals.
- Estimating the parameters in a random effects model is again generally undertaken by maximum likelihood.

```
  1   1   1   1   46   0   0   0   0   0
  2   1   1   1   28   0   0   0   0   0
  3   1   2   1   23   1   1   1   1   1
. . . .
110   2   2   2   63   1   1   1   1   1
111   2   2   1   31   1   1   1   1   1
;
data respl;
  set respw;
  array vs {4} v1-v4;
  do time=1 to 4;
  status=vs{time};
  output;
  end;
run;
```

We first apply GEE with a logistic link function and an independence working correlation matrix to the long form of the data set:

```
proc genmod data=respl desc;
 class centre treat sex id;
 model status=centre treat sex age time bl / d=b;
 repeated subject=id / type=ind;
run;
```

The use of `proc genmod` for generalized linear models was described in Chapter 8. The extension to GEE models involves the use of the `repeated` statement and specification of the subject identifier on it. Note that the subject identifier *must* be named on a `class` statement. The `type=` option specifies the structure of the working correlation matrix.

Proc genmod begins by estimating an ordinary generalized linear model. The parameter estimates from this model, shown in the output under 'Analysis of Initial Parameter Estimate', are used as starting values for the estimation of the GEE model. These are not usually of particular interest. The output for the GEE model is headed 'Analysis of GEE Parameter Estimates'. By default the empirical standard error estimates are calculated and reported. (Model-based standard errors are available via the modelse option on the repeated statement.) In computing the empirical standard errors the dispersion parameter is replaced by an estimate, so the scale option of the model statement will have no effect. The results are shown in Table 13.3.

There is clearly a very substantial treatment effect, with the active treatment increasing the log-odds of having a good respiratory response by between 0.61 and 1.99. This corresponds to an odds ratio 95% confidence interval of 1.84 to 7.32. Amongst the remaining explanatory variables, only baseline respiratory status is significant; a positive response at baseline increases the log-odds of having a positive respiratory response at subsequent visits by between 1.20 and 2.57, corresponding to a 95% confidence interval for the odds ratio of [3.32, 13.07].

Independence is an unrealistic assumption for repeated measures data, so we now fit a model in which we introduce an exchangeable correlation structure by modifying the repeated statement to

```
repeated subject=id / type=exch;
```

The GEE results from this model are shown in Table 13.4.

The results remain very similar to those in Table 13.3 and confirm that the treatment is successful in improving respiratory status and that there is no apparent trend over assessment visits. Other correlation structures could be considered, but this will be left as an exercise for the reader.

Now we will fit a random intercept logistic regression model using proc glimmix. This procedure was introduced, as experimental, in version 9.1 of SAS.* Prior to that, proc nlmixed could be used to fit these models. We use proc glimmix because it has similar syntax to proc mixed and can fit a wider range of models than nlmixed can.

```
proc glimmix data=respl;
 class centre treat sex id;
 model status=centre treat sex age time bl /
s ddfm=bw d=b;
 random int / subject=id type=un;
run;
```

* At the time of writing, the procedure has to be downloaded from the SAS Web site.

TABLE 13.3

Results from GEE with an Independence Working Correlation Matrix for Respiratory Data

```
                         The GENMOD Procedure

                          Model Information

                  Data Set                  WORK.RESPL
                  Distribution                Binomial
                  Link Function                  Logit
                  Dependent Variable            status
                  Observations Used                444


                       Class Level Information

  Class       Levels     Values

  centre           2     1 2
  treat            2     1 2
  sex              2     1 2
  id             111     1 2 3 4 5 6 7 8 9 10 11 12 13 14 15 16 17 18 19 20
                         21 22 23 24 25 26 27 28 29 30 31 32 33 34 35 36 37
                         38 39 40 41 42 43 44 45 46 47 48 49 50 51 52 53 54
                         55 56 57 58 59 60 61 62 63 64 65 66 67 68 69 70 71
                         72 73 74 75 76 77 78 79 80 81 82 83 84 85 86 87
                         ...


                           Response Profile


                     Ordered                   Total
                       Value    Status     Frequency

                           1    1                249
                           2    0                195

PROC GENMOD is modelling the probability that status='1'.


                        Parameter Information

            Parameter       Effect       Centre    Treat    Sex

            Prm1            Intercept
            Prm2            centre       1
            Prm3            centre       2
            Prm4            treat                  1
            Prm5            treat                  2
            Prm6            sex                             1
            Prm7            sex                             2
            Prm8            age
            Prm9            time
            Prm10           bl


                 Criteria for Assessing Goodness of Fit

       Criterion                DF           Value        Value/DF

       Deviance                437        482.8007          1.1048
       Scaled Deviance         437        482.8007          1.1048
       Pearson Chi-Square      437        442.0532          1.0116

                        The GENMOD Procedure

                 Criteria for Assessing Goodness of Fit

       Criterion                DF           Value        Value/DF

       Scaled Pearson X2       437        442.0532          1.0116
       Log Likelihood                    -241.4004
```

TABLE 13.3 (continued)

Results from GEE with an Independence Working Correlation Matrix for Respiratory Data

Algorithm converged.

Analysis of Initial Parameter Estimates

Parameter		DF	Estimate	Standard Error	Wald 95% Confidence Limits		Chi-Square	Pr > ChiSq
Intercept		1	1.3517	0.5537	0.2666	2.4369	5.96	0.0146
centre	1	1	-0.6723	0.2397	-1.1421	-0.2025	7.87	0.0050
centre	2	0	0.0000	0.0000	0.0000	0.0000	.	.
treat	1	1	-1.3006	0.2370	-1.7650	-0.8361	30.12	<.0001
treat	2	0	0.0000	0.0000	0.0000	0.0000	.	.
sex	1	1	-0.1194	0.2948	-0.6972	0.4585	0.16	0.6856
sex	2	0	0.0000	0.0000	0.0000	0.0000	.	.
age		1	-0.0182	0.0089	-0.0356	-0.0008	4.20	0.0403
time		1	-0.0643	0.0995	-0.2593	0.1308	0.42	0.5185
bl		1	1.8841	0.2415	1.4108	2.3574	60.87	<.0001
Scale		0	1.0000	0.0000	1.0000	1.0000		

NOTE: The scale parameter was held fixed.

GEE Model Information

Correlation Structure	Independent
Subject Effect	id (111 levels)
Number of Clusters	111
Correlation Matrix Dimension	4
Maximum Cluster Size	4
Minimum Cluster Size	4

Algorithm converged.

Analysis Of GEE Parameter Estimates
Empirical Standard Error Estimates

Parameter		Estimate	Standard Error	95% Confidence Limits		Z	Pr > |Z|
Intercept		1.3517	0.7770	-0.1711	2.8746	1.74	0.0819
centre	1	-0.6723	0.3572	-1.3725	0.0278	-1.88	0.0598
centre	2	0.0000	0.0000	0.0000	0.0000	.	.
treat	1	-1.3006	0.3510	-1.9885	-0.6126	-3.71	0.0002
treat	2	0.0000	0.0000	0.0000	0.0000	.	.
sex	1	-0.1194	0.4437	-0.9890	0.7503	-0.27	0.7879
sex	2	0.0000	0.0000	0.0000	0.0000	.	.
age		-0.0182	0.0130	-0.0437	0.0073	-1.40	0.1626

The GENMOD Procedure

Analysis Of GEE Parameter Estimates
Empirical Standard Error Estimates

Parameter	Estimate	Standard Error	95% Confidence Limits		Z	Pr > |Z|
time	-0.0643	0.0816	-0.2242	0.0957	-0.79	0.4310
bl	1.8841	0.3502	1.1977	2.5704	5.38	<.0001

In this example, the only difference from the equivalent analysis in `proc mixed` is the `d=b` option on the model statement, which specifies a binomial distribution. Other distributions that can be specified are: exponential

TABLE 13.4

Results from GEE with an Exchangeable Working Correlation Matrix for Respiratory Data

```
                         GEE Model Information

            Correlation Structure                   Exchangeable
            Subject Effect                       id (111 levels)
            Number of Clusters                               111
            Correlation Matrix Dimension                       4
            Maximum Cluster Size                               4
            Minimum Cluster Size                               4


      Algorithm converged.


                   Analysis of GEE Parameter Estimates
                    Empirical Standard Error Estimates

                              Standard   95% Confidence
   Parameter      Estimate     Error          Limits             Z Pr > |Z|

   Intercept        1.3707    0.7769  -0.1520   2.8933     1.76   0.0777
   centre      1   -0.6809    0.3568  -1.3802   0.0183    -1.91   0.0563
   centre      2    0.0000    0.0000   0.0000   0.0000      .       .
   treat       1   -1.2922    0.3505  -1.9793  -0.6052    -3.69   0.0002
   treat       2    0.0000    0.0000   0.0000   0.0000      .       .
   sex         1   -0.1308    0.4441  -1.0012   0.7397    -0.29   0.7684
   sex         2    0.0000    0.0000   0.0000   0.0000      .       .
   age             -0.0184    0.0130  -0.0439   0.0071    -1.41   0.1571
   time            -0.0642    0.0815  -0.2240   0.0956    -0.79   0.4309
   bl               1.8778    0.3501   1.1916   2.5640     5.36   <.0001
```

(`expo`), gamma (`gam`), gaussian or normal (`g` or `n`), geometric (`geom`), inverse gaussian (`ig`), log normal (`logn`), multinomial (`mult`), negative binomial (`nb`), poisson (`p`), and *t* (`t`). The results are shown in Table 13.5.

The significance of the effects as estimated by the random effects model and by the GEE models is generally similar. However, as expected from the discussion in Display 13.2, the estimated regression coefficients are somewhat larger. Thus while the estimated effect of treatment for a randomly selected individual, given the set of observed covariates, was estimated by the marginal models to increase the log-odds of having a good respiratory response by about 1.3, the estimate from the random effects model is 1.5. These are not inconsistent results but reflect the fact that the models are estimating different parameters. The random effects estimator is conditional upon each patient's random effect, a quantity that is rarely known in practice.

13.4 Analysis of Epilepsy Data

To begin we shall examine the data graphically by constructing boxplots of the counts after treatment separately for the two treatment groups:

TABLE 13.5

Results of Fitting a Random Intercept Logistic Regression Model to the Respiratory Data

```
                         The GLIMMIX Procedure

                           Model Information

              Data Set                        WORK.RESPL
              Response Variable               status
              Response Distribution           Binomial
              Link Function                   Logit
              Variance Function               Default
              Variance Matrix Blocked By      id
              Estimation Technique            Residual PL
              Degrees of Freedom Method       Between-Within


                        Class Level Information

      Class      Levels    Values

      centre          2    1 2
      treat           2    1 2
      sex             2    1 2
      id            111    1 2 3 4 5 6 7 8 9 10 11 12 13 14 15 16 17 18
                           19 20 21 22 23 24 25 26 27 28 29 30 31 32 33
                           34 35 36 37 38 39 40 41 42 43 44 45 46 47 48
                           49 50 51 52 53 54 55 56 57 58 59 60 61 62 63
                           64 65 66 67 68 69 70 71 72 73 74 75 76 77 78
                           79 80 81 82 83 84 85 86 87 88 89 90 91 92 93
                           94 95 96 97 98 99 100 101 102 103 104 105 106
                           107 108 109 110 111


                Number of Observations Read          444
                Number of Observations Used          444


                              Dimensions

                   G-side Cov. Parameters            1
                   Columns in X                     10
                   Columns in Z per Subject          1
                   Subjects (Blocks in V)          111
                   Max Obs per Subject               4


                       Optimization Information

             Optimization Technique         Dual Quasi-Newton
             Parameters in Optimization     1
             Lower Boundaries               1
             Upper Boundaries               0
             Fixed Effects                  Profiled
             Starting From                  Data
                        The GLIMMIX Procedure

                          Iteration History

                                          Objective                     Max
 Iteration    Restarts    Subiterations     Function        Change     Gradient

         0           0                4   2006.0075336    0.37823247   6.742E-7
         1           0                5   2071.9584265    0.16661501   1.838E-6
         2           0                3   2098.9940772    0.05552132   0.000041
         3           0                3   2106.2426463    0.01408297   0.000042
         4           0                2   2107.9076507    0.00317825   2.087E-6
         5           0                2   2108.2717014    0.00069116    2.14E-8
         6           0                1   2108.3502455    0.00014911   1.317E-6
         7           0                1   2108.3671604    0.00003200   6.097E-8
         8           0                1   2108.3707892    0.00000688   1.925E-9
         9           0                1   2108.3715692    0.00000148   4.191E-9
        10           0                0    2108.371737    0.00000000   4.617E-6
```

TABLE 13.5 (continued)

Results of Fitting a Random Intercept Logistic Regression Model to the Respiratory Data

```
                 Convergence criterion (PCONV=1.11022E-8) satisfied.

                                 Fit Statistics

                   -2 Res Log Pseudo-Likelihood        2108.37
                   Pseudo-AIC  (smaller is better)     2110.37
                   Pseudo-AICC (smaller is better)     2110.38
                   Pseudo-BIC  (smaller is better)     2113.08
                   Pseudo-CAIC (smaller is better)     2114.08
                   Pseudo-HQIC (smaller is better)     2111.47
                   Pearson Chi-Square                   281.75
                   Pearson Chi-Square / DF                0.64

                         Covariance Parameter Estimates

                    Cov                                 Standard
                    Parm       Subject    Estimate         Error

                    UN(1,1)    id           2.0433        0.5305

                          Solutions for Fixed Effects

                                                 Standard
Effect       Centre     Treat    Sex    Estimate     Error       DF    t Value    Pr > |t|

Intercept                                 1.4908    0.9063      105       1.64      0.1030
centre       1                           -0.7563    0.4114      105      -1.84      0.0689
centre       2                                 0         .        .          .           .
treat                   1                -1.5350    0.3971      105      -3.87      0.0002
treat                   2                      0         .        .          .           .

                             The GLIMMIX Procedure

                          Solutions for Fixed Effects
                                                 Standard
Effect       Centre     Treat    Sex    Estimate     Error       DF    t Value    Pr > |t|

sex                              1       -0.1426    0.5110      105      -0.28      0.7807
sex                              2             0         .        .          .           .
age                                     -0.01891   0.01533      105      -1.23      0.2202
time                                    -0.08012    0.1111      332      -0.72      0.4715
bl                                        2.1967    0.4044      105       5.43      <.0001

                        Type III Tests of Fixed Effects

                                Num       Den
                  Effect         DF        DF     F Value    Pr > F

                  centre          1       105        3.38    0.0689
                  treat           1       105       14.94    0.0002
                  sex             1       105        0.08    0.7807
                  age             1       105        1.52    0.2202
                  time            1       332        0.52    0.4715
                  bl              1       105       29.50    <.0001
```

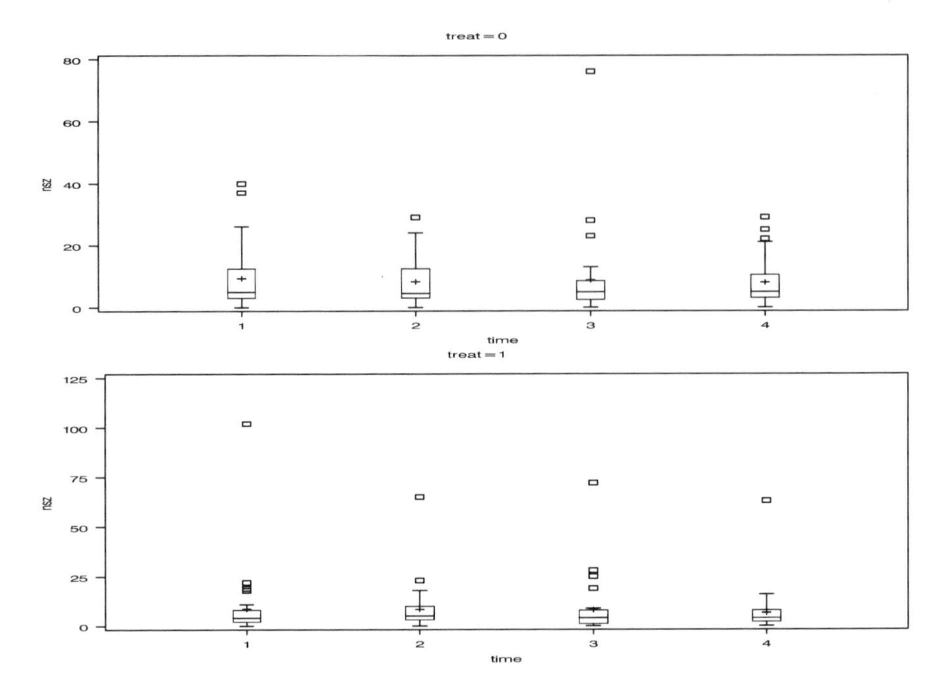

FIGURE 13.1
Boxplots of seizure counts at each time point for each treatment group.

```
data epiw;
  input id  v1-v4 treat bl age;
cards;
15  3   3   3   0   11  31
23  5   3   3   0   11  30
32  4   0   5   0   6   25
. . . .
580 0   0   0   1   13  36
591 4   3   2   1   12  37
;
data epil;
  set epiw;
  array vs {4} v1-v4;
  do time=1 to 4;
  nsz=vs{time};
  output;
  end;
```

```
run;
proc sort data=epil; by treat time; run;
proc boxplot data=epil;
  plot nsz*time / boxstyle=schematic;
  by treat;
run;
```

The resulting plot is shown in Figure 13.1.

The plot indicates that the data contain several outliers. Here, however, we shall not remove such observations but carry on and fit a GEE model with a log link and Poisson errors. (Removal of the outliers as a strategy is left as an exercise for the reader.) As in the previous example we will again consider independence and exchangeable correlation structures. To fit the former we can use the following code:

```
proc genmod data=epil;
 class id;
 model nsz= treat age time bl / d=p;
 repeated subject=id / type=ind;
run;
```

The results from the independence model are shown in Table 13.6.

For the exchangeable structure model we use

```
proc genmod data=epil;
 class id;
 model nsz= treat age time bl / d=p;
 repeated subject=id / type=exch;
run;
```

The GEE results from the exchangeable model are shown in Table 13.7.

For these data the results from the independence model and the exchangeable model are very similar and suggest that there is no significant treatment or time effect, a small age effect, and a large effect of baseline count.

We can fit a random effects model to the epilepsy data using the code that follows:

```
proc glimmix data=epil;
 class id;
 model nsz= treat age time bl /s ddfm=bw d=p;
 random int/ subject=id type=un;
run;
```

TABLE 13.6

Results from GEE Model with Log Link and Poisson Errors Fitted to Epilepsy Data

```
                          The GENMOD Procedure

                           Model Information

                     Data Set                WORK.EPIL
                     Distribution              Poisson
                     Link Function                 Log
                     Dependent Variable            nsz

                 Number of Observations Read         236
                 Number of Observations Used         236


                        Class Level Information

      Class      Levels    Values

      id             59    1 2 3 4 5 6 7 8 9 10 11 12 13 14 15 16 17 18 19 20
                           21 22 23 24 25 26 27 28 29 30 31 32 33 34 35 36 37
                           38 39 40 41 42 43 44 45 46 47 48 49 50 51 52 53 54
                           55 56 57 58 59


                         Parameter Information

                       Parameter       Effect

                       Prm1            Intercept
                       Prm2            treat
                       Prm3            age
                       Prm4            time
                       Prm5            bl


                 Criteria for Assessing Goodness of Fit

        Criterion                   DF          Value        Value/DF

        Deviance                   231       950.0702          4.1129
        Scaled Deviance            231       950.0702          4.1129
        Pearson Chi-Square         231      1178.4937          5.1017
        Scaled Pearson X2          231      1178.4937          5.1017
        Log Likelihood                      2953.7594


     Algorithm converged.


                Analysis of Initial Parameter Estimates

                              Standard   Wald 95% Confidence     Chi-
 Parameter    DF   Estimate      Error         Limits           Square   Pr > ChiSq

 Intercept     1     0.7072     0.1443     0.4244     0.9900     24.03       <.0001
 treat         1    -0.1527     0.0478    -0.2464    -0.0590     10.20       0.0014
 age           1     0.0227     0.0040     0.0149     0.0306     31.94       <.0001
 time          1    -0.0587     0.0203    -0.0985    -0.0190      8.38       0.0038
 bl            1     0.0227     0.0005     0.0217     0.0236   1978.13       <.0001
 Scale         0     1.0000     0.0000     1.0000     1.0000

NOTE: The scale parameter was held fixed.


                         GEE Model Information

                Correlation Structure              Independent
                Subject Effect                   id (59 levels)
                Number of Clusters                          59
                Correlation Matrix Dimension                 4
                Maximum Cluster Size                         4
                Minimum Cluster Size                         4

     Algorithm converged.
```

TABLE 13.6 (continued)

Results from GEE Model with Log Link and Poisson Errors Fitted to Epilepsy Data

Analysis of GEE Parameter Estimates
Empirical Standard Error Estimates

Parameter	Estimate	Standard Error	95% Confidence Limits		Z	Pr > |Z|
Intercept	0.7072	0.3479	0.0253	1.3890	2.03	0.0421
treat	-0.1527	0.1711	-0.4881	0.1827	-0.89	0.3722
age	0.0227	0.0116	0.0000	0.0454	1.96	0.0496
time	-0.0587	0.0350	-0.1273	0.0099	-1.68	0.0934
bl	0.0227	0.0012	0.0202	0.0251	18.33	<.0001

TABLE 13.7

Results from GEE Model with Log Link and Poisson Errors Fitted to Epilepsy Data

GEE Model Information

Correlation Structure	Exchangeable
Subject Effect	id (59 levels)
Number of Clusters	59
Correlation Matrix Dimension	4
Maximum Cluster Size	4
Minimum Cluster Size	4

Algorithm converged.

Exchangeable Working Correlation

Correlation 0.4004432024

Analysis of GEE Parameter Estimates
Empirical Standard Error Estimates

Parameter	Estimate	Standard Error	95% Confidence Limits		Z	Pr > |Z|
Intercept	0.6763	0.3540	-0.0175	1.3701	1.91	0.0561
treat	-0.1479	0.1687	-0.4786	0.1827	-0.88	0.3806
age	0.0236	0.0118	0.0004	0.0467	2.00	0.0459
time	-0.0587	0.0350	-0.1273	0.0099	-1.68	0.0934
bl	0.0227	0.0012	0.0203	0.0252	18.29	<.0001

The results are shown in Table 13.8. The estimated treatment effect is, as expected, larger than in the fitted GEE models but remains nonsignificant. The age effect is smaller and nonsignificant, while the time effect is the same but with a much smaller standard error. If these effects were of substantive interest, we might consider models with more random effects, for example, random slopes in time, and different covariance structures for the random effects.

TABLE 13.8

Random Effects Poisson Model Fitted to Epilepsy Data

```
                         The GLIMMIX Procedure

                           Model Information

              Data Set                      WORK.EPIL
              Response Variable             nsz
              Response Distribution         Poisson
              Link Function                 Log
              Variance Function             Default
              Variance Matrix Blocked By    id
              Estimation Technique          Residual PL
              Degrees of Freedom Method     Between-Within


                        Class Level Information

     Class     Levels    Values

     id            59    1 2 3 4 5 6 7 8 9 10 11 12 13 14 15 16 17 18
                         19 20 21 22 23 24 25 26 27 28 29 30 31 32 33
                         34 35 36 37 38 39 40 41 42 43 44 45 46 47 48
                         49 50 51 52 53 54 55 56 57 58 59


                Number of Observations Read          236
                Number of Observations Used          236


                              Dimensions

                 G-side Cov. Parameters            1
                 Columns in X                      5
                 Columns in Z per Subject          1
                 Subjects (Blocks in V)           59
                 Max Obs per Subject               4


                       Optimization Information

            Optimization Technique        Dual Quasi-Newton
            Parameters in Optimization    1
            Lower Boundaries              1
            Upper Boundaries              0
            Fixed Effects                 Profiled
            Starting From                 Data

                         The GLIMMIX Procedure

                           Iteration History

                                            Objective                        Max
Iteration    Restarts    Subiterations       Function          Change     Gradient

        0           0                3     519.312842      0.19669235      0.00009
        1           0                3    590.0977609      0.03239187      0.00022
        2           0                2   598.52820737      0.00308744     0.000028
        3           0                1   598.69780598      0.00007861     2.373E-6
        4           0                1    598.6988605      0.00000111     1.069E-7
        5           0                0   598.69887364      0.00000000     1.836E-6

           Convergence criterion (PCONV=1.11022E-8) satisfied.


                            Fit Statistics

               -2 Res Log Pseudo-Likelihood          598.70
               Pseudo-AIC  (smaller is better)       600.70
               Pseudo-AICC (smaller is better)       600.72
               Pseudo-BIC  (smaller is better)       602.78
               Pseudo-CAIC (smaller is better)       603.78
               Pseudo-HQIC (smaller is better)       601.51
               Pearson Chi-Square                    408.46
               Pearson Chi-Square / DF                 1.77
```

TABLE 13.8 (continued)

Random Effects Poisson Model Fitted to Epilepsy Data

Covariance Parameter Estimates

Cov Parm	Subject	Estimate	Standard Error
UN(1,1)	id	0.3013	0.06921

Solutions for Fixed Effects

Effect	Estimate	Standard Error	DF	t Value	Pr > |t|
Intercept	0.7030	0.4194	55	1.68	0.0994
treat	-0.2584	0.1574	55	-1.64	0.1064
age	0.01400	0.01283	55	1.09	0.2800
time	-0.05872	0.02028	176	-2.90	0.0043
bl	0.02694	0.002862	55	9.41	<.0001

The GLIMMIX Procedure

Type III Tests of Fixed Effects

Effect	Num DF	Den DF	F Value	Pr > F
treat	1	55	2.69	0.1064
age	1	55	1.19	0.2800
time	1	176	8.38	0.0043
bl	1	55	88.62	<.0001

13.5 Summary

This chapter has illustrated two approaches to the analysis of non-normal longitudinal data, the marginal approach and the conditional/random effects approach. Though less unified than the methods available for normally distributed data, these methods provide powerful and flexible tools to analyse what until relatively recently have been seen as almost intractable data.

14

Survival Analysis

14.1 Introduction

In many medical studies, the main outcome variable is the time to the occurrence of a particular event. In a randomized controlled trial of treatment for cancer, for example, surgery, radiation, and chemotherapy might be compared with respect to time from randomization and the start of therapy until death. In this case the event of interest is the death of a patient, but in other situations, it might be remission from a disease, relief from symptoms, or the recurrence of a particular condition. Such observations are generally referred to by the generic term *survival data* even when the endpoint or event being considered is not death but something else. Such data generally require special techniques for their analysis for two main reasons:

- Survival data are generally not symmetrically distributed — they will often appear positively skewed, with a few people surviving a very long time compared with the majority. Thus, assuming a normal distribution will not be reasonable.
- At the completion of the study, some patients may not have reached the endpoint of interest (death, relapse, etc.). Consequently, the exact survival times are not known. All that is known is that the survival times are greater than the length of time the individual has been in the study. The survival times of these individuals are said to be *censored* (more precisely, they are right-censored).

14.2 The Survivor Function and the Hazard Function

Of central importance in the analysis of survival data are two functions used to describe the distribution of survival times, namely the *survivor* (or *survival*) *function* and the *hazard function*.

14.2.1 Survivor Function

The survivor function, $S(t)$, is defined as the probability that the survival time, T, is greater than or equal to t, i.e.,

$$S(t) = \Pr(T > t) \tag{14.1}$$

A plot of an estimate of $S(t)$ against t is often a useful way of describing the survival experience of a group of individuals. When there are no censored observations in the sample of survival times, a nonparametric estimate of the survivor function is given by

$$\hat{S}(t) = \frac{\text{number of individuals with survival times} \geq t}{\text{number of individuals in the data set}} \tag{14.2}$$

Because this is simply a proportion, confidence intervals can be obtained for each time t by using the variance estimate

$$\hat{S}(t)\left(1 - \hat{S}(t)\right)/n \tag{14.3}$$

where n is the total number of individuals.

The method above cannot be used to estimate the survivor function when the data contain censored observations. In the presence of censoring, the survivor function is generally estimated using the Kaplan–Meier estimator, which is based on the calculation and use of conditional probabilities. A short description of the Kaplan–Meier estimator is given in Display 14.1.

To illustrate the use of the Kaplan-Meier estimator we shall use the small data set shown in Table 14.1, which gives survival times in weeks for 20 patients with stage 3 and 4 melanoma. We can find and plot the estimated survivor function and its 95% confidence interval for these data using the following SAS code:

```
data melanoma;
  input weeks status$;
  censor=status='alive';
cards;
12.8    dead
15.6    dead
24.0    alive
....
140.0   alive
168.0   alive
;
```

DISPLAY 14.1

The Kaplan–Meier Estimator of the Survival Function

- The Kaplan-Meier estimator is a nonparametric estimator that may be used to estimate the survivor function from censored data.
- Assume we have a sample of n observations from the population for which we wish to estimate the survivor function. Some of the survival times in the sample are right censored — for those individuals we know only that their true survival times exceed the censoring time.
- We denote by $t_1 < t_2 \ldots$ the times when deaths are observed and let d_j, be the number of individuals who 'die' at t_j.
- The Kaplan-Meier estimator for the survival function then takes the form

$$\hat{S}(t) = \prod_{t_j \le t} \left(1 - \frac{d_j}{r_j}\right)$$

where r_j is the number of individuals at risk, i.e., alive and not censored, just prior to time t_j. If there are no censored observations the estimator reduces to that given in Equation (14.2).

- The essence of the Kaplan–Meier estimator is the use of the continued product of a series of conditional probabilities. For example, to find the probability of surviving 2 years we use

Pr(surviving two years) = Pr (surviving one year)
× Pr(surviving two years | having survived one year)

and the probability of surviving three years

$$\Pr(3) = \Pr(3 \mid 2) \times \Pr(2) = \Pr(3 \mid 2) \times \Pr(2 \mid 1) \times \Pr(1)$$

In this way censored observations can be accommodated correctly.

- The variance of the Kaplan–Meier estimator is given by

$$V\left[\hat{S}(t)\right] = \left[\hat{S}(t)\right]^2 \sum_{t_j \le t} \frac{d_j}{r_j\left(r_j - d_j\right)}$$

- When there is no censoring this reduces to the standard binomial variance estimator given in Equation (14.3).

TABLE 14.1

Ordered Survival Times for 20 Patients with Stage 3 and 4 Melanoma and Status of Patients at the End of the Study

Survival Time (weeks)	Status
12.8	Dead
15.6	Dead
24.0	Alive
26.4	Dead
29.2	Dead
30.8	Alive
39.2	Dead
42.0	Dead
58.4	Alive
72.0	Alive
77.2	Dead
82.4	Dead
87.2	Alive
94.4	Alive
97.2	Alive
106.0	Alive
114.8	Alive
117.2	Alive
140.0	Alive
168.0	Alive

```
proc lifetest data=melanoma plots=(s);
  time weeks*censor(0);
run;
```

`Proc lifetest` is used to estimate and plot the survivor function as well as for testing differences in survival between groups. A range of plots are available with the `plots=` option; here we simply request the survivor function plot. The `time` statement is used to specify survival time and censoring. The variable containing the survival times comes first, then an asterisk and the censoring variable with a value, or list of values, indicating censored observations in parentheses. The censoring variable needs to be numeric, so a new variable is computed for the purpose in the preceding data step.

The resulting plot is shown in Figure 14.1. The estimated median survival time is 97.2 with 95% confidence interval 87.2 to 117.2.

14.2.2 The Hazard Function

In the analysis of survival data it is often of interest to assess which periods have high or low chances of death (or whatever the event of interest may

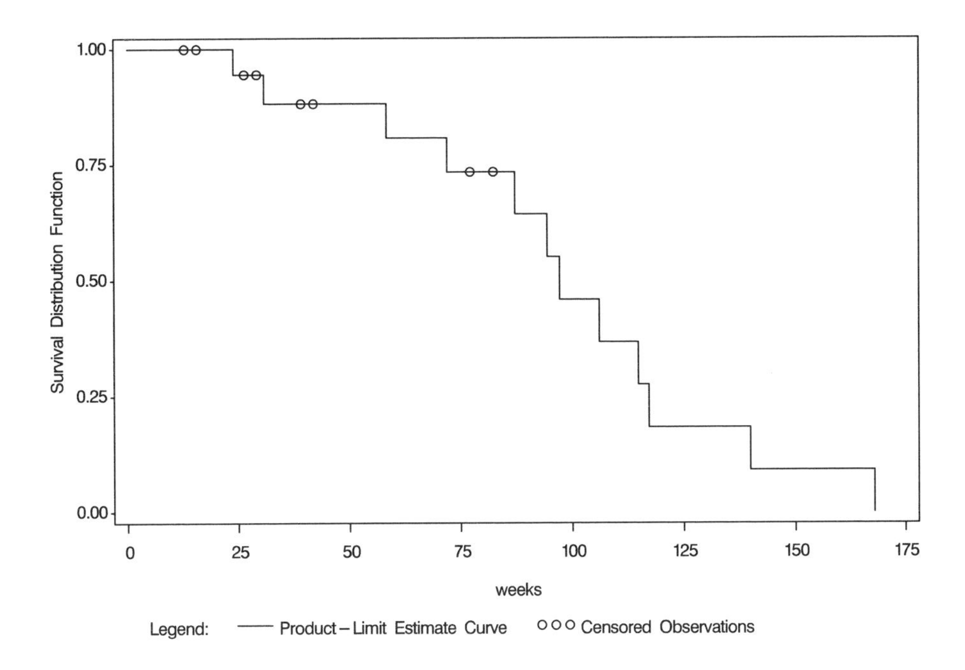

FIGURE 14.1
Kaplan-Meir estimated survival function for melanoma data in Table 14.1.

be), among those still active at the time. A suitable approach to characterize such risks is the hazard function, $h(t)$, defined as the probability that an individual experiences the event in a small time interval s, given that the individual has survived up to the beginning of the interval, when the size of the time interval approaches zero; mathematically this is written as

$$h(t) = \lim_{s \to 0} \frac{\Pr(t \le T \le t + s \mid T \ge t)}{S} \tag{14.5}$$

where T is the individual's survival time. The conditioning feature of this definition is very important. For example, the probability of dying at age 100 is very small because most people die before that age; in contrast, the probability of a person dying at age 100 who has reached that age is much greater.

The hazard function is a measure of how likely an individual is to experience an event as a function of the age of the individual; it is often known as the *instantaneous death rate*.

The hazard function and survivor function are related by the formula

$$S(t) = \exp[-H(t)] \tag{14.6}$$

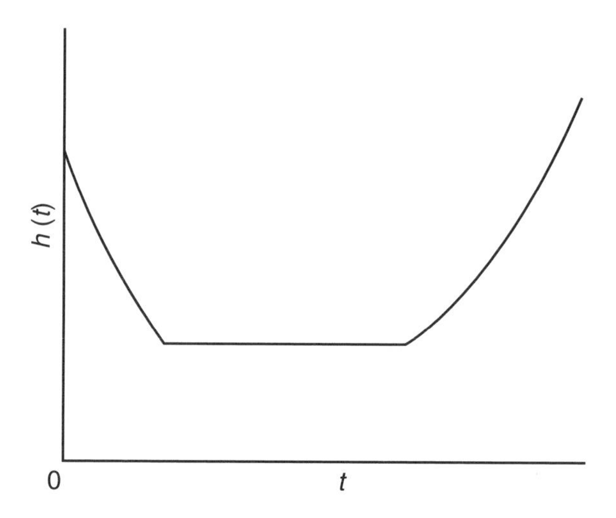

Figure 14.2
Bathtub hazard function.

where $H(t)$ is known as the *integrated hazard* or *cumulative hazard*, and is defined as follows:

$$H(t) = \int_0^t h(u)\,du \tag{14.7}$$

(Details of how this relationship arises are given in Everitt and Pickles, 2004.)

In practice the hazard function may increase, decrease, remain constant, or have a more complex shape. The hazard function for death in human beings, for example, has the 'bathtub' shape shown in Figure 14.2. It is relatively high immediately after birth, declines rapidly in the early years and then remains approximately constant before beginning to rise again during late middle age.

14.3 Comparing Survival Functions

Although the survival function of a single group of patients is a useful description of their survival times, it is often the comparison of the survival functions of different groups of patients that is of greater interest. For example, a clinician may wish to compare the survival times of males and females suffering from some particular condition, or a researcher may need to compare the retinopathy-free time of two groups of diabetic patients or, in a clinical trial, the survival times of patients given an active treatment may need to be compared with those of patients receiving a placebo.

TABLE 14.2

Initial Remission Times (days) for Leukemia Patients

Treatment 1
4, 5, 9, 10, 11, 12, 13, 23, 28, 28, 28, 29, 31, 32, 37, 41, 41, 57, 62, 74, 100, 139, 200+, 258+, 269+
Treatment 2
8, 10, 10, 12, 14, 20, 48, 70, 75, 99, 103, 162, 169, 195, 220, 161+, 199+, 217,+ 245
Treatment 3
8, 10, 11, 23, 25, 25, 28, 28, 31, 31, 40, 48, 89, 124, 143, 12+, 159+, 190+, 196+, 197+, 205+, 219+

Note: + indicates right censoring.

An example of a data set in which a comparison of survival functions is needed is shown in Table 14.2. These data give the initial remission times in days for leukemia patients randomly allocated to three different treatments. What is needed here is a formal test of the hypothesis

$$H_0 : S_1 = S_2 = S_3$$

where S_1, S_2, and S_3 are the survival functions of the three treatments.

A number of nonparametric tests are available for assessing the equality of survivor functions. The original developers of these tests sought ways to extend tests used with noncensored data to the censored data setting. Lawless (1982) presents a concise summary of the various tests, and in Andersen et al. (1993) the tests are reexamined from the counting process point of view. A further excellent overview of the tests is given in Hosmer and Lemeshow (1999). Although the tests may lead to different conclusions in some circumstances, in general they will not. All the tests have an associated normal approximation, but these need to be used with caution since they are strictly only applicable to large sample sizes.

With a small data set like that in Table 14.2 it would be easy to reformat with a text editor, for example, the SAS editor so that it can be read in relatively simply. Here, however, we read the data directly as they appear in Table 14.2 for illustrative purposes:

```
data leukemia;
 infile cards dsd missover;
  treatment=_n_;
  do until(days=.);
    input number$ @;
    censor=0;
    if indexc(number,'+') then censor=1;
    number=compress(number,'+');
```

```
      days=input(number,3.);
      if days~=. then output;
    end;
  cards;
  4, 5, 9, 10, ...... 74, 100, 139, 200+, 258+, 269+
  8, 10, 10, ..... 195, 220, 161+, 199+, 217+, 245
  8, 10, 11, .....12+, 159+, 190+, 196+, 197+, 205+, 219
  +
  ;
  proc lifetest data=leukemia plots=(s);
    time days*censor(1);
    strata treatment / test=(all);
  run;
```

Using proc lifetest to compare the survival functions of different groups is achieved by including the strata statement and specifying the variable(s) that define the subgroups on it. The test=(all) option gives all the available nonparametric tests. The results are shown in Table 14.3.

The conclusions from all the tests are the same; there is no evidence of a difference in the survivor functions of the three treatments. With such small sample sizes the power of all the tests will, of course, be rather low.

TABLE 14.3

Tests for the Equality of the Survivor Function of the Three Groups in Table 14.2

Test of Equality over Strata

Test	Chi-Square	DF	Pr > Chi-Square
Log-Rank	2.2797	2	0.3199
Wilcoxon	3.0028	2	0.2228
Tarone	3.1466	2	0.2074
Peto	2.8168	2	0.2445
Modified Peto	2.8666	2	0.2385
Fleming(1)	2.7208	2	0.2566

14.4 Cox's Regression; the Proportional Hazards Model

Models in which the aim is to identify explanatory variables most associated with a response variable of interest have featured in several earlier chapters (see Chapter 6 and Chapter 7). And in studies involving survival times there is often a similar aim of assessing the effects of explanatory variables on these times. But the models considered in earlier chapters not suitable are for survival time data because of the likely presence of censored observations. Instead a form of regression developed by Sir David Cox in his now-classic 1972 paper (Cox, 1972) is used. One of the essential features of this approach is that it is the hazard function rather than the mean or some other measure of location that is modeled. Since the hazard function is restricted to being positive this might suggest a model of the form

$$\log\left[h(t)\right] = \beta_0 + \beta_1 x_1 \ldots + \beta_p x_p \tag{14.8}$$

where $x_1 \ldots x_p$ are the explanatory variables of interest. But this would only be suitable for a hazard function that is constant over time, corresponding to an exponential distribution for the survival times. Such a model is very restrictive since hazards that increase or decrease with time or have some more complex form are far more likely to occur in practice, but it may be difficult to find the appropriate explicit function of time to include in Equation (14.8). How this problem is overcome in Cox's regression and further details of the technique are given in Display 14.2.

To illustrate the use of Cox's regression we shall apply it to the data shown in Table 14.4. These data give the survival times of 51 adult patients with acute myeloblastic leukemia along with the values of five explanatory variables.

We can apply Cox's regression using `proc phreg`. The necessary code for the data in Table 14.4 is

```
data leukemia2;
 input age p_blasts p_inf p_lab maxtemp months status;
cards;
20   78   39    7    990   18   0
25   64   61   16   1030   31   1
.....
75   60   60   17    990   13   0
77   69   69    9    986   13   0
80   73   73    7    986    1   0
;
proc phreg data=leukemia2;
 model months*status(1)=age p_blasts p_inf p_lab maxte
mp;
run;
```

The survival times are specified on the `model` statement in the same way as on the time statement in `proc lifetest`. The survival time variable comes first, then an asterisk and the censoring variable with censoring

DISPLAY 14.2

Cox's Regression Model

- In Cox's regression model an arbitrary baseline hazard function $h_0(t)$ is introduced giving the model

$$\log[h(t)] = \log[h_0(t)] + \beta_1 x_1 \ldots + \beta_p x_p$$

- The function $h_0(t)$ is the hazard function for individuals with all explanatory variables equal to zero. This function is left unspecified.
- The model can be rewritten as

$$h(t) = h_0(t)\exp(\beta_1 x_1 + \cdots \beta_p x_p)$$

- Written in this way, we see that the model forces the hazard ratio between two individuals to be constant over time since

$$\frac{h(t \mid \mathbf{x}_1)}{h(t \mid \mathbf{x}_2)} = \frac{\exp(\boldsymbol{\beta}'\mathbf{x}_1)}{\exp(\boldsymbol{\beta}'\mathbf{x}_2)}$$

  where $\mathbf{x}_1$ and $\mathbf{x}_2$ are vectors of covariate values for two individuals and β is the vector or regression coefficients.
- So if an individual has a risk of death at some initial time point that is twice as high as that of another individual, then at all later time points the risk of death remains twice as high. Hence the term *proportional hazards model* as an alternative name for the technique.
- Proportionality of hazards is an assumption of the model that needs to be checked in any application.
- In the Cox model, the baseline hazard describes the common slope of the survival time distribution for all individuals, while the relative risk, $\exp(\boldsymbol{\beta}'\mathbf{x})$, gives the relative level of each individual's hazard.
- The interpretation of the parameter, β_j, is that $\exp(\beta_j)$ gives the relative risk associated with an increase of one unit in x_j, all other explanatory variables remaining constant.

DISPLAY 14.2 (continued)

Cox's Regression Model

- Cox's proportional hazards model is semiparametric; it makes a parametric assumption concerning the effect of the predictors on the hazard function, but makes no assumption regarding the nature of the hazard function itself. In many situations, either the form of the true hazard function is unknown or it is complex and more interest centres on the effects of the predictors than the exact nature of the hazard function — in such a situation Cox's method has the distinct advantage of allowing the shape of the hazard function to be ignored.
- Details of how the parameters in Cox's regression are estimated are given in Kalbfleisch and Prentice (1980). One problem with estimation is that the continuous survival times are assumed, whereas in reality, survival times are measured in discrete units and there are often ties. There are a variety of approaches to dealing with ties — see Hosmer and Lemeshow (1999) for details.
- If we do not wish to assume proportionality among groups of individuals defined by a certain predictor, we can estimate a *stratified Cox model* with distinct baseline hazards for the groups but common values of the coefficient vector $\boldsymbol{\beta}$.

TABLE 14.4

Data for 51 Leukemia Patients

Variable						
1	2	3	4	5	6	7
20	78	39	7	990	18	0
25	64	61	16	1030	31	1
26	61	55	12	982	31	0
26	64	64	16	100	31	0
27	95	95	6	980	36	0
27	80	64	8	1010	1	0
28	88	88	20	986	9	0
28	70	70	14	1010	39	1
31	72	72	5	988	20	1
33	58	58	7	986	4	0
33	92	92	5	980	45	1
33	42	38	12	984	36	0
34	26	26	7	982	12	0
36	55	55	14	986	8	0

TABLE 14.4 (continued)

Data for 51 Leukemia Patients

Variable						
1	2	3	4	5	6	7
37	71	71	15	1020	1	0
40	91	91	9	986	15	0
40	52	49	12	988	24	0
43	74	63	4	986	2	0
45	78	47	14	980	33	0
45	60	36	10	992	29	1
45	82	32	10	1016	7	0
45	79	79	4	1030	0	0
47	56	28	2	990	1	0
48	60	54	10	1002	2	0
50	83	66	19	996	12	0
50	36	32	14	992	9	0
51	88	70	8	982	1	0
52	87	87	7	986	1	0
53	75	68	13	980	9	0
53	65	65	6	982	5	0
56	97	92	10	992	27	1
57	87	83	19	1020	1	0
59	45	45	8	999	13	0
59	36	34	5	1038	1	0
60	39	33	7	988	5	0
60	76	53	12	982	1	0
61	46	37	4	1006	3	0
61	39	8	8	990	4	0
61	90	90	11	990	1	0
62	84	84	19	1020	18	0
63	42	27	5	1014	1	0
65	75	75	10	1004	2	0
71	44	22	6	990	1	0
71	63	63	11	986	8	0
73	33	33	4	1010	3	0
73	93	84	6	1020	4	0
74	58	58	10	1002	14	0
74	32	30	16	988	3	0
75	60	60	17	990	13	0
77	69	69	9	986	13	0
80	73	73	7	986	1	0

Note: Variables are as follows: 1, age at diagnosis; 2, smear differential percentage of blasts; 3, percentage of absolute marrow leukemia infiltrate; 4, percentage labeling index of the bone marrow leukemia cells; 5, highest temperature prior to treatment (degrees F, decimal points omitted); survival time from diagnosis (months); 7, status (0 = dead, 1 = alive).

value(s) in parentheses. Both variables need to be numeric. Although `proc phreg` does not support the `class` statement, so all explanatory variables need to the continuous, in SAS version 9.1 there is an experimental version, `proc tphreg`, which has a `class` statement with a syntax similar to the `class` statement in `proc logistic`. The results are shown in Table 14.5.

The three tests of the hypothesis that the regression coefficients in the model are zero each have associated p values less than 0.05, and so the hypothesis can be rejected. Examining the results for each variable strongly suggests that age alone is predictive of the hazard function. The relative risk is exp(0.03359) = 1.034, with 95% confidence interval [exp(0.03359 + 1.96 × 0.01036), exp (0.03359 – 1.96 × 0.01036)] i.e., 1.01 to 1.06. So each increase of a year in age leads to an increase in the hazard function of between 1 and 6%.

As with the regression methods described in Chapter 6 and Chapter 7, important subsets of covariates in a Cox's regression model can be chosen by one of a variety of stepwise procedures, although the selection criterion used in this case is the score or Wald statistic.

```
proc phreg data=leukemia2;
 model months*status(1)=age p_blasts p_inf p_lab maxte
mp / selection=b;
run;
```

This example uses backwards elimination, and only age is selected, as we might have predicted from the results given in Table 14.5.

As with the other regression models discussed in earlier chapters, the next stage in the analysis of survival times using Cox's regression is to examine residual and diagnostic plots for evidence of outliers, influential observations or departures from assumptions such as that of proportional hazards. Some possible diagnostics for the Cox regression model are described in Display 14.3.

Lin et al. (1993) extend the use of the martingale residuals and also suggest some numerical measures for the lack of fit of a model. These measures are now incorporated into SAS, and we will illustrate their use to check the required functional form of age in the Cox model and assess the proportional hazards assumptions when modeling the data in Table 14.4.

```
ods html;
ods graphics on;
proc phreg data=leukemia2;
 model months*status(1)=age;
 assess var=(age) ph / resample;
run;
ods graphics off;
ods html close;
```

TABLE 14.5

Results of Applying Cox's Regression to the Data in Table 14.4

Results

```
                    The PHREG Procedure

                     Model Information

        Data Set                    WORK.LEUKEMIA2
        Dependent Variable          months
        Censoring Variable          status
        Censoring Value(s)          1
        Ties Handling               BRESLOW

        Number of Observations Read          51
        Number of Observations Used          51

     Summary of the Number of Event and Censored Values

                                                Percent
         Total         Event     Censored      Censored

            51            45            6         11.76

                    Convergence Status

      Convergence criterion (GCONV=1E-8) satisfied.

                  Model Fit Statistics

                          Without              With
        Criterion       Covariates       Covariates

        -2 LOG L           291.106          276.086
        AIC                291.106          286.086
        SBC                291.106          295.120

        Testing Global Null Hypothesis: BETA=0

 Test                  Chi-Square       DF     Pr > ChiSq

 Likelihood Ratio         15.0194        5         0.0103
 Score                    14.8274        5         0.0111
 Wald                     14.0130        5         0.0155

The PHREG Procedure

          Analysis of Maximum Likelihood Estimates

                 Parameter     Standard                                      Hazard
Variable    DF    Estimate        Error    Chi-Square    Pr > ChiSq           Ratio

age          1     0.03359      0.01036       10.5140        0.0012           1.034
p_blasts     1     0.00928      0.01473        0.3968        0.5287           1.009
p_inf        1    -0.01613      0.01267        1.6195        0.2032           0.984
p_lab        1    -0.05386      0.03899        1.9086        0.1671           0.948
maxtemp      1  -0.0003663      0.00128        0.0820        0.7746           1.000
```

The `assess` statement (experimental in version 9.1) is used to perform the checks of functional form and the proportional hazards assumption. The variables whose functional form is to be checked are named in parentheses after `var=`, and `ph` results in a check of the proportional hazards assumption for *all* variables in the model. The `resample` option requests the Kolmogorov-type supremum test for these. By default it is based on 1000 simulations,

DISPLAY 14.3

Diagnostics for Cox Regression

- The *Cox–Snell residual* is defined as

$$r_{Ci} = \exp\left(\hat{\beta}'\hat{H}_0(t_i)\right)$$

  where $\hat{H}_0(t_i)$ is the estimated integrated hazard function at time t_i, the observed survival time of subject i. If the model is correct, r_{Ci} follows an exponential distribution with mean 1.
- The *martingale residual* is the difference between the event indicator δ_i (equal to 1 if the person died and 0 otherwise) and the Cox-Snell residual

$$r_{Mi} = \delta_i - r_{Ci}$$

- The *deviance residual* is defined as

$$r_{Di} = \text{sign}\left(r_{Mi}\sqrt{-2\left[r_{Mi} + \delta_i \log\left(\delta_i - r_{Mi}\right)\right]}\right)$$

- Subjects with large positive or negative deviance residuals are poorly predicted by the model.
- The partial score residual, also known as the *Schoenfeld residual* or *efficient score residual*, is defined as the first derivative of the partial log-likelihood function with respect to an explanatory variable. For the jth explanatory variable,

$$r_{Sij} = \frac{x_{ij} - \sum_{r(i)} x_{rj} \exp(\beta' \mathbf{x}_r)}{\sum_{r(i)} x_{rj} \exp(\beta' \mathbf{x}_r)}$$

  The score residual is large in absolute value if a case's explanatory variable differs substantially from the explanatory variables of subjects whose estimated risk of failure is large at the case's time of failure or censoring. This residual can be used to detect potentially influential points.

DISPLAY 14.3 (continued)

Diagnostics for Cox Regression

- For each explanatory variable, there is one score residual for each event. A rescaled score residual can be defined whose expected value is equal to the corresponding regression coefficient (Grambsch and Therneau, 1994). If the hazards are proportional, the regression coefficient is constant over time and the plot of the rescaled Schoenfeld residuals against time should form a horizontal line. Grambsch and Therneau (1994) proposed a test of proportional hazards based on these rescaled residuals.
- Influence statistics are defined as for linear regression. For example, we can compute the change in scaled coefficient associated with the removal of each observation from the data set.

but this can be controlled with `resample=n`. The graphs produced by the `assess` statement are part of the ods graphics feature (also experimental in version 9.1). The `ods graphics` statement switches the feature on and off. The resulting graphs are not displayed in the graph window but need a suitable ods output destination to be defined. Here we illustrate the html destination. The resulting html output is stored in the current directory — indicated at the bottom left of the screen — and the graphs will be in GIF files in that directory. These are shown in Figure 14.3 and Figure 14.4.

```
                    Supremum Test for Functional Form
                              Maximum
                             Absolute
              Pr >
         Variable            Value     Replications
Seed     MaxAbsVal
         age                4.1631              1000      51185
9001        0.2330
                   Supremum Test for Proportionals Hazards
Assumption
                              Maximum
                             Absolute
              Pr >
         Variable            Value     Replications
Seed     MaxAbsVal
         age                0.7187              1000      51185
9001        0.9290
```

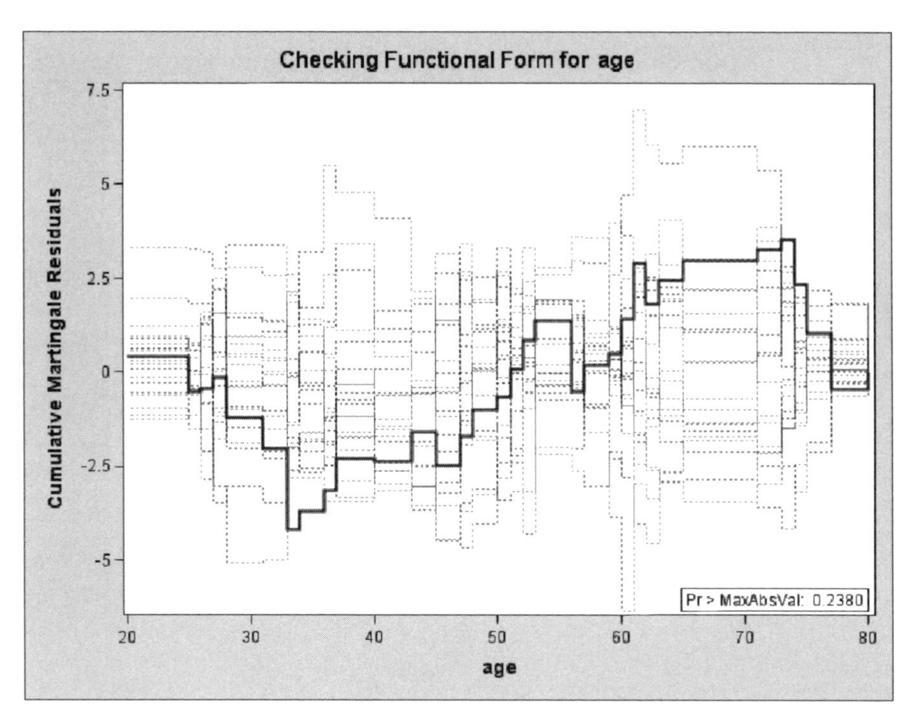

FIGURE 14.3
Plot of cumulative martingale residuals versus age for the myeloblastic leukemia data.

14.5 Time Varying Covariates

Studies in which survival data are collected often include covariates with values that do not remain fixed over time. Individuals might, for example, have laboratory measurements made repeatedly during the time they were observed. A small hypothetical data set of this kind in shown in Table 14.6.

How can we now fit a Cox's regression model that makes allowance for the changes in such variables? In essence it is very simple; the survival period of each individual is divided up into a sequence of shorter survival spells, each characterized by an entry and exit time, and within which covariate values remain fixed. Thus the data for each individual are represented by a number of shorter censored intervals and possibly one interval ending with the occurrence of the event of interest (death, for example). Table 14.7 shows the data in Table 14.6 rearranged in this way.

It may be thought that the observations in Table 14.6 that arise from the same individual are 'correlated' and so not suitable for Cox's regression as described in the previous chapter. Fortunately, this is not an issue, since the partial likelihood on which estimation is based has a term for each unique

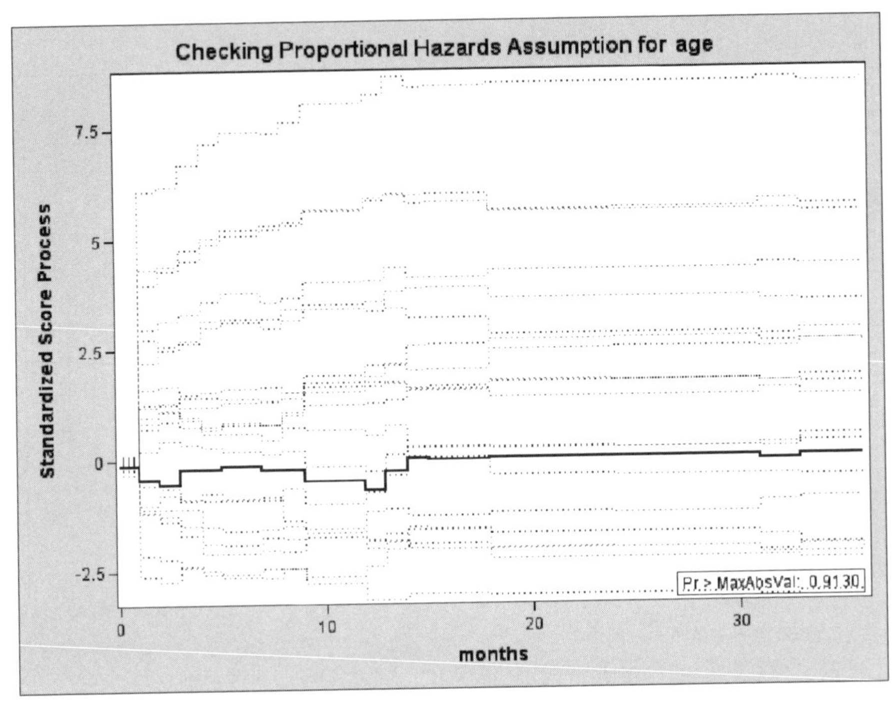

FIGURE 14.4
Plot of standardized score process versus time for age.

TABLE 14.6
Hypothetical Survival Data with a Time Varying Covariate

Individual	Laboratory Measurement (day) 0	60	120	Survival Time	Status
1	0.5	0.7	0.8	130	1
2	0.2	0.6	0.3	190	1
3	0.2	0.4	—	70	0

Note: Status: 1 = dead; 2 = censored.

death or event time and involves sums over those observations that are available or at risk at the actual event date. Since the intervals for a particular individual do not overlap, the likelihood will involve at most only one of the observations for the individual, and so will still be based on independent observations. The values of the covariates between event times do not enter the partial likelihood. So applying Cox's model to survival data with time-varying covariates is little more complex than for time-fixed covariates.

One circumstance where the use of time-varying covariates may be helpful is where the timing of the delivery of one or both treatments is not under complete experimental control. Such circumstances frequently arise in organ and tissue transplantation, where at the time of randomisation, no suitably

TABLE 14.7

Rearranged Data from Table 14.6

Individual	Interval (T_1, T_2)	Lab Measurement	Status
1	0, 60	0.5	0
1	61, 120	0.7	0
1	121, 130	0.8	1
2	0, 60	0.2	0
2	61, 120	0.6	0
2	121, 130	0.3	1
3	0, 60	0.2	0
3	61, 170	0.4	1

Note: The survival time for each interval is calculated as $T_2 - T_1$.

well-matched donors may be available for all patients. Two comparisons then become of interest. The first essentially defines the treatment as that given, i.e., a waiting time of unknown duration followed by transplantation, and compares survival over both waiting and posttransplant survival periods combined. The second defines the treatment as transplantation for which only the posttransplant survival is relevant. These correspond to the two rather different clinical circumstances of considering the treatment alternatives of a patient for whom a well-matched donor is already available (the second case) and a patient for whom one is yet to be found (the first case). Without a very rigorous protocol, it is often unreasonable to assume that the waiting time to find a well-matched donor is independent of transplant survival, since matching criteria are likely to be relaxed as the waiting time increases, and transplantation may only be possible if the patient is fit enough to survive surgery. Despite this potential difficulty we shall now illustrate the use of Cox's regression with time varying covariates with an example of this type, using the well-known set of survival times of potential heart transplant recipients from their date of acceptance into the Stanford heart transplant program. The data are shown in Table 14.8 in the form described previously. So, for example, patient 3 waited a single day for a transplant and then died after 15 days. In these data, patients change treatment status during the course of the study. Specifically, a patient is part of the control group until a suitable donor is located and transplantation takes place, at which time that individual joins the treatment group. So treatment is a time-dependent covariate. The other covariates to be considered are age (in years minus 48), whether the patient had had previous heart surgery, and waiting time for acceptance into the program (years since October 1, 1967).

The necessary SAS code to read in the data and apply a series of Cox's regression models, the first with a single covariate, Transplant, the second with all four covariates, and the third with an interaction between Year and Transplant, is as follows:

TABLE 14.8

Stanford Heart Transplant Data

ID	Start	Stop	Event	Age	Year	Surgery	Transplant
1	0.0	50.0	1	–17.155	0.123	0	0
2	0.0	6.0	1	3.836	0.255	0	0
3	0.0	1.0	0	6.297	0.266	0	0
3	1.0	16.0	1	6.297	0.266	0	1
4	0.0	36.0	0	–7.737	0.490	0	0
4	36.0	39.0	1	–7.737	0.490	0	1
5	0.0	18.0	1	–27.214	0.608	0	0
6	0.0	3.0	1	6.5955	0.701	0	0
7	0.0	51.0	0	2.8693	0.780	0	0
7	51.0	675.0	1	2.8693	0.780	0	1
8	0.0	40.0	1	–2.650	0.835	0	0
9	0.0	85.0	1	–0.838	0.857	0	0
10	0.0	12.0	0	–5.498	0.862	0	0
10	12.0	58.0	1	–5.498	0.862	0	1
11	0.0	26.0	0	–0.019	0.873	0	0
11	26.0	153.0	1	–0.019	0.873	0	1
12	0.0	8.0	1	5.194	0.964	0	0
13	0.0	17.0	0	6.574	0.969	0	0
13	17.0	81.0	1	6.574	0.969	0	1
14	0.0	37.0	0	6.012	0.972	0	0
14	37.0	1387.0	1	6.012	0.972	0	1
15	0.0	1.0	1	5.815	0.991	1	0
16	0.0	28.0	0	1.448	1.070	0	0
16	28.0	308.0	1	1.448	1.070	0	1
17	0.0	36.0	1	–27.669	1.076	0	0
18	0.0	20.0	0	8.849	1.087	0	0
18	20.0	43.0	1	8.849	1.087	0	1
19	0.0	37.0	1	11.124	1.133	0	0
20	0.0	18.0	0	7.280	1.331	0	0
20	18.0	28.0	1	7.280	1.331	0	1
21	0.0	8.0	0	–4.657	1.339	0	0
21	8.0	1032.0	1	–4.657	1.339	0	1
22	0.0	12.0	0	–5.216	1.462	0	0
22	12.0	51.0	1	–5.216	1.462	0	1
23	0.0	3.0	0	10.357	1.528	0	0
23	3.0	733.0	1	10.357	1.528	0	1
24	0.0	83.0	0	3.800	1.566	0	0
24	83.0	219.0	1	3.800	1.566	0	1
25	0.0	25.0	0	–14.776	1.574	0	0
25	25.0	1800.0	0	–14.776	1.574	0	1
26	0.0	1401.0	0	–17.465	1.582	0	0
27	0.0	263.0	1	–39.214	1.591	0	0
28	0.0	71.0	0	6.023	1.684	0	0
28	71.0	72.0	1	6.023	1.684	0	1
29	0.0	35.0	1	2.434	1.785	0	0
30	0.0	16.0	0	–3.088	1.884	0	0
30	16.0	852.0	1	–3.088	1.884	0	1
31	0.0	16.0	1	6.886	1.895	0	0
32	0.0	17.0	0	16.408	1.911	0	0
32	17.0	77.0	1	16.408	1.911	0	1

TABLE 14.8 (continued)

Stanford Heart Transplant Data

ID	Start	Stop	Event	Age	Year	Surgery	Transplant
33	0.0	51.0	0	0.903	2.157	0	0
33	51.0	1587.0	0	0.903	2.157	0	1
34	0.0	23.0	0	–7.447	2.198	0	0
34	23.0	1572.0	0	–7.447	2.199	0	1
35	0.0	12.0	1	–4.534	2.308	0	0
36	0.0	46.0	0	0.925	2.508	0	0
36	46.0	100.0	1	0.925	2.508	0	1
37	0.0	19.0	0	13.500	2.565	0	0
37	19.0	66.0	1	13.500	2.565	0	1
38	0.0	4.5	0	–6.530	2.593	0	0
38	4.5	5.0	1	–6.530	2.593	0	1
39	0.0	2.0	0	2.519	2.634	0	0
39	2.0	53.0	1	2.519	2.634	0	1
40	0.0	41.0	0	0.482	2.648	1	0
40	41.0	1408.0	0	0.482	2.648	1	1
41	0.0	58.0	0	–2.697	2.883	1	0
41	58.0	1322.0	0	–2.697	2.883	1	1
42	0.0	3.0	1	–11.559	2.888	0	0
43	0.0	2.0	1	–4.608	3.058	1	0
44	0.0	40.0	1	–5.421	3.165	1	0
45	0.0	1.0	0	–11.817	3.264	0	0
45	1.0	45.0	1	–11.817	3.264	0	1
46	0.0	2.0	0	0.611	3.277	1	0
46	2.0	996.0	1	0.611	3.277	1	1
47	0.0	21.0	0	–0.901	3.340	0	0
47	21.0	72.0	1	–0.901	3.340	0	1
48	0.0	9.0	1	8.036	3.348	0	0
49	0.0	36.0	0	–11.346	3.376	1	0
49	36.0	1142.0	0	–11.346	3.376	1	1
50	0.0	83.0	0	–2.114	3.376	1	0
50	83.0	980.0	1	–2.114	3.376	1	1
51	0.0	32.0	0	0.734	3.477	0	0
51	32.0	285.0	1	0.734	3.477	0	1
52	0.0	102.0	1	–6.752	3.565	0	0
53	0.0	41.0	0	–0.657	3.751	0	0
53	41.0	188.0	1	–0.657	3.751	0	1
54	0.0	3.0	1	–0.208	3.751	0	0
55	0.0	10.0	0	4.454	3.855	0	0
55	10.0	61.0	1	4.454	3.855	0	1
56	0.0	67.0	0	–9.257	3.923	0	0
56	67.0	942.0	0	–9.257	3.923	0	1
57	0.0	149.0	1	–6.735	3.951	0	0
58	0.0	21.0	0	0.016	3.978	1	0
58	21.0	343.0	1	0.016	3.978	1	1
59	0.0	78.0	0	–6.617	3.995	1	0
59	78.0	916.0	0	–6.617	3.995	1	1
60	0.0	3.0	0	1.054	4.131	0	0
60	3.0	68.0	1	1.054	4.131	0	1
61	0.0	2.0	1	4.564	4.175	0	0
62	0.0	69.0	1	–8.646	4.189	0	0

TABLE 14.8 (continued)

Stanford Heart Transplant Data

ID	Start	Stop	Event	Age	Year	Surgery	Transplant
63	0.0	27.0	0	–15.340	4.197	0	0
63	27.0	842.0	0	–15.340	4.197	0	1
64	0.0	33.0	0	0.816	4.337	1	0
64	33.0	584.0	1	0.816	4.337	1	1
65	0.0	12.0	0	3.294	4.430	0	0
65	12.0	78.0	1	3.294	4.430	0	1
66	0.0	32.0	1	5.213	4.468	0	0
67	0.0	57.0	0	–28.449	4.476	0	0
67	57.0	285.0	1	–28.449	4.476	0	1
68	0.0	3.0	0	–2.760	4.517	0	0
68	3.0	68.0	1	–2.760	4.517	0	1
69	0.0	10.0	0	–0.011	4.668	0	0
69	10.0	670.0	0	–0.011	4.668	0	1
70	0.0	5.0	0	5.002	4.712	0	0
70	5.0	30.0	1	5.002	4.712	0	1
71	0.0	31.0	0	–0.591	4.805	0	0
71	31.0	620.0	0	–0.591	4.805	0	1
72	0.0	4.0	0	–21.273	4.871	0	0
72	4.0	596.0	0	–21.273	4.871	0	1
73	0.0	27.0	0	8.331	4.947	0	0
73	27.0	90.0	1	8.331	4.947	0	1
74	0.0	5.0	0	–18.834	4.966	0	0
74	5.0	17.0	1	–18.834	4.966	0	1
75	0.0	2.0	1	4.181	4.997	0	0
76	0.0	46.0	0	4.085	5.010	1	0
76	46.0	545.0	0	4.085	5.010	1	1
77	0.0	21.0	1	–6.888	5.016	0	0
78	0.0	210.0	0	0.704	5.092	0	0
78	210.0	515.0	0	0.704	5.092	0	1
79	0.0	67.0	0	5.782	5.166	0	0
79	67.0	96.0	1	5.782	5.166	0	1
80	0.0	26.0	0	–1.555	5.183	1	0
80	26.0	482.0	0	–1.555	5.183	1	1
81	0.0	6.0	0	4.893	5.284	0	0
81	6.0	445.0	0	4.893	5.284	0	1
82	0.0	428.0	0	–18.798	4.085	0	0
83	0.0	32.0	0	5.309	5.317	0	0
83	32.0	80.0	1	5.309	5.317	0	1
84	0.0	37.0	0	–5.281	5.333	0	0
84	37.0	334.0	1	–5.281	5.333	0	1
85	0.0	5.0	1	–0.019	5.352	0	0
86	0.0	8.0	0	0.920	5.415	0	0
86	8.0	397.0	0	0.920	5.415	0	1
87	0.0	60.0	0	–1.747	5.470	0	0
87	60.0	110.0	1	–1.747	5.470	0	1
88	0.0	31.0	0	6.363	5.489	0	0
88	31.0	370.0	0	6.363	5.489	0	1
89	0.0	139.0	0	3.047	5.511	0	0
89	139.0	207.0	1	3.047	5.511	0	1
90	0.0	160.0	0	4.033	5.514	1	0

TABLE 14.8 (continued)

Stanford Heart Transplant Data

ID	Start	Stop	Event	Age	Year	Surgery	Transplant
90	160.0	186.0	1	4.033	5.514	1	1
91	0.0	340.0	1	–0.405	5.533	0	0
92	0.0	310.0	0	–3.017	5.572	0	0
92	310.0	340.0	0	–3.017	5.572	0	1
93	0.0	28.0	0	–0.249	5.777	0	0
93	28.0	265.0	0	–0.249	5.777	0	1
94	0.0	4.0	0	–4.159	5.955	1	0
94	4.0	165.0	1	–4.158	5.955	1	1
95	0.0	2.0	0	–7.718	5.977	0	0
95	2.0	16.0	1	–7.718	5.977	0	1
96	0.0	13.0	0	–21.350	6.010	0	0
96	13.0	180.0	0	–21.350	6.010	0	1
97	0.0	21.0	0	–24.383	6.144	0	0
97	21.0	131.0	0	–24.383	6.144	0	1
98	0.0	96.0	0	–19.370	6.204	0	0
98	96.0	109.0	0	–19.370	6.204	0	1
99	0.0	21.0	1	1.834	6.234	0	0
100	0.0	38.0	0	–12.939	6.396	1	0
100	38.0	39.0	0	–12.939	6.396	1	1
101	0.0	31.0	0	1.517	6.418	0	0
102	0.0	11.0	0	–7.608	6.472	0	0
103	0.0	6.0	1	–8.684	–0.049	0	0

Note: Surgery: 0 = no previous surgery, 1 = previous surgery; Transplant: 0 = no transplant, 1 = transplant; Event: 0 = censored, 1 = died.

```
data SHTD;
input ID Start Stop Event Age Year Surgery Transplant;
duration=stop-start;
cards;
  1   0.0   50.0  1  -17.155   0.123  0  0
  2   0.0    6.0  1    3.836   0.255  0  0
  3   0.0    1.0  0    6.297   0.266  0  0
  3   1.0   16.0  1    6.297   0.266  0  1
....
102   0.0   11.0  0   -7.608   6.472  0  0
103   0.0    6.0  1   -8.684  -0.049  0  0
;
proc phreg data=SHTD;
  model (start,stop)*event(0)=Transplant / rl;
run;
proc phreg data=SHTD;
```

```
  model (start,stop)*event(0)=Age Year Surgery
Transplant / rl;
run;
proc tphreg data=SHTD;
  model (start,stop)*event(0)=Age Year Surgery
Transplant year*transplant / rl;
run;
```

`Proc phreg` has an alternative version of the `model` statement designed for data in this format, which SAS refers to as the 'counting process style of input'. Instead of a single variable for the survival time, two variables are named (in parentheses), which define the beginning and end of a period during which the subject is at risk. The example also illustrates the use of the `rl` (`risklimits`) option to include the confidence limits in the output.

For the last model we illustrate the use of `proc tphreg`. This is a version of `proc phreg` introduced on a trial basis in version 9.1. It includes a number of features found in `proc logistic`; a similar `class` statement, specification of effects (e.g., interactions and polynomial terms) using the asterisk and vertical bar, and variable selection methods that preserve the hierarchy of effects. To fit this model with `proc phreg,` a new variable would have to be computed for the interaction term.

Selected output from these three models is shown in Table 14.9. In the first model there is no evidence that transplantation affects the hazard function. In the second model the regression coefficients for both age and year are significant, implying that each is associated with survival. The results from the last model appear to imply that survival time depends on the time of acceptance into the study; as this increases, the hazard function for the death of a patient decreases. But this claim become less clear-cut if we examine the Transplant × time of acceptance interaction, which approaches significance, with an effect that is in the opposite direction. According to Kalbfleisch and Prentice (1980), taken together these results imply that the overall quality of patients being admitted to the study may be improving with time (possibly due to the relaxation of admission requirements or to improved patient management), but the survival time of the transplanted patients is not improving at the same rate.

A further model that might be considered is one which allows separate baseline hazards for the after-transplanted and before- or not-transplanted patients, but common coefficients in each group. To fit this model we can use the following code:

```
proc phreg data=SHTD;
  model (start,stop)*event(0)=Age Year Surgery  / rl;
  strata transplant;
run;
```

TABLE 14.9

Results from Fitting Three Cox Regression Models to the Heart Transplant Data

Analysis of Maximum Likelihood Estimates

Model 1

Variable	DF	Parameter Estimate	Standard Error	Chi-Square	Pr > ChiSq	Hazard Ratio	95% Hazard Ratio Confidence Limits	
Transplant	1	0.12567	0.30108	0.1742	0.6764	1.134	0.628	2.046
Model 2								
Age	1	0.02715	0.01372	3.9158	0.0478	1.028	1.000	1.056
Year	1	-0.14611	0.07047	4.2994	0.0381	0.864	0.753	0.992
Surgery	1	-0.63582	0.36721	2.9980	0.0834	0.530	0.258	1.088
Transplant	1	-0.01189	0.31364	0.0014	0.9698	0.988	0.534	1.827
Model 3								
Age	1	0.02988	0.01374	4.7307	0.0296	1.030	1.003	1.058
Year	1	-0.25211	0.10482	5.7848	0.0162	0.777	0.633	0.954
Surgery	1	-0.66270	0.36811	3.2410	0.0718	0.515	0.251	1.061
Transplant	1	-0.62153	0.53092	1.3704	0.2417	0.537	0.190	1.521
Year*Transplant	1	0.19697	0.13944	1.9953	0.1578	.	.	

Model Fit Statistics

	Criterion	Without Covariates	With Covariates
Model 1	-2 LOG L	596.651	596.475
Model 2	-2 LOG L	596.651	581.589
Model 3	-2 LOG L	596.651	579.569

The results are shown in Table 14.10.

Plotting the graph of the predicted survival curves in each stratum, with all covariates equal to their mean values using the following code:

```
proc phreg data=SHTD;
  model (start,stop)*event(0)=Age Year Surgery  / rl;
  strata transplant;
  baseline out=phout survival=sfest / method=ch;
run;
symbol1 v=none i=join;
symbol2 v=none i=join l=2;
proc gplot data=phout;
  plot sfest*stop=transplant;
run;
```

results in Figure 14.5. The `baseline` statement saves the survival function estimates as the variable `sfest` in the `phout` data set. The product limit estimator is the default, and `method=ch` requests the alternative empirical cumulative hazard estimate. The estimates are then plotted using different linetypes for the transplant and control groups.

TABLE 14.10

Results from a Stratified Cox's Model for Heart Transplant Data

The PHREG Procedure

Model Information

Data Set	WORK.SHTD
Dependent Variable	Start
Dependent Variable	Stop
Censoring Variable	Event
Censoring Value(s)	0
Ties Handling	BRESLOW

Number of Observations Read	172
Number of Observations Used	172

Summary of the Number of Event and Censored Values

Stratum	Transplant	Total	Event	Censored	Percent Censored
1	0	103	30	73	70.87
2	1	69	45	24	34.78
Total		172	75	97	56.40

Convergence Status

Convergence criterion (GCONV=1E-8) satisfied.

Model Fit Statistics

Criterion	Without Covariates	With Covariates
-2 LOG L	525.608	510.000
AIC	525.608	516.000
SBC	525.608	522.952

Testing Global Null Hypothesis: BETA=0

Test	Chi-Square	DF	Pr > ChiSq
Likelihood Ratio	15.6082	3	0.0014
Score	15.4010	3	0.0015
Wald	14.8433	3	0.0020

The PHREG Procedure

Analysis of Maximum Likelihood Estimates

Variable	DF	Parameter Estimate	Standard Error	Chi-Square	Pr > ChiSq	Hazard Ratio	95% Hazard Ratio Confidence Limits	
Age	1	0.02931	0.01391	4.4370	0.0352	1.030	1.002	1.058
Year	1	-0.15201	0.07099	4.5849	0.0323	0.859	0.747	0.987
Surgery	1	-0.61681	0.37067	2.7690	0.0961	0.540	0.261	1.116

Figure 14.5 demonstrates the longer survival experience of patients who have a transplant.

As this example illustrates, time varying covariates can be introduced into a Cox model for survival data very simply. But this apparent simplicity should not disguise the potential problems; in particular, the inclusion of such covariates runs the risk of biasing the estimated treatment effect if they themselves reflect the development of the disease process and so may be

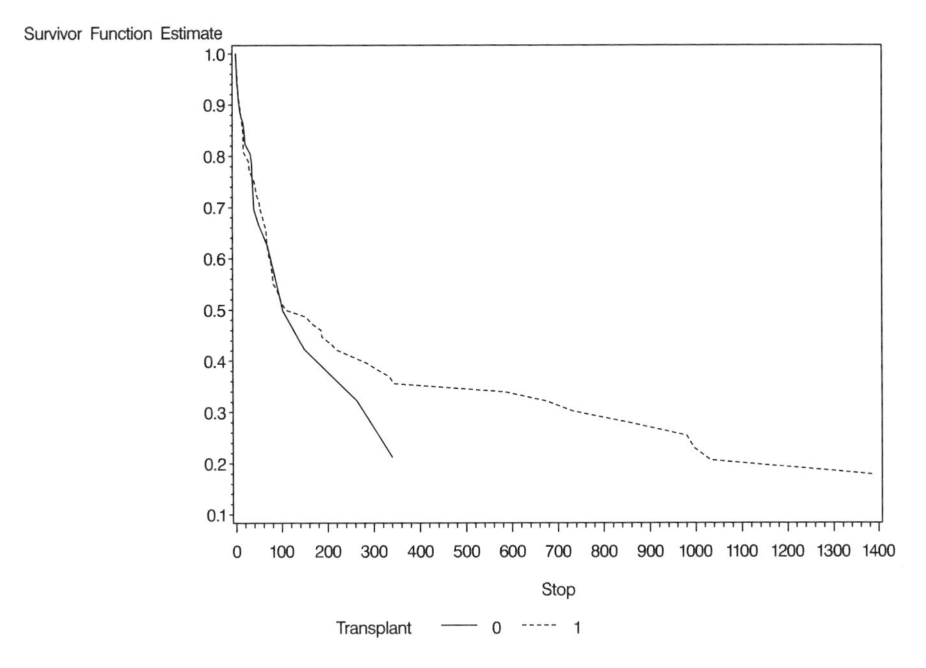

FIGURE 14.5
Predicted survival curves for heart transplant data.

partly influenced by treatment. Biochemical or physical measures of disease are obvious examples. This is well illustrated in an example given by Altman and DeStavola (1994). High levels of bilirubin and low levels of albumin reflect advanced biliary cirrhosis and are highly prognostic. A treatment that improves cirrhosis will tend to reduce bilirubin levels and increase those of albumin. Altman and DeStavola showed how much of the significant and substantial estimate of treatment effect could be removed by the inclusion into the model of updated values of either of these variables. From the point of view of treatment effect estimation, updating these variables is most unwise, casting unnecessary doubt on treatment differences. From the point of view of a scientific investigation of the development of the process and for constructing prognostic indices, their inclusion will be of more interest.

Thus, it is important that *internal* or *endogenous* variables should be distinguished from *external* or *exogenous* variables. External variables are either predetermined, e.g., a patient's age, or vary independently of survival, e.g., the weather. However, the status of many time varying variables as internal or external is uncertain, which explains our caution. It is perhaps most helpful to think of internal variables as being those that are 'causally downstream' of treatment, but the link between treatment and the internal variable does not have to be a direct one. Thus if the poor health of those on the worse or placebo treatment results in their choosing to move to a more pleasant and health-promoting climate, then not even the weather is external.

14.6 Summary

Survival analysis is the study of the distribution of times to some terminating event (death, relapse, etc.). A distinguishing feature of survival data is the presence of censored observations, and this has led to the development of a wide range of techniques for analyzing survival times. Of the available methods, the most widely used is Cox's proportional hazards model, which allows the investigation of the effects of multiple covariates on the hazard function. Time varying covariates can be handled relatively easily in the Cox's model, although care is needed to ensure that it is sensible to include such covariates in the modeling process. Correlated survival times can be dealt with by introducing random effects (frailties) into the model.

15

Analysing Multivariate Data: Principal Components and Cluster Analysis

15.1 Introduction

Multivariate data arise when researchers measure several variables on each individual in their sample. This would appear to imply that in previous chapters of this book we have already been concerned with multivariate data. But this is not the case; previously, the data sets have involved a single response variable and a set of explanatory variables or covariates and, as explained in several places, it is strictly only the response that is considered to be a random variable. With multivariate data, *all* the measurements are regarded as random variables, with a particular multivariate probability distribution, for example, the *multivariate normal* (see Everitt, 2001).

Many of the data sets collected by researchers in medicine are multivariate. Most multivariate data sets have a common form and consist of a data matrix, the rows of which contain the units in the sample, and the columns of which refer to the variables measured on each unit. Symbolically, a set of multivariate data can be represented by the matrix, **X**, given by

$$\mathbf{X} = \begin{bmatrix} x_{11} & x_{12} & x_{1p} \\ \vdots & \vdots & \vdots \\ x_{n1} & \cdots & x_{np} \end{bmatrix}$$

where n is the number of units in the sample, p is the number of variables measured on each unit, and x_{ij} denotes the value of the jth variable for the ith unit. A hypothetical example of a multivariate data matrix is given in Table 15.1. Here $n = 10$, $p = 7$ and, for example, $x_{34} = 135$. These data illustrate that the variables that make up a set of multivariate data will not necessarily all be of the same type.

Although in some cases it may make sense to isolate each variable and study it separately, in the main it does not. In most instances the variables

TABLE 15.1

Hypothetical Set of Multivariate Data

Individual	Sex	Age (yr)	IQ	Depression	Health	Weight (lb)
1	Male	21	120	Yes	Very good	150
2	Male	43	NK	No	Very good	160
3	Male	22	135	No	Average	135
4	Male	86	150	No	Very poor	140
5	Male	60	92	Yes	Good	110
6	Female	16	130	Yes	Good	110
7	Female	NK	150	Yes	Very good	120
8	Female	43	NK	Yes	Average	120
9	Female	22	84	No	Average	105
10	Female	80	70	No	Good	100

Note: NK = not known.

are related in such a way that when analyzed in isolation they may often fail to reveal the full structure of the data. With the great majority of multivariate data sets *all* the variables need to be examined simultaneously in order to uncover the patterns and key features in the data.

Multivariate analysis includes methods that are largely descriptive and others that are primarily inferential. The aim of all the procedures, in a very general sense, is to display or extract any 'signal' in the data in the presence of noise and to discover what the data have to tell us. Comprehensive accounts of multivariate analysis are given in, for example, Everitt and Dunn (2001) and Timm (2002). In this chapter we concentrate on two particular techniques, *principal component analysis* and *cluster analysis*.

15.2 Principal Components Analysis

The basic aim of principal components analysis is to describe variation in a set of correlated variables, $x_1, x_2, ..., x_p$, in terms of a new set of uncorrelated variables, $y_1, y_2, ..., y_p$, each of which is a linear combination of the x variables. The new variables are derived in decreasing order of 'importance' in the sense that y_1 accounts for as much as possible of the variation in the original data amongst all linear combinations of $x_1, x_2, ..., x_p$. Then y_2 is chosen to account for as much as possible of the remaining variation, subject to being uncorrelated with y_1 — and so on. The new variables defined by this process, $y_1, y_2, ..., y_p$, are the principal components.

The general hope of principal components analysis is that the first few components will account for a substantial proportion of the variation in the original variables, $x_1, x_2, ..., x_p$, and can, consequently, be used to provide a convenient lower-dimensional summary of these variables that might prove useful for a variety of reasons:

- The investigator may want to use the components to infer something about the structure of the relationships between the original variables; for example, the first principal component derived from say clinical psychiatric scores on patients may provide an index of the severity of symptoms, and the remaining components might give the psychiatrist important information about the 'pattern' of symptoms.
- More often the components are obtained for use as a means of constructing an informative graphical representation of the data (see later in the chapter) or as input to some other analysis. One example of the latter is provided by regression analysis; principal components may be useful here when there are too many explanatory variables relative to the number of observations, or when the explanatory variables are highly correlated. (See Rencher, 1995, for an example of using principal component analysis in this way.)

The first principal component of the observations is that linear combination of the original variables whose sample variance is greatest amongst all possible such linear combinations. The second principal component is defined as that linear combination of the original variables that accounts for a maximal proportion of the remaining variance subject to being uncorrelated with the first principal component. Subsequent components are defined similarly. The question now arises as to how the coefficients specifying the linear combinations of the original variables defining each component are found. The algebra of *sample* principal components is summarized in Display 15.1.

In geometrical terms it is easy to show that the first principal component defines the line of best fit (in the least squares sense) to the p-dimensional observations in the sample. These observations may therefore be represented in one dimension by taking their projection onto this line, that is, finding their first principal component score. If the observations happen to be collinear in p dimensions, this representation would account completely for the variation in the data, and the sample covariance matrix would have only one nonzero eigenvalue. In practice, of course, such collinearity is extremely unlikely, and an improved representation would be given by projecting the p-dimensional observations onto the space of the best fit, defined by the first two principal components. Similarly, the first m components give the best fit in m dimensions. If the observations fit exactly into a space of m-dimensions, it would be indicated by the presence of $p - m$ zero eigenvalues of the covariance matrix. This would imply the presence of $p - m$ linear relationships between the variables. Such constraints are sometimes referred to as *structural relationships*.

The account of principal components given in Display 15.1 is in terms of the eigenvalues and eigenvectors of the covariance matrix, $\mathbf{S}$. In practice, however, it is far more usual to extract the components from the correlation matrix, $\mathbf{R}$. The reasons are not difficult to identify. If we imagine a set of

DISPLAY 15.1

Algebraic Basis of Principal Components Analysis

- The first principal component of the observations, y_1, is the linear combination

$$y_1 = a_{11}x_1 + a_{12}x_2 + \ldots a_{1p}x_p$$

whose sample variance is greatest among all such linear combinations.

- Since the variance of y_1 could be increased without limit simply by increasing the coefficients $a_{11}, a_{12}, \ldots a_{1p}$ (which we will write as the vector $\mathbf{a}_1$), a restriction must be placed on these coefficients. As we shall see later, a sensible constraint is to require that the sum of squares of the coefficients, $\mathbf{a}_1'\mathbf{a}_1$, should take the value one, although other constraints are possible.
- The second principal component y_2 is the linear combination

$$y_2 = a_{21}x_1 + a_{22}x_2 + \ldots + a_{2p}x_p$$

(i.e. $y_2 = \mathbf{a}_2'\mathbf{x}$ where $\mathbf{a}_2' = \left[a_{21}, a_{22}, \ldots, a_{2p}\right]$ and $\mathbf{x}' = \left[x_1, x_2, \ldots, x_p\right]$

which has the greatest variance subject to the following two conditions:

$$\mathbf{a}_2'\mathbf{a}_2 = 1,$$

$$\mathbf{a}_2'\mathbf{a}_1 = 0.$$

The second condition ensures that y_1 and y_2 are uncorrelated.

- Similarly, the jth principal component is that linear combination $y_1 = \mathbf{a}_j'\mathbf{x}$ that has the greatest variance subject to the conditions

$$\mathbf{a}_j'\mathbf{a}_j = 1,$$

$$\mathbf{a}_j'\mathbf{a}_i = 0 \qquad (i < j).$$

- To find the coefficients defining the first principal component we need to choose the elements of the vector $\mathbf{a}_1$ so as to maximize the variance of y_1 subject to the constraint $\mathbf{a}_1'\mathbf{a}_1 = 1$.

DISPLAY 15.1 (continued)

Algebraic Basis of Principal Components Analysis

- To maximize a function of several variables subject to one or more constraints, the method of *Lagrange multipliers* is used. In this case this leads to the solution that $\mathbf{a}_1$ is the eigenvector of the sample covariance matrix, **S**, corresponding to its largest eigenvalue; full details are given in Morrison (1990).
- The other components are derived in similar fashion, with $\mathbf{a}_j$ the eigenvector of **S** associated with its *j*th largest eigenvalue.
- If the eigenvalues of **S** are $\lambda_1, \lambda_2, \ldots, \lambda_p$, then since $\mathbf{a}_i'\mathbf{a}_i = 1$, the variance of the *i*th principal component is given by λ_i.
- The total variance of the *q* principal components will equal the total variance of the original variables so that

$$\sum_{i=1}^{p} \lambda_i = s_1^2 + s_2^2 \ldots + s_p^2$$

where s_i^2 is the sample variance of x_i. We can write this more concisely as

$$\sum_{i=1}^{p} \lambda_i = \mathrm{trace}(S)\ .$$

- Consequently, the *j*th principal component accounts for a proportion P_j of the total variation of the original data, where

$$P_j = \frac{\lambda_j}{\mathrm{trace}(\mathbf{S})}.$$

- The first *m* principal components, where $m < p$ accounts for a proportion $P(m)$ of the total variation in the original data, where

$$P^{(m)} = \frac{\sum_{i=1}^{m} \lambda_i}{\mathrm{trace}(\mathbf{S})}$$

multivariate data where the variables $x_1, x_2, \ldots, x_p$ are of completely different types, for example, length, temperature, blood pressure, anxiety rating, etc., then the structure of the principal components derived from the covariance matrix will depend upon the essentially arbitrary choice of units of measurement; for example, changing lengths from centimetres to inches will alter the derived components. Additionally, if there are large differences between the variances of the original variables, those whose variances are largest will tend to dominate the early components; an example illustrating this problem is given in Jolliffe (2002). Extracting the components as the eigenvectors of **R**, which is equivalent to calculating the principal components from the original variables after each has been standardized to have unit variance, overcomes these problems. It should be noted, however, that there is rarely any simple correspondence between the components derived from **S** and those derived from **R**. And choosing to work with **R** rather than with **S** involves a definite but possibly arbitrary decision to make variables 'equally important'.

Principal components analysis is seen to be a technique for transforming a set of observed variables into a new set of variables, which are uncorrelated with one another. But the variation in the original q variables is only *completely* accounted for by *all* q principal components. The usefulness of these transformed variables, however, stems from their property of accounting for the variance in decreasing proportions. The first component, for example, accounts for the maximum amount of variation possible for any linear combination of the original variables. But how useful is this artificial variate constructed from the observed variables? To answer this question we would first need to know the proportion of the total variance of the original variables for which it accounted. If, for example, 80% of the variation in a multivariate data set involving six variables could be accounted for by a simple weighted average of the variable values, then almost all the variation can be expressed along a single continuum rather than in six-dimensional space. The principal components analysis would have provided a highly parsimonious summary (reducing the dimensionality of the data from six to one) that might be useful in later analysis.

So the question we need to ask is how many components are needed to provide an adequate summary of a given data set? A number of informal and more formal techniques are available. Here we shall concentrate on the former; examples of the use of formal inferential methods are given in Jolliffe (2002) and Rencher (1995).

The most common of the relatively *ad hoc* procedures that have been suggested are the following:

- Retain just enough components to explain some specified, large percentage of the total variation of the original variables. Values between 70 and 90% are usually suggested, although smaller values might be appropriate as q or n, the sample size, increases.

- Exclude those principal components whose eigenvalues are less than the average, $\sum_{i=1}^{p} \lambda_i / p$. Since $\sum_{i}^{p} \lambda_i = \text{trace}(\mathbf{S})$ the average eigenvalue is also the average variance of the original variables. This method then retains those components that account for more variance than the average for the variables.
- When the components are extracted from the correlation matrix, $\text{trace}(\mathbf{R}) = p$, and the average is therefore one; components with eigenvalues less than one are therefore excluded. This rule was originally suggested by Kaiser (1958) but Jolliffe (1972), on the basis of a number of simulation studies, proposes that a more appropriate procedure would be to exclude components extracted from a correlation matrix whose associated eigenvalues are less than 0.7.
- Cattell (1965) suggests examination of the plot of the λ_i against i, the so-called *scree diagram*. The number of components selected is the value of i corresponding to an 'elbow' in the curve, this point being considered to be where 'large' eigenvalues cease and 'small' eigenvalues begin. A modification described by Jolliffe (2002) is the *log-eigenvalue diagram* consisting of a plot of $\log(\lambda_i)$ against i.

If we decide that we need say m principal components to adequately represent our data (using one or other of the methods described in the previous subsection), then we will generally wish to calculate the scores on each of these components for each individual in our sample. If, for example, we have derived the components from the covariance matrix, $\mathbf{S}$, then the m principal component scores for individual i with original $p \times 1$ vector of variable values $\mathbf{x}_i$, are obtained as

$$y_{i1} = \mathbf{a}_1'\mathbf{x}_i$$

$$y_{i2} = \mathbf{a}_2'\mathbf{x}_i$$

$$\vdots$$

$$y_{im} = \mathbf{a}_m'\mathbf{x}_i$$

If the components are derived from the correlation matrix, then $\mathbf{x}_i$ would contain individual i's standardized scores for each variable.

15.3 Examples of Principal Components Analysis

15.3.1 Head Measurements

To begin, we will illustrate the application of principal component analysis on part of a data set reported over 80 years ago by Frets (1921). The data are

TABLE 15.2

Head Lengths of Pairs of Sons (mm)

x_1	x_2
191	179
195	201
181	185
183	188
176	171
208	192
189	190
197	189
188	197
192	187
179	186
183	174
174	185
190	195
188	187
163	161
195	183
186	173
181	182
175	165
192	185
174	178
176	176
197	200
190	187

Note: x_1 = head length of first son;
x_2 = head length of second son.

given in Table 15.2 and give head lengths (in mm) for each of the first two adult sons in 25 families. Here the family is the 'individual' in our data set, and the two head measurements the variables. A principal component analysis of the correlation 'matrix' (a single scalar in this case) is obtained using

```
data heads;
  input x1-x2;
cards;
191   179
195   201
. . . .
176   176
197   200
190   187
;
proc princomp data=heads;
 var x1 x2;
run;
```

TABLE 15.3

Results of a Principal Components Analysis on Head Size Data

```
                    The PRINCOMP Procedure
                   Observations          25
                   Variables              2


                      Simple Statistics

                                x1                    x2

           Mean       185.7200000           151.1200000
           StD          9.7618304             7.3729234


                      Correlation Matrix

                               x1          x2

                   x1      1.0000      0.7346
                   x2      0.7346      1.0000


              Eigenvalues of the Correlation Matrix

          Eigenvalue    Difference    Proportion    Cumulative

     1    1.73455554    1.46911107        0.8673        0.8673
     2    0.26544446                      0.1327        1.0000


                         Eigenvectors

                          Prin1         Prin2

                 x1    0.707107      0.707107
                 x2    0.707107      -.707107
```

The results are shown in Table 15.3. Here the first component is essentially the sum of the two head size measurements and the second the difference of these two measurements. Note that the components do not depend on the size of the correlation, r; the size affects only the proportion of variance accounted for by each. The first component accounts for a proportion, $(1 + r)/2$, and the second $(1 - r)/2$. As r tends to one, the proportion of variance accounted for by the first components also tends to 1.

15.3.2 Expectations of Life

The data in Table 15.4 show life expectancy in years by country, age, and sex. The data come from Keyfitz and Flieger (1972) and relate to life expectancies in the 1960s. Here we will apply principal component analysis to both the covariance matrix and the correlation matrix so that we can compare the results. The analysis is carried out using the following code:

```
data lifeexp;
  input country $ 1-21 x1-x8;
cards;
Algeria 63  51  30  13  67  54  34  15
```

TABLE 15.4

Life Expectancies for Different Countries by Age and Sex

	Male				Female			
	0	25	50	75	0	2	50	75
Age	(m0)	(m25)	(m50)	(m75)	(w0)	(w25)	(w50)	(w75)
Algeria	63	51	30	13	67	54	34	15
Cameroon	34	29	13	5	38	32	17	6
Madagascar	38	30	17	7	38	34	20	7
Mauritius	59	42	20	6	64	46	25	8
Reunion	56	38	18	7	62	46	25	10
Seychelles	62	44	24	7	69	50	28	14
South Africa (C)	50	39	20	7	55	43	23	8
South Africa (W)	65	44	22	7	72	50	27	9
Tunisia	56	46	24	11	63	54	33	19
Canada	69	47	24	8	75	53	29	10
Costa Rica	65	48	26	9	68	50	27	10
Dominican Republic	64	50	28	11	66	51	29	11
El Salvador	56	44	25	10	61	48	27	12
Greenland	60	44	22	6	65	45	25	9
Grenada	61	45	22	8	65	49	27	10
Guatemala	49	40	22	9	51	41	23	8
Honduras	59	42	22	6	61	43	22	7
Jamaica	63	44	23	8	67	48	26	9
Mexico	59	44	24	8	63	46	25	8
Nicaragua	65	48	28	14	68	51	29	13
Panama	65	48	26	9	67	49	27	10
Trinidad (62)	64	63	21	7	68	47	25	9
Trinidad (67)	64	43	21	6	68	47	24	8
United States (66)	67	45	23	8	74	51	28	10
United States (NW66)	61	40	21	10	67	46	25	11
United States (W66)	68	46	23	8	75	52	29	10
United States (67)	67	45	23	8	74	51	28	10
Argentina	65	46	24	9	71	51	28	10
Chile	59	43	23	10	66	49	27	12
Colombia	58	44	24	9	62	47	25	10
Ecuador	57	46	28	9	60	49	28	11

```
Cameroon        34   29   13    5   38   32   17    6
. . . .
Chile           59   43   23   10   66   49   27   12
Colombia        58   44   24    9   62   47   25   10
Ecuador         57   46   28    9   60   49   28   11
;
proc princomp data=lifeexp cov;
 var x1-x8;
run;
```

As we saw in the previous example, SAS analyses the correlation matrix by default. The `cov` option on the `proc princomp` statement specifies that the covariance matrix is to be analysed. The principal component results for the covariance matrix are shown in Table 15.5.

To analyse the correlation matrix and produce some diagnostic plots, we can use ods graphics as follows:

```
ods rtf style=minimal;
ods graphics on;
proc princomp data=lifeexp;
 var x1-x8;
run;
ods graphics off;
ods rtf close;
```

The numerical results are shown in Table 15.6. The graphical output appears in Figure 15.1 to Figure 15.4.

The principal components of the covariance matrix and those obtained for the correlation matrix are a little different. The first two components of the covariance matrix account for over 91% of the variance in the observations. The first component is essentially a weighted average of all eight life expectancies, with the weights decreasing from younger to older age groups within both sexes. The second component contrasts the younger age group in both men and women with the average of the three older age groups.

The first two components of the correlation matrix account for 87% of the variance of the observations (the scree diagram in Figure 15.1 also reflects that two components are probably sufficient for these data). The first component is again a weighted average of all eight life expectancies, but with the eight weights being very similar. The second component now contrasts the first two life expectancies within each sex with the last two. (Figure 15.3 shows a graphical representation of the makeup of each component in terms of the coefficients that define the components.)

We could try to give 'labels' to the components we have found, but there are dangers in this as reflected in the following quotation from Marriott (1974)

> It must be emphasized that no mathematical method is, or could be, designed to give physically meaningful results. If a mathematical expression of this sort has an obvious physical meaning, it must be attributed to a lucky chance, or to the fact that the data have a strongly marked structure that shows up in analysis. Even in the latter case, quite small sampling fluctuations can upset the interpretation; for example, the first two principal components may appear in reverse order, or may become confused altogether. Reification then requires considerable skill and experience if it is to give a true picture of the physical meaning of the data.

TABLE 15.5

Principal Components of the Life Expectancy Data Based on the Covariance Matrix

The PRINCOMP Procedure

Observations	31
Variables	8

Simple Statistics

	x1	x2	x3	x4
Mean	59.61290323	44.12903226	22.93548387	8.387096774
StD	7.91907999	5.90334332	3.40524580	2.027764275

Simple Statistics

	x5	x6	x7	x8
Mean	64.19354839	47.51612903	26.29032258	10.12903226
StD	8.82201547	4.98578625	3.33859799	2.57865515

Covariance Matrix

	x1	x2	x3	x4
x1	62.71182796	34.98494624	17.14086022	4.65483871
x2	34.98494624	34.84946237	13.40860215	4.68172043
x3	17.14086022	13.40860215	11.59569892	5.19247312
x4	4.65483871	4.68172043	5.19247312	4.11182796
x5	68.47741935	36.10752688	16.74623656	4.42258065
x6	34.50645161	21.33118280	13.10107527	5.52688172
x7	18.41612903	12.76129032	9.11935484	4.65053763
x8	6.48494624	5.98279570	5.20860215	3.71505376

Covariance Matrix

	x5	x6	x7	x8
x1	68.47741935	34.50645161	18.41612903	6.48494624
x2	36.10752688	21.33118280	12.76129032	5.98279570
x3	16.74623656	13.10107527	9.11935484	5.20860215
x4	4.42258065	5.52688172	4.65053763	3.71505376
x5	77.82795699	39.03010753	20.90860215	8.30752688
x6	39.03010753	24.85806452	15.64516129	8.79784946
x7	20.90860215	15.64516129	11.14623656	7.12795699
x8	8.30752688	8.79784946	7.12795699	6.64946237

Total Variance 233.75053763

Eigenvalues of the Covariance Matrix

	Eigenvalue	Difference	Proportion	Cumulative
1	193.942282	173.492404	0.8297	0.8297
2	20.449878	7.608019	0.0875	0.9172
3	12.841860	8.642563	0.0549	0.9721
4	4.199296	3.069301	0.0180	0.9901
5	1.129996	0.537974	0.0048	0.9949
6	0.592022	0.217205	0.0025	0.9975
7	0.374817	0.154430	0.0016	0.9991
8	0.220387		0.0009	1.0000

Eigenvectors

	Prin1	Prin2	Prin3	Prin4	Prin5	Prin6	Prin7	Prin8
x1	0.557660	-.280538	-.066515	0.360961	0.105495	0.056922	0.669952	-.111322
x2	0.342718	0.415342	-.803343	-.245107	0.022156	-.023086	-.058624	0.011757
x3	0.172229	0.414378	0.080866	0.699441	-.267315	0.353687	-.309644	0.102175
x4	0.057439	0.320169	0.158547	0.240856	0.787608	-.414396	-.125900	-.056057
x5	0.616689	-.409299	0.157986	-.203449	0.131610	0.094961	-.547658	0.244029
x6	0.336979	0.235138	0.313908	-.173682	-.360590	-.319526	-.086411	-.680340
x7	0.192922	0.339341	0.301687	-.169401	-.259602	-.364621	0.285566	0.667852
x8	0.086711	0.369602	0.322531	-.402674	0.286106	0.674793	0.216919	-.073809

TABLE 15.6

Principal Components for Life Expectancy Data Based on the Correlation Matrix

The PRINCOMP Procedure

Observations	31
Variables	8

Simple Statistics

	x1	x2	x3	x4
Mean	59.61290323	44.12903226	22.93548387	8.387096774
StD	7.91907999	5.90334332	3.40524580	2.027764275

Simple Statistics

	x5	x6	x7	x8
Mean	64.19354839	47.51612903	26.29032258	10.12903226
StD	8.82201547	4.98578625	3.33859799	2.57865515

Correlation Matrix

	x1	x2	x3	x4	x5	x6	x7	x8
x1	1.0000	0.7484	0.6356	0.2899	0.9802	0.8740	0.6966	0.3176
x2	0.7484	1.0000	0.6670	0.3911	0.6933	0.7247	0.6475	0.3930
x3	0.6356	0.6670	1.0000	0.7520	0.5574	0.7717	0.8021	0.5932
x4	0.2899	0.3911	0.7520	1.0000	0.2472	0.5467	0.6869	0.7105
x5	0.9802	0.6933	0.5574	0.2472	1.0000	0.8874	0.7099	0.3652
x6	0.8740	0.7247	0.7717	0.5467	0.8874	1.0000	0.9399	0.6843
x7	0.6966	0.6475	0.8021	0.6869	0.7099	0.9399	1.0000	0.8280
x8	0.3176	0.3930	0.5932	0.7105	0.3652	0.6843	0.8280	1.0000

Eigenvalues of the Correlation Matrix

	Eigenvalue	Difference	Proportion	Cumulative
1	5.60241029	4.24422874	0.7003	0.7003
2	1.35818155	0.85885454	0.1698	0.8701
3	0.49932700	0.19120110	0.0624	0.9325
4	0.30812590	0.15343627	0.0385	0.9710
5	0.15468962	0.09605584	0.0193	0.9903
6	0.05863378	0.04581216	0.0073	0.9977
7	0.01282163	0.00701139	0.0016	0.9993
8	0.00581023		0.0007	1.0000

The PRINCOMP Procedure

Eigenvectors

	Prin1	Prin2	Prin3	Prin4	Prin5	Prin6	Prin7	Prin8
x1	0.357304	-.432363	-.003143	-.250233	0.163128	0.241465	0.360147	-.638864
x2	0.335191	-.227614	0.497028	0.750693	0.138585	-.059124	-.023806	0.044646
x3	0.365020	0.177514	0.479770	-.293359	-.644082	0.292138	-.010077	0.136832
x4	0.285148	0.542410	0.320106	-.304141	0.646254	-.100410	-.039654	0.014654
x5	0.351253	-.433576	-.229867	-.207197	0.238954	0.189863	0.003472	0.706898
x6	0.410576	-.094551	-.236581	-.067987	-.100882	-.268268	-.786019	-.248848
x7	0.400357	0.151529	-.256454	0.038834	-.233062	-.664853	0.497207	0.076905
x8	0.305280	0.464377	-.495710	0.382389	-.010217	0.541042	0.054780	-.058110

Even if we do not care to label the three components, they can still be used as the basis of various graphical displays of the countries. In fact this is often the most useful aspect of a principal components analysis because regarding the principal components analysis as a means to providing an informative view of multivariate data has the advantage of making it less urgent or

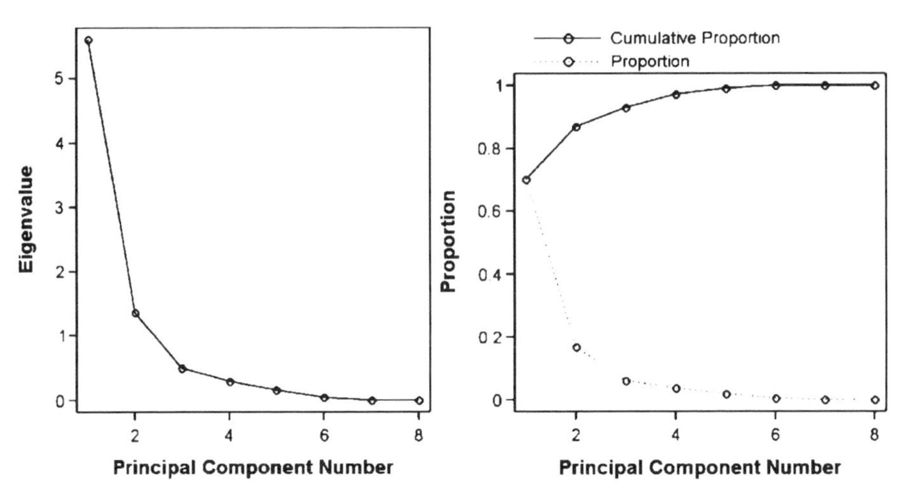

FIGURE 15.1
Scree plot and proportion of variance plot for life expectancy data.

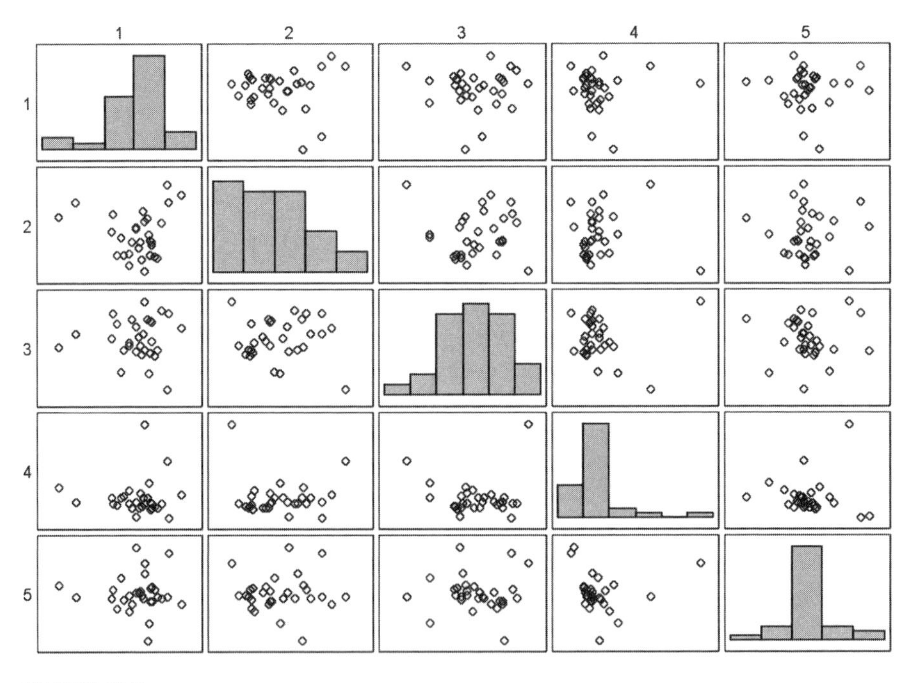

FIGURE 15.2
Scatterplot matrix of principal component scores from analyzing the correlation matrix of the life expectancy data.

tempting to try to interpret and label the components. The first few component scores provide a low-dimensional "map" of the observations, in which the Euclidean distances between the points representing the individuals best

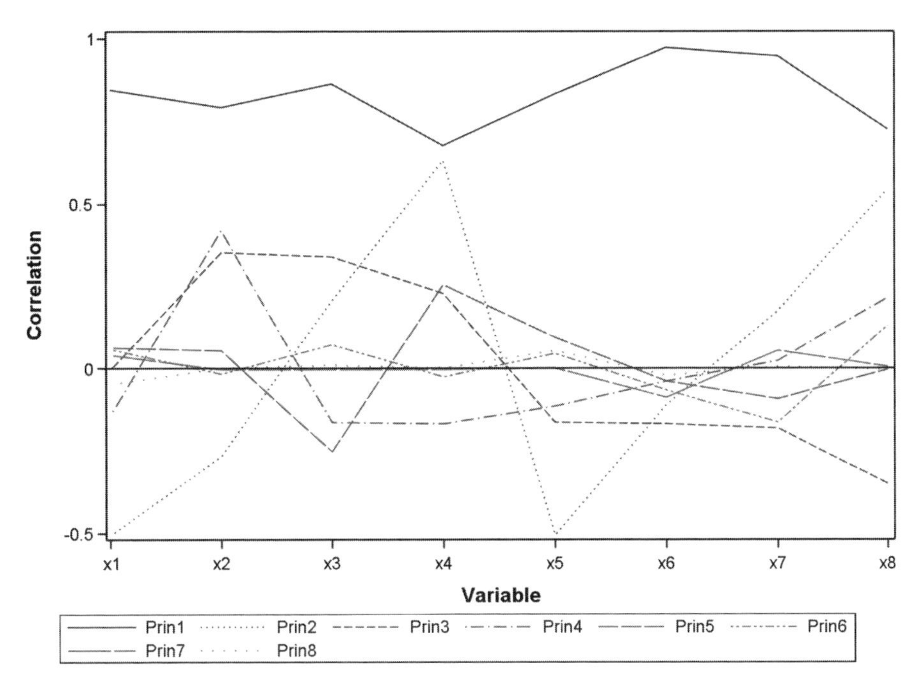

FIGURE 15.3
Profiles of the values defining each principal component of the life expectancy data.

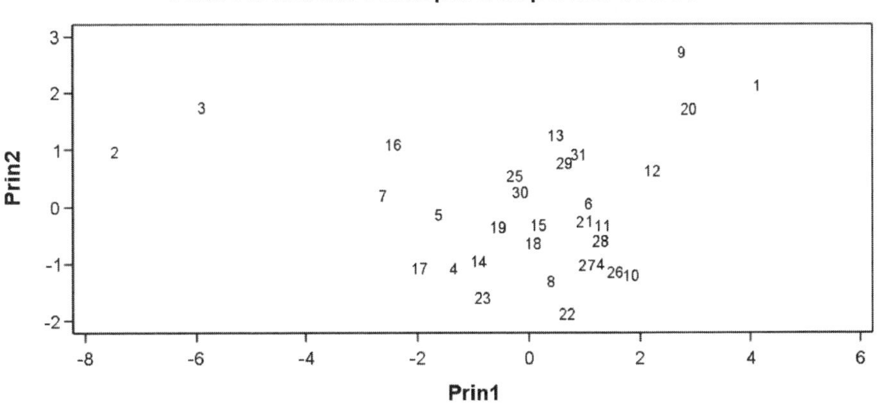

FIGURE 15.4
Plot of the life expectancy data in the space of the first two principal components of the correlation matrix (note the axes are scaled to reflect the "importance" of each component).

approximate in some sense the Euclidean distances between the individuals based on the original variables. Explicitly, the low dimensional representation achieved by principal component analysis is such that the function ϕ given by

$$\phi = \sum_{r,s}^{n} \left(d_{rs}^2 - \hat{d}_{rs}^2 \right)$$

is minimized. In this expression, d_{rs} is the Euclidean distance between observations r and s in the original q-dimensional space, and $\hat{d}_{rs}$ is the corresponding distance in k-dimensional space $(k < q)$, i.e., for the first k components.

The ODS graphics output shown above includes a scatterplot matrix of the first five component scores (Figure 15.2) and a plot of the data in the space of the first two principal components (Figure 15.4). There the points are simply labelled with the observation number. To produce a plot labelled with the country name, the principal component scores can be saved and plotted with `proc gplot`, as follows:

```
proc princomp data=lifeexp noprint out=pcout;
  var x1-x8;
run;
proc gplot data=pcout;
  plot prin2*prin1;
  symbol1 v=dot pointlabel=(j=r position=middle '#coun
try');
run;
```

The `out=` option on the proc statement saves the original variables plus the principal component scores to the named data set. The `pointlabel` option on the `symbol` statement specifies that the variable country supplies the labels and can also specify the formatting of the labels. Here it is just the positioning of labels relative to the points that is illustrated, with the `justify(j)` and `position` options. Note that the entire description is enclosed in parentheses and that the variable name must be in quotes and preceded by hash. The result is shown in Figure 15.5.

The first component largely ranks the countries according to their average life expectancy over all eight age categories. The second component shows the contrast between life expectancy for the two younger age groups and that for the two older age groups.

15.3.3 Drug Usage by American Students

The majority of adult and adolescent Americans use psychoactive substances at some time during their lifetimes. Various forms of licit and illicit psychoactive substance use are prevalent, suggesting that patterns of psychoactive substance taking are a major part of the individual's behavioural repertory and have pervasive implications on the performance of other behaviours. In

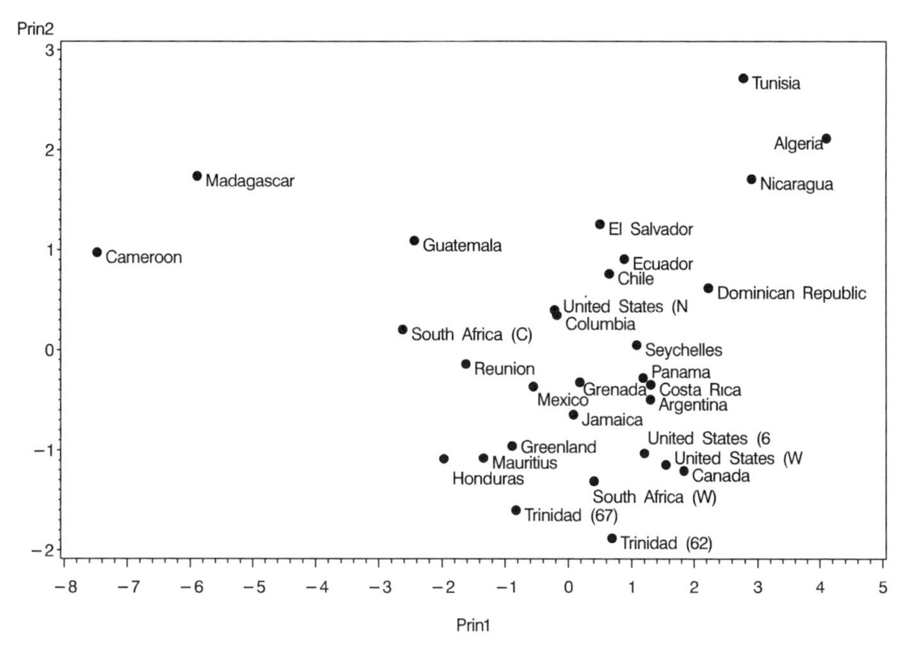

FIGURE 15.5
Plot of the life expectancy data in the space of the first two principal components with points labelled with country name.

an investigation of these phenomena, Huba et al. (1981) collected data on drug usage rates for 1634 adolescents in the seventh to ninth grades in 11 schools in the greater metropolitan area of Los Angeles. Each participant completed a questionnaire about the number of times a particular substance had ever been used. The substances asked about were as follows:

X1 Cigarettes
X2 Beer
X3 Wine
X4 Liquor
X5 Cocaine
X6 Tranquillizers
X7 Drugstore medications used to get high
X8 Heroin and other opiates
X9 Marijuana
X10 Hashish
X11 Inhalants (glue, gasoline, etc.)
X12 Hallucinogenics (LSD, mescaline, etc.)
X13 Amphetamine stimulants

TABLE 15.7

Correlation Matrix for Drug Usage Data

	X1	X2	X3	X4	X5	X6	X7	X8	X9	X10	X11	X12	X13
X1	1												
X2	0.447	1											
X3	0.442	0.619	1										
X4	0.435	0.604	0.583	1									
X5	0.114	0.068	0.053	0.115	1								
X6	0.203	0.146	0.139	0.258	0.349	1							
X7	0.091	0.103	0.110	0.122	0.209	0.221	1						
X8	0.082	0.063	0.066	0.097	0.321	0.355	0.201	1					
X9	0.513	0.445	0.365	0.482	0.186	0.315	0.150	0.154	1				
X10	0.304	0.318	0.240	0.368	0.303	0.377	0.163	0.219	0.534	1			
X11	0.245	0.203	0.183	0.255	0.272	0.323	0.310	0.288	0.301	0.302	1		
X12	0.101	0.088	0.074	0.139	0.279	0.367	0.232	0.320	0.204	0.368	0.304	1	
X13	0.245	0.199	0.184	0.293	0.278	0.545	0.232	0.314	0.394	0.467	0.392	0.511	1

Responses were recorded on a five-point scale:

1. Never tried
2. Only once
3. A few times
4. Many times
5. Regularly

The correlations between the usage rates of the 13 substances are shown in Table 15.7.

A principal component analysis can be applied to this correlation matrix using

```
data druguse (type=corr);
  infile cards missover;
  input _name_ $ x1-x13;
  _type_='CORR';
cards;
X1   1
X2   0.447 1
X3   0.442 0.619 1
X4   0.435 0.604 0.583 1
X5   0.114 0.068 0.053 0.115 1
X6   0.203 0.146 0.139 0.258 0.349 1
X7   0.091 0.103 0.110 0.122 0.209 0.221 1
X8   0.082 0.063 0.066 0.097 0.321 0.355 0.201 1
X9   0.513 0.445 0.365 0.482 0.186 0.315 0.150 0.154 1
X10 0.304 0.318 0.240 0.368 0.303 0.377 0.163 0.219 0.534 1
X11 0.245 0.203 0.183 0.255 0.272 0.323 0.310 0.288 0.301 0.302 1
X12 0.101 0.088 0.074 0.139 0.279 0.367 0.232 0.320 0.204 0.368 0.304 1
X13 0.245 0.199 0.184 0.293 0.278 0.545 0.232 0.314 0.394 0.467 0.392 0.511 1
;
proc princomp data=druguse;
run;
```

For princomp to recognise that the data are in the form of a correlation matrix the `type=corr` option is used when the data set is created. As the correlation matrix is in lower triangular format the `missover` option on the `infile` statement sets the upper triangular elements to missing. The special variable `_name_` identifies the row of the matrix. This enables a subset of the matrix to be analysed, if required. The other special variable, `_type_`, specifies the type of entry in that observation, as datasets of type=corr can also contain entries with `_type_` = '`mean`,' '`std`,' or '`n`,' which contain the means, standard deviations, and sample sizes for the variables. The results are shown in Table 15.8.

The first three components account for 52% of the variation in the data. The first component is clearly a measure of overall drug usage, as might be expected since all the correlations in Table 15.7 are positive. The second component contrasts "legal" with "illegal" substances (with the exception of marijuana, which has the same sign as the legal substances).* Alternatively this component might be seen as contrasting "soft" and "hard" drug usage. So after overall usage has been accounted for, the main source of variation is between the different patterns of consumption of these two types of substances. The third component is essentially a contrast of drugstore and inhalant substance usage on the one hand with marijuana, hashish, and amphetamine usage on the other.

15.4 Cluster Analysis

Cluster analysis is a generic term for a wide range of numerical methods for examining multivariate data with a view to uncovering or discovering groups or clusters of observations that are homogeneous and separated from other groups. In medicine, for example, discovering that a sample of patients with measurements on a variety of characteristics and symptoms actually consists of a small number of groups within which these characteristics are relatively similar and between which they are different might have important implications both in terms of future treatment and for investigating the aetiology of a condition. More recently, cluster analysis techniques have been applied to microarray data (Alon et al., 1999) and image analysis (Everitt and Bullmore, 1999).

Clustering techniques essentially try to formalize what human observers do so well in two or three dimensions. Consider, for example, the scatterplot shown in Figure 15.6. The conclusion that there are three natural groups or clusters of dots is reached with no conscious effort or thought. Clusters are identified by the assessment of the relative distances between points and in this example, the relative homogeneity of each cluster and the degree of their separation makes the task relatively simple.

* We are including cigarettes, beer, and wine as the "legal" category although in the USA they cannot be bought legally by people in the age range considered.

TABLE 15.8

Principal Components of Drug Usage Correlations

The PRINCOMP Procedure

Observations	10000
Variables	13

Eigenvalues of the Correlation Matrix

	Eigenvalue	Difference	Proportion	Cumulative
1	4.37971830	2.33359919	0.3369	0.3369
2	2.04611911	1.09092819	0.1574	0.4943
3	0.95519092	0.14114066	0.0735	0.5678
4	0.81405026	0.04922120	0.0626	0.6304
5	0.76482906	0.07355922	0.0588	0.6892
6	0.69126984	0.06201151	0.0532	0.7424
7	0.62925833	0.00955260	0.0484	0.7908
8	0.61970574	0.04629490	0.0477	0.8385
9	0.57341083	0.17139536	0.0441	0.8826
10	0.40201547	0.01003193	0.0309	0.9135
11	0.39198355	0.01654061	0.0302	0.9437
12	0.37544294	0.01843729	0.0289	0.9725
13	0.35700565		0.0275	1.0000

Eigenvectors

	Prin1	Prin2	Prin3	Prin4	Prin5	Prin6	Prin7
x1	0.280121	-.282629	-.043397	0.031391	-.300127	-.386878	-.124035
x2	0.286610	-.393937	0.120193	0.097135	0.186565	0.161472	0.113823
x3	0.267087	-.393023	0.206557	0.138872	0.308694	0.140546	0.040886
x4	0.318333	-.321882	0.045674	0.058261	0.180778	0.141897	-.021635
x5	0.207913	0.290111	0.066889	0.582239	-.432238	0.416079	0.185154
x6	0.292682	0.261794	-.164872	0.074391	0.122376	-.035893	-.628825
x7	0.175849	0.190270	0.723125	-.372180	-.178067	0.276730	-.308688
x8	0.201284	0.317035	0.152564	0.533930	0.326952	-.359086	-.049665
x9	0.339613	-.160462	-.228014	-.112054	-.364862	-.128550	-.095511
x10	0.328807	0.054179	-.352225	-.125101	-.255565	0.243499	0.166978

Eigenvectors

	Prin8	Prin9	Prin10	Prin11	Prin12	Prin13
x1	0.137129	0.655208	0.139034	0.136157	-.168568	-.263178
x2	0.004567	-.093756	0.060324	0.035909	0.695202	-.409763
x3	-.091297	0.107101	0.421436	-.210201	-.188118	0.564396
x4	-.164030	-.213859	-.563127	0.180774	-.519478	-.209767
x5	-.244021	0.204137	-.097632	-.154117	0.019893	-.000801
x6	-.399145	-.041932	0.123675	0.420872	0.169986	0.137841
x7	0.252887	0.015248	0.002652	-.007027	-.032880	-.050492
x8	0.524627	-.169355	-.015642	-.046311	-.055149	-.054449
x9	0.285184	-.149143	-.418442	-.154463	0.285482	0.501568
x10	0.273719	-.400257	0.496217	0.186764	-.239738	-.151781

The PRINCOMP Procedure

Eigenvectors

	Prin1	Prin2	Prin3	Prin4	Prin5	Prin6	Prin7
x11	0.273764	0.162692	0.329973	-.158688	-.152308	-.531126	0.465520
x12	0.245408	0.327223	-.143952	-.271700	0.379139	0.210365	0.413337
x13	0.328273	0.234984	-.235411	-.267497	0.203350	-.047619	-.132293

Detailed accounts of clustering techniques are available in Everitt et al. (2001) and Gordon (1999). Here we concentrate on one class of clustering procedures, those generally called *agglomerative hierarchical methods.*

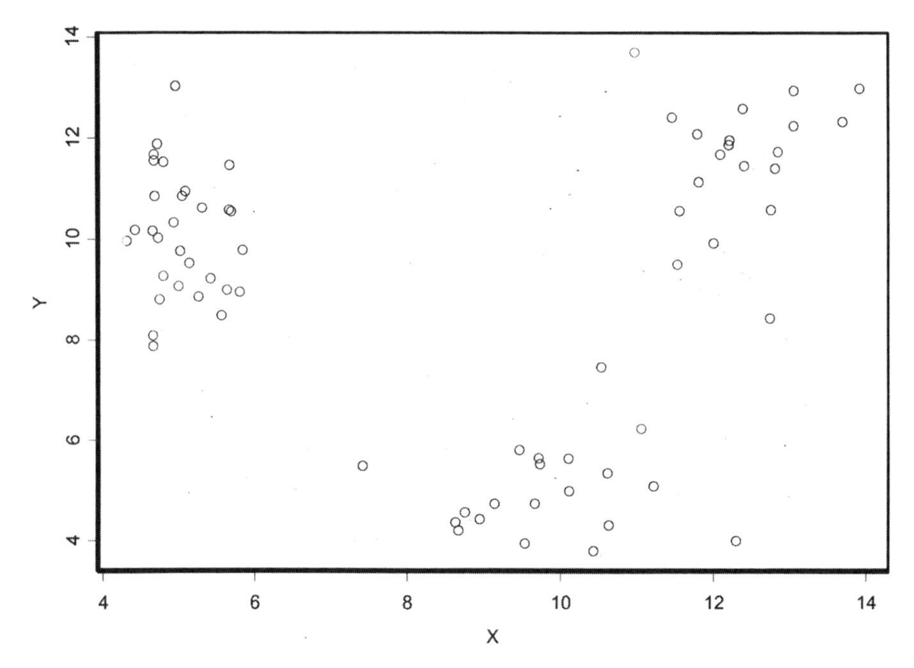

FIGURE 15.6
Bivariate data showing the presence of three clusters.

15.5 Agglomerative Hierarchical Clustering

In a hierarchical classification the data are not partitioned into a particular number of classes or clusters at a single step. Instead the classification consists of a series of partitions that may run from a single 'cluster' containing all individuals to n clusters each containing a single individual. Agglomerative hierarchical clustering techniques produce partitions by a series of successive fusions of the n individuals into groups. With such methods fusions, once made, are irreversible, so that when an agglomerative algorithm has placed two individuals in the same group they cannot subsequently appear in different groups. Since all agglomerative hierarchical techniques ultimately reduce the data to a single cluster containing all the individuals, the investigator seeking the solution with the 'best' fitting number of clusters will need to decide which division to choose. The problem of deciding on the 'correct' number of clusters is a difficult one and is discussed in detail in Everitt et al. (2001). We shall mention one informal approach later.

An agglomerative hierarchical clustering procedure produces a series of partitions of the data, $P_n, P_{n-1}, \ldots, P_1$. The first, P_n, consists of n single-member clusters, and the last, P_1, consists of a single group containing all n individuals. The basic operation of all methods is similar:

(START) Clusters $C_1, C_2, \ldots, C_n$ each containing a single individual.

(1) Find the nearest pair of distinct clusters, say C_i and C_j, merge C_i and C_j, delete C_j and decrease the number of clusters by one.

(2) If number of clusters equals one then stop, else return to 1.

At each stage in the process the methods fuse individuals or groups of individuals which are closest (or most similar). The methods begin with an interindividual distance matrix; for example, one containing Euclidean distances defined for two observations i and j as follows;

$$d_{ij} = \left[\sum_{k=1}^{p} \left(x_{ik} - x_{jk} \right)^2 \right]^{\frac{1}{2}}$$

where x_{ik} and x_{jk} $k = 1, \ldots, p$ are the variables' values for each observation. (Many other distance measures might be used — for details see Everitt et al., 2001.)

As groups are formed, the distance between an individual and a group containing several individuals or between two groups of individuals will need to be calculated. How such distances are defined leads to a variety of different techniques as we shall see below.

Hierarchic classifications may be represented by a two-dimensional diagram known as a *dendrogram*, which illustrates the fusions made at each stage of the analysis. An example of such a diagram is given in Figure 15.7.

Large changes between particular fusion levels in a dendrogram can sometimes be taken to indicate the "optimal" number of clusters for a data set, although the method is far from foolproof and is, of course, very subjective.

Agglomerative hierarchical clustering techniques differ primarily in how they measure the distances between or similarity of two clusters (where a cluster may, at times, consist of only a single individual). Two simple intergroup measures are

$$d_{AB} = \min_{\substack{i \in A \\ i \in B}} \left(d_{ij} \right),$$

$$d_{AB} = \max_{\substack{i \in A \\ i \in B}} \left(d_{ij} \right),$$

where d_{AB} is the distance between two clusters A and B, and d_{ij} is the distance between individuals i and j. This will often be Euclidean distance.

The first intergroup dissimilarity measure above is the basis of *single linkage* clustering, the second that of *complete linkage* clustering. Both these techniques have the desirable property that they are invariant under monotone transformations of the original interindividual dissimilarities or distances.

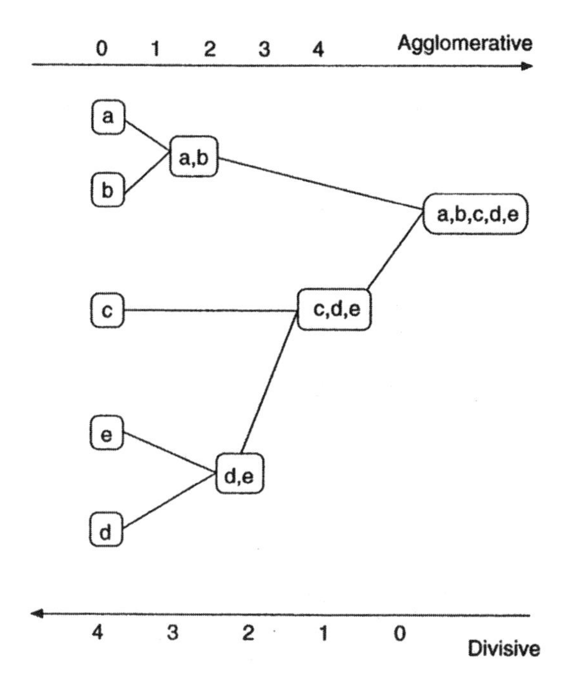

FIGURE 15.7
Example of a dendrogram. (Kaufman, L. and Rousseeuw, P.J. (1990). *Finding Groups in Data: An Introduction to Cluster Analysis*, Wiley.)

A further possibility for measuring intercluster distance or dissimilarity is

$$d_{AB} = \frac{1}{n_A n_B} \sum_{i \in A} \sum_{i \in B} d_{ij}$$

where n_A and n_B are the number of individuals in clusters A and B. This measure is the basis of a commonly used procedure known as *group average* clustering. All three intergroup measures described here are illustrated in Figure 15.8.

To illustrate the use of single linkage, complete linkage, and group average clustering we shall apply each method to the data shown in Table 15.9. These data were collected in an investigation of environmental causes of disease. They show the annual mortality rate per 100,000 for males, averaged over the years 1958 to 1964, and the calcium concentration (in parts per million) in the drinking water supply for 61 large towns in England and Wales. (The higher the calcium concentration, the harder the water.) Also identified in the table are towns as far north as Derby.

Here we shall base the clustering on the Euclidean distances between each pair of towns based on the two variable values, mortality and calcium concentration. The following code reads in the data and then applies single linkage, complete linkage, and average linkage:

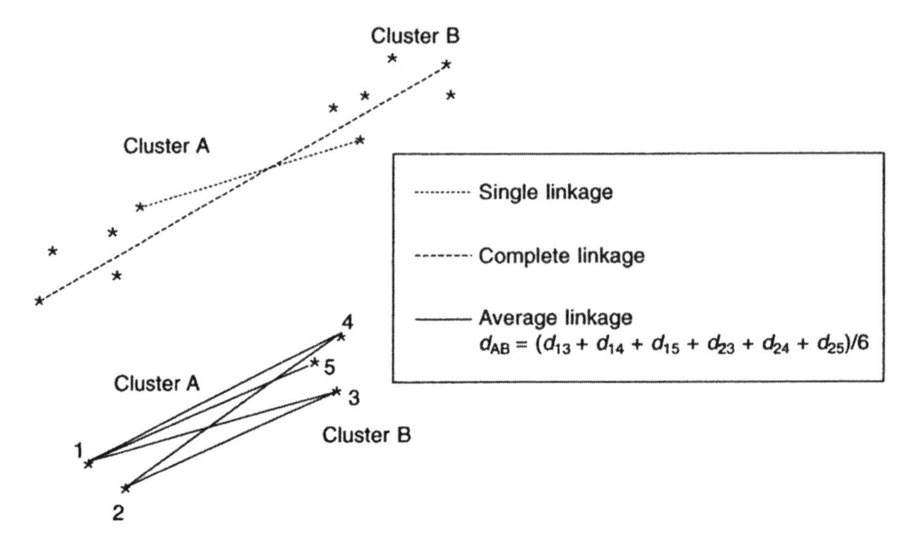

FIGURE 15.8
Three inter-cluster distance measures.

TABLE 15.9
Mortality and Water Hardness Data

Location	Town	Mortal	Hardness
S	Bath	1247	105
N	Birkenhead	1668	17
S	Birmingham	1466	5
N	Blackburn	1800	14
N	Blackpool	1609	18
N	Bolton	1558	10
N	Bootle	1807	15
S	Bournemouth	1299	78
N	Bradford	1637	10
S	Brighton	1359	84
S	Bristol	1392	73
N	Burnley	1755	12
S	Cardiff	1519	21
S	Coventry	1307	78
S	Croydon	1254	96
N	Darlington	1491	20
N	Derby	1555	39
N	Doncaster	1428	39
S	East Ham	1318	122
S	Exeter	1260	21
N	Gateshead	1723	44
N	Grimsby	1379	94
N	Halifax	1742	8
N	Huddersfield	1574	9
N	Hull	1569	91
S	Ipswich	1096	138

TABLE 15.9 (continued)

Mortality and Water Hardness Data

Location	Town	Mortal	Hardness
N	Leeds	1591	16
S	Leicester	1402	37
N	Liverpool	1772	15
N	Manchester	1828	8
N	Middlesbrough	1704	26
N	Newcastle	1702	44
S	Newport	1581	14
S	Northampton	1309	59
S	Norwich	1259	133
N	Nottingham	1427	27
N	Oldham	1724	6
S	Oxford	1175	107
S	Plymouth	1486	5
S	Portsmouth	1456	90
N	Preston	1696	6
S	Reading	1236	101
N	Rochdale	1711	13
N	Rotherham	1444	14
N	St. Helens	1591	49
N	Salford	1987	8
N	Sheffield	1495	14
S	Southampton	1369	68
S	Southend	1257	50
N	Southport	1587	75
N	South Shields	1713	71
N	Stockport	1557	13
N	Stoke	1640	57
N	Sunderland	1709	71
S	Swansea	1625	13
N	Wallasey	1625	20
S	Walsall	1527	60
S	West Bromwich	1627	53
S	West Ham	1486	122
S	Wolverhampton	1485	81
N	York	1378	71

```
data water;
   input location $ 1 Town $ 3-19 Mortal Hardness;
cards;
S Bath              1247  105
N Birkenhead        1668  17
. . . .
S West Ham          1486  122
S Wolverhampton     1485  81
```

```
N York                1378  71
;
proc cluster data=water method=single std outtree=
single;
 var mortal hardness;
 id town;
 copy location;
run;
axis1 value=(h=.7) label=(a=90);
proc tree data=single hor vaxis=axis1;
run;
proc cluster data=water method=complete std outtree=
complete;
 var mortal hardness;
 id town;
 copy location;
run;
proc tree data=complete hor vaxis=axis1;
run;
proc cluster data=water method=average std outtree=
average;
 var mortal hardness;
 id town;
 copy location;
run;
proc tree data=average hor vaxis=axis1;
run;
```

As the mortality and hardness variables are measured on very different scales, the `std` option on the `proc cluster` statement is used to standardise them to zero mean and unit standard deviation. In addition to the three clustering methods illustrated here, proc cluster supports a further eight methods, selectable with the `method` option. The `outtree` option names the data set to be used by `proc tree` to create a dendrogram. The `id` statement specifies a variable that identifies the observations. The `copy` statement is used to copy the `location` variable to the `outtree` data set.

`Proc tree` constructs the dendrogram and can also be used to divide the observations into a specified number of clusters. The `horizontal` (`hor`) option draws the tree horizontally, and the `vaxis` option has been used to decrease the font size of the axis values (i.e., town names) and to rotate the axis label.

The details of single linkage clustering are shown in Table 15.10, complete linkage in Table 15.11, and average linkage in Table 15.12. The corresponding dendrograms are shown in Figure 15.9, Figure 15.10, and Figure 15.11. The dendrogram from single linkage shows the phenomenon usually labelled "chaining", in which separated clusters with "noise" points in between them tend to be joined together. Consequently, we will concentrate on the results from the other two methods.

The dendrogram from complete linkage suggests a broad division of the towns into two groups along with some possible subgrouping of each of the main groups. The dendrogram for average linkage suggests a similar, although not identical, structure. The two groups given by complete linkage and average linkage can be displayed graphically by placing appropriate cluster labels on a scatterplot of the data. The required code is

```
proc tree data=complete n=2 noprint out=comp2c;
 copy mortal hardness location town;
run;
proc tree data=average n=2 noprint out=avge2c;
 copy mortal hardness location town;
run;
symbol1 v=none pointlabel=(position=middle '#cluster')
;
proc gplot data=comp2c;
  plot mortal*hardness;
run;
proc gplot data=avge2c;
  plot mortal*hardness;
run;
```

In addition to producing dendrograms, `proc tree` is also used to assign observations to clusters. The number of clusters is specified with the `n=` option on the `proc` statement. The `noprint` option suppresses the dendrogram and the `out=` option specifies the data set that will contain the cluster assignments in a variable named `cluster`. The `copy` statement is used to add variables to this data set. The `cluster` variable can then be used in the scatterplots, via the `pointlabel` option on a symbol statement. Since `justify=centre(j=c)` is the default for the `pointlabel` option, only `position=middle` is needed to ensure that the cluster numbers are plotted in the correct position. The resulting plots are shown in Figure 15.12 and Figure 15.13. We now see that the clusters produced by average linkage are more similar in size than those

TABLE 15.10

Single Linkage Clustering on Mortality and Water Hardness Data

```
                 The CLUSTER Procedure
             Single Linkage Cluster Analysis

          Eigenvalues of the Correlation Matrix

       Eigenvalue    Difference    Proportion    Cumulative

  1    1.65484862    1.30969725        0.8274        0.8274
  2    0.34515138                      0.1726        1.0000

The data have been standardized to mean 0 and variance 1
Root-Mean-Square Total-Sample Standard Deviation =         1
Mean Distance Between Observations               =   1.73315

                     Cluster History

                                                           Norm    T
                                                            Min    i
NCL    -----------Clusters Joined------------     FREQ     Dist    e

 60    South Shields        Sunderland               2   0.0123
 59    Bournemouth          Coventry                 2   0.0246
 58    Blackburn            Bootle                   2   0.0263
 57    Leeds                Newport                  2   0.0432
 56    Bolton               Stockport                2   0.0455
 55    CL56                 Huddersfield             3   0.0515
 54    Bristol              York                     2   0.0526
 53    CL54                 Southampton              3   0.0532
 52    Blackpool            Wallasey                 2   0.0578
 51    Bradford             Swansea                  2   0.0585
 50    Birmingham           Plymouth                 2   0.0615
 49    CL52                 CL57                     4   0.0631    T
 48    Halifax              Oldham                   2   0.0631
 47    Gateshead            Newcastle                2   0.0646
 46    Burnley              Liverpool                2   0.0693
 45    Bath                 Reading                  2   0.0694
 44    CL46                 CL48                     4   0.0726    T
 43    Stoke                West Bromwich            2   0.0726
 42    CL49                 CL55                     7   0.0753
 41    Doncaster            Leicester                2   0.0855
 40    CL44                 Preston                  5   0.0861
 39    CL58                 CL40                     7   0.0874    T
 38    Cardiff              Darlington               2   0.0874
 37    CL42                 CL51                     9   0.0903
 36    CL38                 Sheffield                3   0.0917
 35    CL45                 Croydon                  3   0.0938
 34    CL39                 Rochdale                 8   0.1133
 33    CL34                 Manchester               9   0.1241
 32    St Helens            CL43                     3   0.1262
 31    CL50                 CL36                     5   0.1391
 30    Birkenhead           CL37                    10   0.1398
 29    CL30                 CL33                    19   0.1454
 28    CL31                 Rotherham                6   0.1522
 27    Portsmouth           Wolverhampton            2   0.1629
 26    Brighton             Grimsby                  2   0.1635

                 The CLUSTER Procedure
             Single Linkage Cluster Analysis

                     Cluster History

                                                           Norm    T
                                                            Min    i
NCL    -----------Clusters Joined------------     FREQ     Dist    e

 25    CL29                 CL28                    25   0.1683
 24    CL41                 Nottingham               3   0.1698
 23    CL25                 Middlesbrough           26   0.1756
 22    CL59                 CL26                     4   0.1839
 21    Derby                CL32                     4   0.1876
 20    CL22                 CL53                     7   0.1951
 19    CL23                 CL24                    29   0.2037
 18    CL35                 Oxford                   4   0.2084
 17    Northampton          Southend                 2   0.2101
```

TABLE 15.10 (continued)

Single Linkage Clustering on Mortality and Water Hardness Data

16	CL20	CL17	9	0.2294
15	CL16	CL27	11	0.2444
14	East Ham	Norwich	2	0.2463
13	Hull	Southport	2	0.2486
12	CL21	Walsall	5	0.2578
11	CL12	CL47	7	0.2679
10	CL19	CL11	36	0.2727
9	CL10	CL13	38	0.2927
8	CL9	CL15	49	0.2994
7	CL8	CL60	51	0.2999
6	CL18	CL7	55	0.3057
5	CL6	CL14	57	0.3376
4	CL5	Exeter	58	0.4393
3	CL4	Salford	59	0.4888
2	CL3	West Ham	60	0.4934
1	CL2	Ipswich	61	0.5068

TABLE 15.11

Complete Linkage Clustering on Mortality and Water Hardness Data

```
                 The CLUSTER Procedure
            Complete Linkage Cluster Analysis

          Eigenvalues of the Correlation Matrix

       Eigenvalue    Difference    Proportion    Cumulative

  1    1.65484862    1.30969725        0.8274        0.8274
  2    0.34515138                      0.1726        1.0000

The data have been standardized to mean 0 and variance 1
Root-Mean-Square Total-Sample Standard Deviation =        1
Mean Distance Between Observations               =  1.73315
```

Cluster History

NCL	Clusters Joined		FREQ	Norm Max Dist	Tie
60	South Shields	Sunderland	2	0.0123	
59	Bournemouth	Coventry	2	0.0246	
58	Blackburn	Bootle	2	0.0263	
57	Leeds	Newport	2	0.0432	
56	Bolton	Stockport	2	0.0455	
55	Bristol	York	2	0.0526	
54	Blackpool	Wallasey	2	0.0578	
53	Bradford	Swansea	2	0.0585	
52	Birmingham	Plymouth	2	0.0615	
51	Halifax	Oldham	2	0.0631	
50	Gateshead	Newcastle	2	0.0646	
49	Burnley	Liverpool	2	0.0693	
48	Bath	Reading	2	0.0694	
47	Stoke	West Bromwich	2	0.0726	
46	CL56	Huddersfield	3	0.08	
45	Doncaster	Leicester	2	0.0855	
44	Cardiff	Darlington	2	0.0874	
43	CL55	Southampton	3	0.1036	
42	Preston	Rochdale	2	0.1156	
41	CL58	Manchester	3	0.1252	
40	CL44	Sheffield	3	0.1292	
39	CL46	CL57	5	0.1362	
38	CL48	Croydon	3	0.138	
37	CL51	CL42	4	0.1446	
36	Birkenhead	CL53	3	0.1454	
35	Portsmouth	Wolverhampton	2	0.1629	
34	Brighton	Grimsby	2	0.1635	

TABLE 15.11 (continued)

Complete Linkage Clustering on Mortality and Water Hardness Data

33	CL45	Nottingham	3	0.1818	
32	CL36	CL54	5	0.182	
31	Derby	St Helens	2	0.1876	
30	CL52	Rotherham	3	0.1878	
29	Northampton	Southend	2	0.2101	
28	CL41	CL49	5	0.2325	
27	East Ham	Norwich	2	0.2463	
26	Hull	Southport	2	0.2486	

The CLUSTER Procedure
Complete Linkage Cluster Analysis

Cluster History

NCL	----------Clusters Joined-----------		FREQ	Norm Max Dist	Tie
25	CL50	Middlesbrough	3	0.2788	
24	CL30	CL40	6	0.292	
23	CL38	Oxford	4	0.2945	
22	CL59	CL43	5	0.2958	
21	CL31	Walsall	3	0.3295	
20	CL32	CL39	10	0.3544	
19	CL21	CL47	5	0.3777	
18	CL34	CL35	4	0.39	
17	CL28	CL37	9	0.407	
16	CL26	CL60	4	0.5364	
15	CL22	CL29	7	0.5419	
14	CL24	CL33	9	0.5492	
13	CL23	CL27	6	0.5606	
12	CL17	CL25	12	0.6689	
11	CL18	West Ham	5	0.6955	
10	CL19	CL16	9	0.7888	
9	CL14	Exeter	10	0.7963	
8	CL13	Ipswich	7	0.8004	
7	CL20	CL12	22	0.8366	
6	CL9	CL15	17	1.2462	
5	CL11	CL10	14	1.2749	
4	CL7	Salford	23	1.3242	
3	CL6	CL5	31	1.7732	
2	CL8	CL3	38	2.3443	
1	CL2	CL4	61	3.3736	

TABLE 15.12

Average Linkage Clustering on Mortality and Water Hardness Data

The CLUSTER Procedure
Average Linkage Cluster Analysis

Eigenvalues of the Correlation Matrix

	Eigenvalue	Difference	Proportion	Cumulative
1	1.65484862	1.30969725	0.8274	0.8274
2	0.34515138		0.1726	1.0000

The data have been standardized to mean 0 and variance 1
Root-Mean-Square Total-Sample Standard Deviation = 1
Root-Mean-Square Distance Between Observations = 2

Cluster History

TABLE 15.12 (continued)

Average Linkage Clustering on Mortality and Water Hardness Data

NCL	Clusters Joined		FREQ	Norm RMS Dist	Tie
60	South Shields	Sunderland	2	0.0107	
59	Bournemouth	Coventry	2	0.0213	
58	Blackburn	Bootle	2	0.0228	
57	Leeds	Newport	2	0.0374	
56	Bolton	Stockport	2	0.0395	
55	Bristol	York	2	0.0456	
54	Blackpool	Wallasey	2	0.0501	
53	Bradford	Swansea	2	0.0507	
52	Birmingham	Plymouth	2	0.0533	
51	Halifax	Oldham	2	0.0547	
50	Gateshead	Newcastle	2	0.0559	
49	CL56	Huddersfield	3	0.0583	
48	Burnley	Liverpool	2	0.06	
47	Bath	Reading	2	0.0601	
46	Stoke	West Bromwich	2	0.0629	
45	CL55	Southampton	3	0.0714	
44	Doncaster	Leicester	2	0.0741	
43	Cardiff	Darlington	2	0.0757	
42	CL49	CL57	5	0.0909	
41	CL43	Sheffield	3	0.0971	
40	Preston	Rochdale	2	0.1002	
39	CL47	Croydon	3	0.1022	
38	CL51	CL40	4	0.1025	
37	CL58	Manchester	3	0.108	
36	CL54	CL53	4	0.1111	
35	Birkenhead	CL36	5	0.1329	
34	Portsmouth	Wolverhampton	2	0.1412	
33	St Helens	CL46	3	0.1415	
32	Brighton	Grimsby	2	0.1417	
31	CL37	CL48	5	0.1423	
30	CL52	Rotherham	3	0.1481	
29	CL44	Nottingham	3	0.1524	
28	Northampton	Southend	2	0.1821	
27	CL35	CL42	10	0.1877	

The CLUSTER Procedure
Average Linkage Cluster Analysis

Cluster History

NCL	Clusters Joined		FREQ	Norm RMS Dist	Tie
26	CL30	CL41	6	0.1889	
25	CL39	Oxford	4	0.2123	
24	East Ham	Norwich	2	0.2134	
23	Hull	Southport	2	0.2154	
22	CL31	CL38	9	0.228	
21	CL59	CL45	5	0.229	
20	CL50	Middlesbrough	3	0.239	
19	CL21	CL32	7	0.2486	
18	Derby	CL33	4	0.2608	
17	CL18	Walsall	5	0.2753	
16	CL23	CL34	4	0.3157	
15	CL27	CL26	16	0.3496	
14	CL25	CL24	6	0.3965	
13	CL19	CL28	9	0.3996	
12	CL17	CL20	8	0.4148	
11	CL12	CL60	10	0.4435	
10	CL29	Exeter	4	0.4646	
9	CL16	West Ham	5	0.5338	
8	CL14	Ipswich	7	0.5777	
7	CL15	CL22	25	0.5827	
6	CL13	CL9	14	0.6252	
5	CL7	CL11	35	0.6477	
4	CL6	CL10	18	0.7539	
3	CL8	CL4	25	0.8992	
2	CL5	Salford	36	1.0282	
1	CL3	CL2	61	1.2748	

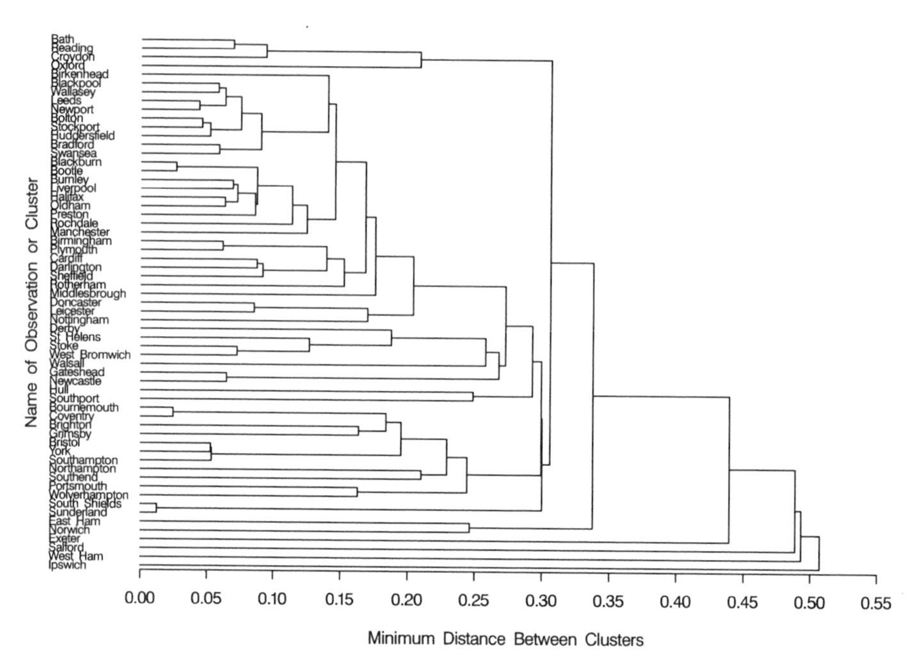

FIGURE 15.9
Single linkage dendrogram for mortality and water hardness data.

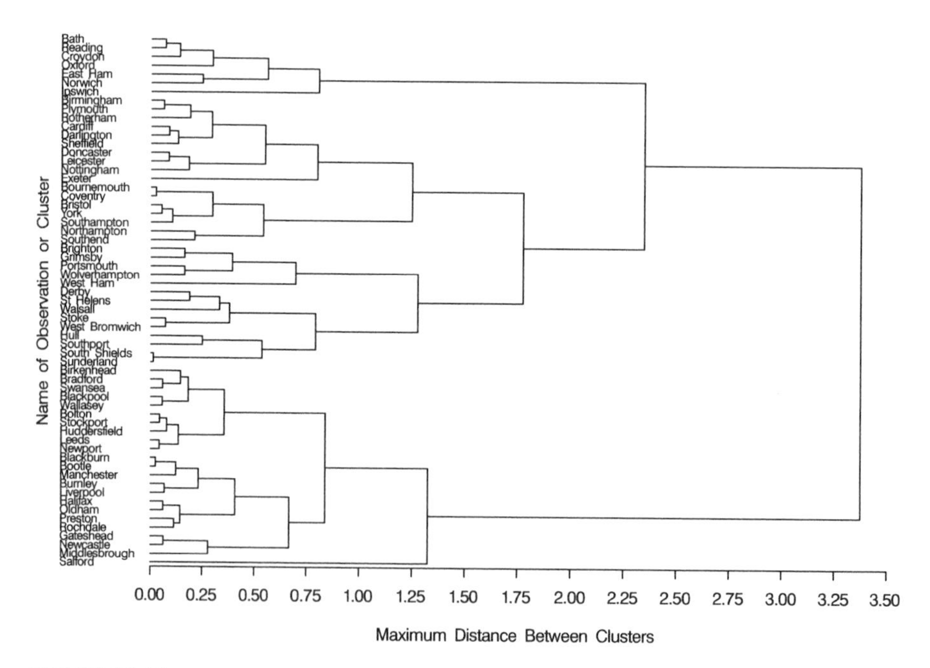

FIGURE 15.10
Complete linkage data on mortality and water hardness data.

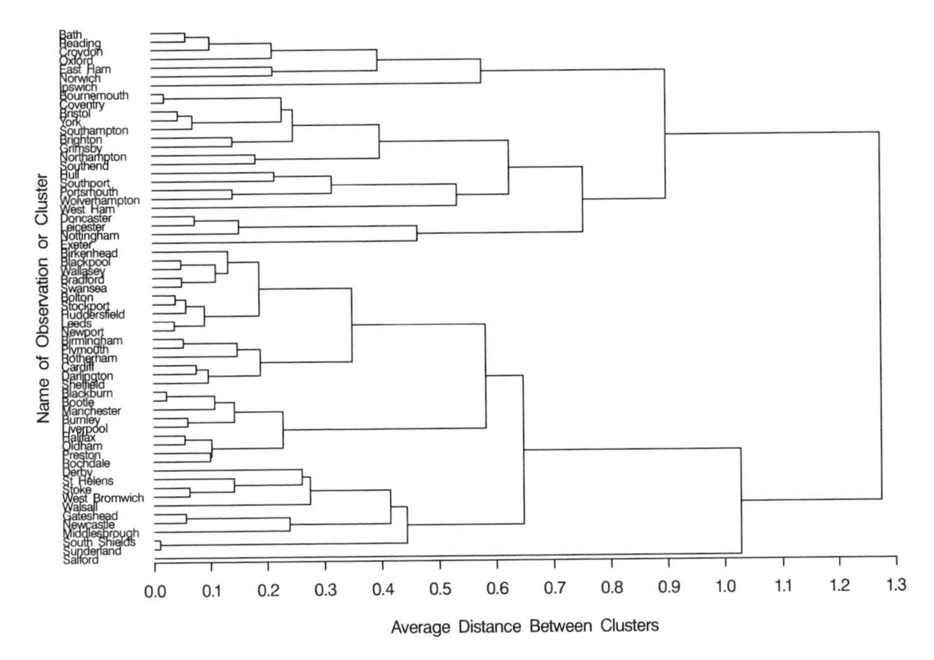

FIGURE 15.11
Average linkage dendrogram on mortality and water hardness data.

produced by complete linkage; the two solutions are similar but do differ a little at the 'boundary' between the two groups.

The difference between the average linkage and complete linkage two-group solutions becomes clearer if we construct a plot with both cluster number and the town name for, say, the average linkage solution as follows:

```
symbol1 v='1' pointlabel=(h=.7 '#town');
symbol2 v='2' pointlabel=(h=.7 '#town');
 proc gplot data=avge2c;
  plot mortal*hardness=cluster /noleglend;
run;
```

The resulting plot is shown in Figure 15.14. The size of the font for the town names has been reduced slightly to reduce the overlap. We see that the average linkage solution places several towns in the Midlands, such as West Bromwich, Nottingham, and Stoke, in the same group as towns farther north and west, whereas it is the latter towns alone that form one of the two clusters from the complete linkage solution. But the division into clusters from both methods reflects a geographical division of the towns related to decreasing water hardness and decreasing mortality as we move from the north to the south of the United Kingdom.

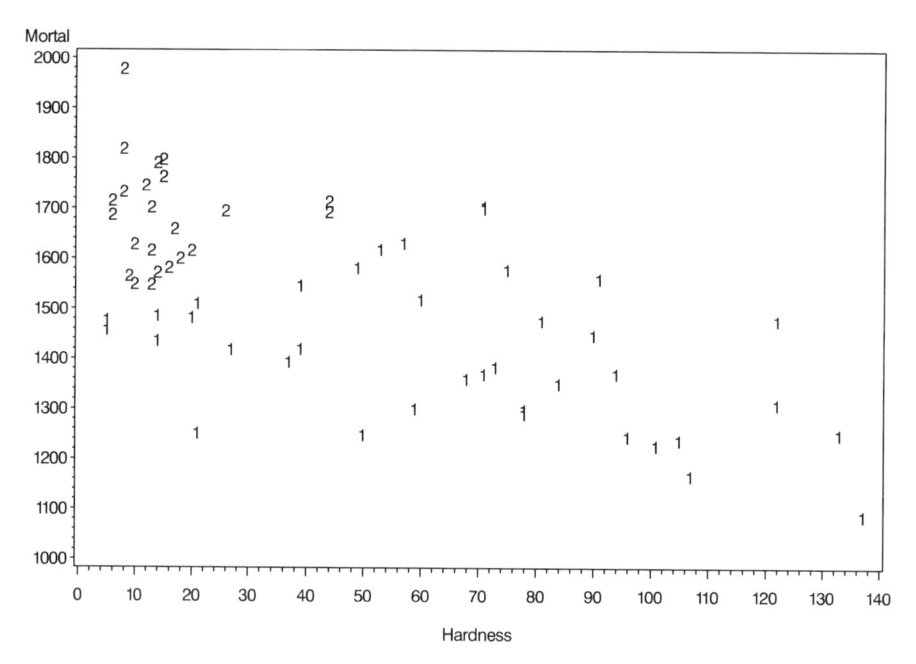

FIGURE 15.12
Scatterplot of mortality and water hardness data showing the two-cluster solution from complete linkage.

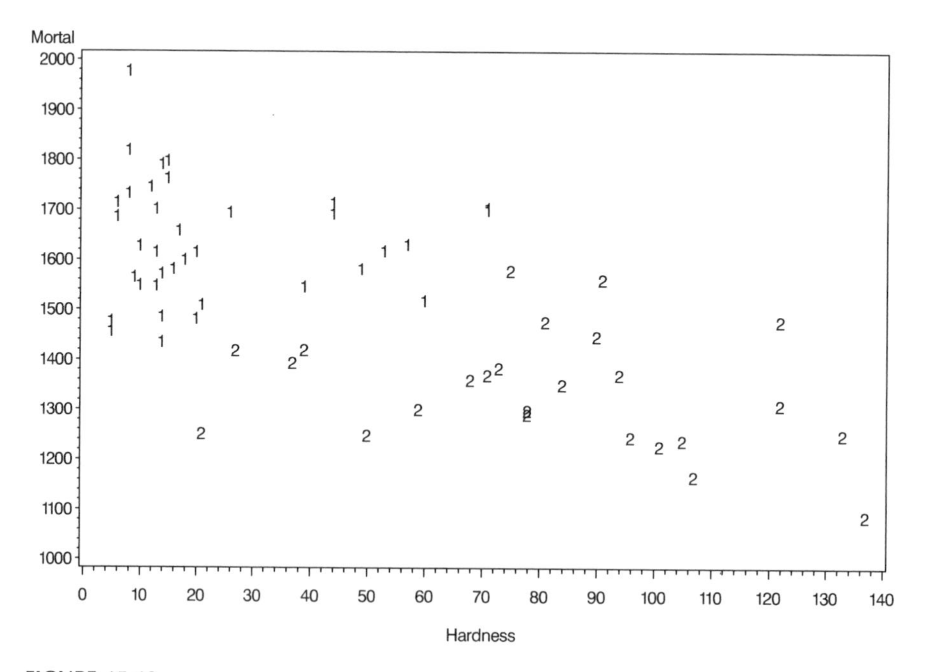

FIGURE 15.13
Scatterplot of mortality and water hardness data showing the two-cluster solution from average linkage.

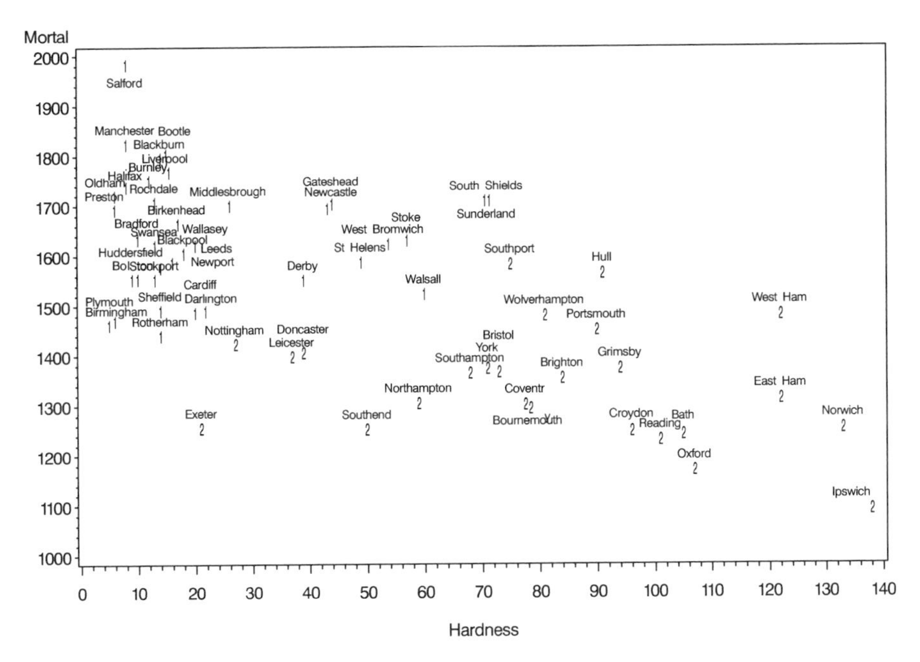

FIGURE 15.14
Scatterplot of mortality and water hardness data showing the two-cluster solution from average linkage with town names added.

Here it is of interest to compare the two groups' solutions with the *a priori* classification of the data into "northern" and "southern" towns.

```
proc freq data=comp2c;
  tables cluster*location;
run;
proc freq data=avge2c;
  tables cluster*location;
run;
```

The results are shown in Table 15.13. The average linkage solution more closely matches the geographical division; the complete linkage solution has one cluster that consists primarily of northern towns and one that is a mix of towns from both north and south.

15.6 Summary

Principal components analysis is among the oldest of multivariate techniques, having been introduced originally by Pearson (1901) and independently by

TABLE 15.13

Cross Classification of Cluster Analysis Solutions for Two Groups from Complete Linkage and Average Linkage against Geographical Location of Towns

```
(1) Complete linkage

                      The FREQ Procedure

                   Table of CLUSTER by location

                 CLUSTER     location

                 Frequency,
                 Percent  ,
                 Row Pct  ,
                 Col Pct  ,N       ,S       ,  Total
                 --------- -------- --------
                        1 ,     14 ,     24 ,     38
                          ,  22.95 ,  39.34 ,  62.30
                          ,  36.84 ,  63.16 ,
                          ,  40.00 ,  92.31 ,
                 --------- -------- --------
                        2 ,     21 ,      2 ,     23
                          ,  34.43 ,   3.28 ,  37.70
                          ,  91.30 ,   8.70 ,
                          ,  60.00 ,   7.69 ,
                 --------- -------- --------
                 Total          35       26       61
                             57.38    42.62   100.00

(2) Average linkage

                      The FREQ Procedure

                   Table of CLUSTER by location

                 CLUSTER     location

                 Frequency,
                 Percent  ,
                 Row Pct  ,
                 Col Pct  ,N       ,S       ,  Total
                 --------- -------- --------
                        1 ,     29 ,      7 ,     36
                          ,  47.54 ,  11.48 ,  59.02
                          ,  80.56 ,  19.44 ,
                          ,  82.86 ,  26.92 ,
                 --------- -------- --------
                        2 ,      6 ,     19 ,     25
                          ,   9.84 ,  31.15 ,  40.98
                          ,  24.00 ,  76.00 ,
                          ,  17.14 ,  73.08 ,
                 --------- -------- --------
                 Total          35       26       61
                             57.38    42.62   100.00
```

Hotelling (1933). It remains, however, one of the most widely employed methods of multivariate analysis useful both for providing a convenient method of displaying multivariate data in a lower dimensional space and for possibly simplifying other analyses of the data. Modern competitors to principal components analysis that may offer more powerful analyses of complex multivariate data are *projection pursuit* (Jones and Sibson, 1987), and *independent components analysis* (Hyvarinen et al., 2001). The former is a technique for finding "interesting" directions in multidimensional data sets; a brief account of the method is given in Everitt and Dunn (2001). The latter is a statistical and computational technique for revealing hidden factors that underlie sets of random variables, measurements, or signals.

Cluster analysis techniques provide a rich source of possible stategies for exploring complex multivariate data. They have been used widely in medical investigations; examples include Everitt et al. (1971), and Wastell and Gray (1987). In this chapter we have described only one class of clustering technique. Some more complex procedures are described in Banfield and Raftery (1993) and Peel and McLachlan (2000).

References

Agresti, A. (1996). *Introduction to Categorical Data Analysis.* New York, Wiley.

Aitkin, M. (1978). The analysis of unbalanced cross classifications. *Journal of the Royal Statistical Society Series A* **141**: 195–223.

Afon, U., N. Barkai, D.A. Notternam, K. Gish, S. Ybarra, D. Mack, and A. J. Levine (1999). Broad patterns of gene expressions revealed by clustering analysis of tumour and normal colon tissues probed by oligonucleotide arrays. *Cell Biology* **99**: 6750–6754.

Altman, D.G. (1991). *Practical Statistics for Medical Research.* London, CRC/Chapman & Hall.

Altman, D.G. and B.L. De Stavola (1994). Practical problems in fitting proportional hazards model to data with updated measurements of the covariates. *Statistics in Medicine* **13**: 301–341.

Andersen, P.K., Ø. Borgan, R.D. Gill, and N. Keiding (1993). *Statistical Models Based on Counting Processes*, New York, Springer-Verlag.

Banfield, J.D. and A.E. Raftery (1993). Model-based Gaussian and non-Gaussian clustering. *Biometrics* **49**: 803–821.

Beck, A.T., A. Steer, and G.K. Brown (1996). *Beck Depression Inventory Manual.* San Antonio, The Pyschological Corporation.

Begg, T.B. and J.B. Hearns (1966). Components in blood viscosity: The relative contribution of haematocrit, plasma fibrinogen and other proteins, *Clinical Science*, **31**, 87–93.

Burman, P. (1996). Model fitting via testing. *Statistica Sinica* **6**: 589–601.

Carpenter, J., S.J. Pocock, and C.J. Lamm, (2002). Coping with missing data in clinical trials: a model-based approach to asthma trials. *Statistics in Medicine* **21**: 1043–1066.

Cattell, R.B. (1965). Factor analysis: an introduction to essentials. *Biometrics* **21**: 190–215.

Chambers, J.M. and T.J. Hastie (1993). *Statistical Models in S.* New York, CRC/Chapman & Hall.

Chatterjee, S. and B. Price (1991). *Regression Analysis by Example.* New York, Wiley.

Cleveland, W.S. (1979). Robust locally weighted regression and smoothing scatterplots. *Journal of the American Statistical Association* **74**: 829–836.

Collett, D. (2003). *Modelling Binary Data*, 2nd ed., Boca Raton, Chapman & Hall/CRC.

Cook, R.D. and S. Weisberg (1982). *Residuals and Influence in Regression.* London, CRC/Chapman & Hall.

Cook, R.D. and S. Weisberg (1994). *Residuals and Influence in Regression.* London, CRC/Chapman & Hall.

Cox, D.R. (1959). The analysis of exponentially distributed life-times with two types of failure. *Journal of the Royal Statistical Society Series B* **21**: 411.

Cox, D.R. (1972). Regression models and life tables. *Journal of the Royal Statistical Society Series B* **34**: 187–200.
Cullen, B.F. and G. van Belle (1975). Lymphocyte transformation and changes in leukocyte count: Effects of anesthesia and operation. *Anesthesiology* **43**: 577–583.
Davis, C.S. (1991). Semiparametric and nonparametric methods for the analysis of repeated measurements with applications to clinical trials. *Statistics in Medicine* **16**: 1959–1980.
Davis, C.S. (2002). *Statistical Methods for the Analysis of Repeated Measurements.* New York, Springer.
Diggle, P.J. (1998). Dealing with missing values in longitudinal studies, In B.S. Everitt and G. Dunn (Eds.), *Statistical Analysis of Medical Data*, London, Arnold.
Diggle, P. J. and M.G. Kenward (1994). Informative drop-out in longitudinal analysis (with discussion). *Applied Statistics* **43**: 49–93.
Diggle, P.L., K. Liang, and S.L. Zeger (1994). *Analysis of Longitudinal Data.* Oxford, Oxford University Press.
Dizney, H. and L. Groman (1967). Predictive validity and differential achievement in three MLA comparative foreign language tests. *Educational and Psychological Measurement* **27**: 1127–1130.
Dobson, A.J. (2001). *An Introduction to Generalized Linear Models.* London, CRC/Chapman & Hall.
Draper, N. R. and H. Smith (1998). *Applied Regression Analysis.* New York, Wiley.
Everitt, B.S. (1987). *An Introduction to Optimization Methods and Their Application in Statistics.* London, CRC/Chapman & Hall.
Everitt, B.S. (1992). *The Analysis of Contingency Tables.* Boca Raton, FL, CRC/Chapman & Hall.
Everitt, B.S. (2001). *Statistics for Psychologists.* New Jersey, Lawrence Erlbaum.
Everitt, B.S. (2002). *Modern Medical Statistics.* London, Arnold.
Everitt, B.S. and E.T. Bullmore (1999). Mixture model mapping of brain activation in functional magnetic resonance images. *Human Brain Mapping* **7**: 1–14.
Everitt, B.S. and G. Dunn (2001). *Applied Multivariate Data Analysis.* London, Arnold.
Everitt, B.S., J. Gourlay, and R.E. Kendall (1971). An attempt at validation of traditional psychiatric syndromes by cluster analysis. *British Journal of Psychiatry* **119**: 299–412.
Everitt, B.S., S. Landau, and M. Leese (2001). *Cluster Analysis.* 4th ed., London, Arnold.
Everitt, B.S. and A. Pickles (2004). *Statistical Aspects of the Design and Analysis of Clinical Trials,* revised ed., London, Imperial College Press.
Fisher, L.D. and G. van Belle (1993). *Biostatistics: A Methodology for the Health Sciences.* New York, Wiley.
Frets, G.P. (1921). Heredity of head form in man. *Genetica* **3**: 193–384.
Frison, L. and S.J. Pocock (1992). Repeated measures in clinical trials: analysis using mean summary statistics and its implications for design. *Statistics in Medicine* **11**: 1685–1704.
Gehan, E. (1965). A generalized Wilcoxon test for comparing arbitrarily singly censored data. *Biometrika* **52**: 650–654.
Goldberg, D. (1972). *The Detection of Psychiatric Illness by Questionnaire.* Oxford, Oxford University Press.
Gordon, A.D. (1999). *Classification*, 2nd ed., Boca Raton, Chapman & Hall.
Grambsch, P.M. and T.M. Therneau (1994). Proportional hazard tests and diagnostics based on weighted residuals, *Biometrika*, **81**, 515–526.

Greenwood, M. and C.V. Yule (1920). An inquiry into the nature of frequency distributions representative of multiple happenings, with particular reference to the occurrence of multiple attacks of disease or repeated accidents. *Journal of the Royal Statistical Society Series A* **89**: 255–279.

Hancock, B. W. , M. Aitkin, J. Martin, I. R. Dunsmore, C. M. Ross, I. Carr, and I. G. Emmanuel (1979). Hodgkin's disease in Sheffield (1971–76) with computer analysis of variables. *Clinical Oncology* **5**: 283–297.

Hartigan, J. (1975). *Clustering Algorithms*, New York, Wiley.

Hand, D.J., F. Daly, A.D. Lunn, K.J. McConway, and E. Ostrowski (1994). *Small Data Sets*, London, Chapman & Hall.

Hastie, T. J. and R. J. Tibshirani (1990). *Generalized Additive Models.* London, CRC/ Chapman & Hall.

Heitjan, D. F. (1997). Annotation: what can be done about missing data? Approaches to imputation. *American Journal of Public Health* **87**: 548–550.

Hollander, M. and D. A. Wolf (1999). *Nonparametric Statistical Methods.* New York, Wiley.

Hosmer, D.W. and S. Lemeshow (1989). *Applied Logistic Regression.* New York, Wiley.

Hosmer, D.W. and S. Lemeshow (1999). *Applied Survival Analysis*, New York, Wiley.

Hotelling, H. (1933). Analysis of a complex of statistical variables into principal components. *Journal of Educational Psychology* **24**: 417–441.

Howell, D. C. (1992). *Statistical Methods for Psychologists.* Belmont, CA, Duxbury Press.

Huby, G.J., J.A. Wingard, and P.M. Bentler (1981). A comparison of two latent variable causal models for adolescent drug use. *Journal of Personality and Social Psychology*, **40**, 180–193.

Huet, S., A. Bouvier, A.-M. Poursat, and E. Jolivet (2004). *Statistical Tools for Nonlinear Regression: A Practical Guide with R and S-PLUS Examples.* New York, Springer Verlag.

Hyvarinen, A., J. Karhunen, and E. Oja (2000). *Independent Component Analysis.* New York, Wiley.

Jolliffe, I.T. (1972). Discarding variables in a principal components analysis I: Artificial data. *Applied Statistics* **21**: 160–173.

Jolliffe, I.T. (2002). *Principal Component Analysis.* New York, Springer.

Jones, M. C. and R. Sibson (1987). What is projection pursuit? *Journal of the Royal Statistical Society Series A* **150**: 1–36.

Kalbfleisch, J. D. and J. L. Prentice (1980). *The Statistical Analysis of Failure Time Data.* New York, Wiley.

Kaufman, L. and Rousseeuw, P.J. (1990). *Finding Groups in Data: An Introduction to Cluster Analysis*, New York, Wiley.

Kelsey, J. L. and R. J. Hardy (1975). Driving of motor vehicles as a risk factor for acute lumbar inter-vertebral disc. *American Journal of Epidemiology* **102**: 63–73.

Keyfitz, N. and W. Flieger (1972). *Population: Facts and Methods of Demography.* San Francisco, W. H. Freeman.

Kolkiewicz, A.W. (2005). Nonlinear regression, in P. Armitage and T. Colton, Eds., *Encyclopedia of Biostatistics*, 2nd ed. Chichester, Wiley.

Kontula, K., L. C. Anderrson, T. Paavonen, G. Myllyla, L. Terrenharr, and P. Kuopio (1980). Glucocorticord receptors and glucocorticord sensitivity of human leukaemia cells. *International Journal of Cancer* **26**: 177–783.

Krzanowski, W.J. and F.H.C. Marriott (1995). *Multivariate Analysis, Part 2.* London, Arnold.

Larner, M. (1996). *Mass and Its Relationship to Physical Measurements.* Department of Mathematics, University of Queensland.
Kaiser, H.E. (1958). The Varimax criterion for analytic rotation in factor analysis, *Psychometrika*, **23**, 187–200.
Liang, K.Y. and S.L. Zeger (1986). Longitudinal data analysis using generalized linear models. *Biometrika* **73**: 13–22.
Lin, D.Y., L.J. Wei, and Z. Ying (1993). Checking the Cox model with cumulative sums of martingale-based residuals, *Biometrika*, **80**. 557–572.
Longford, N.T. (1993). *Random Coefficient Model.* Oxford, Oxford University Press.
Mallows, C.L. (1973). Some comments on Cp. *Technometrics* **15**: 661–675.
Mallows, C.L. (1995). More comments on Cp. *Technometrics* **37**: 362–372.
Mantel, N. (1966). Evaluation of survival data and two new rank order statistics arising in its considerations. *Cancer Chemotherapy Reports* **50**: 163–170.
Marriott, F. H. C. (1974). *The Interpretation of Multiple Observations.* London, Academic Press.
Matthews, J.N.S., D.G. Altman, M.J. Campbell, and P. Royston (1990). Analysis of serial measurements in medical research. *British Medical Journal* **300**: 230–235.
Matthews, J.N.S. (1993). Arefinement to the analysis of serial data using summary measures, *Statistics in Medicine*, **12**, 27–37.
Matthews, J.N.S. (2005) Summary measure analysis of longitudinal data, in P. Armitage and T. Colton, Eds., *Encyclopedia of Biostatistics*, 2nd ed., Chichester, Wiley.
Maxwell, S. E. and H. D. Delaney (1990). *Designing Experiments and Analysing Data.* Belmont, CA, Wadsworth.
McCullagh, P. (1980). Regression models for ordinal data (with discussion). *Journal of the Royal Statistical Society Series B* **42**: 109–142.
McCullagh, P. and J. A. Nelder (1989). *Generalized Linear Models.* 2nd ed., London, CRC/Chapman & Hall.
Mehta, C.R. and N.R. Patel (1986). A hybrid algorithm for Fisher's exact test on unordered r × c contingency tables. *Communications in Statistics* **15**: 387–403.
Morrison, D.F. (1990). *Multivariate Statistical Methods.* New York, McGraw-Hill.
Murray, G.D. and J.G. Findlay (1988). Correcting for the bias caused by drop-outs in hypertension trials. *Statistics in Medicine* **7**: 941–946.
Nelder, J.A. and R.W.M. Wederburn (1972). Generalized linear models, *Journal Of The Royal Statistical Society, Series A*, 135, 370–384.
Nelder, J.A. (1977). A reformulation of linear models. *Journal of the Royal Statistical Society Series A* **140**: 48–63.
Oldham, P.D. (1962). A note on the analysis of repeated measurements of the same subjects. *Journal of Chronic Disease* **15**: 969–977.
O'Neill, S., F. Leahy, M. Pasterkamp, and A. Tal (1983). The effects of chronic hyperinflation, nutritional status, and posture on respiratory muscle strength in cystic fibrosis. *American Review of Respiratory Disease* **128**: 1051–1054.
Pearson, K. (1901). On lines and planes of closest fit to systems of points in space. *Philosophical Magazine* **2**: 559–572.
Peel, D. and G.J. McLachlan (2000). Robust mixture modelling using the *t* distribution. *Statistics and Computing* **10**: 335–344.
Piantadosi, S. (1997). *Clinical Trials: A Methodologic Perspective.* New York, Wiley.
Proudfoot, J., D. Goldberg, A. Mann, B.S. Everitt, I. Marks, and J. Gray (2003). Computerised, interactive, multimedia cognitive behavioural therapy for anxiety and depression in general practice. *Psychological Medicine* **33**: 217–227.
Rencher, A.C. (1995). *Methods of Multivariate Analysis.* New York, Wiley.

Rifland, A. B., V. Canale and M. I. New (1976). Antipyrine clearance in homozygenous beta-thalassemia. *Clinical Pharmaceuticals and Therapeutics* **20**: 476–483.

Rubin, D. B. (1976). Inference and missing data. *Biometrika* **63**: 581–592.

Scheffe, H. (1953). A method for judging all contrasts in the analysis of variance. *Biometrika* **40**: 87–104.

Seeber, G.U.H. (1989). On the regression analysis of tumour recurrence rates. *Statistics in Medicine* **8**: 1363–1369.

Seeber, G.U.H. (1998). Poisson regression, in P. Armitage and T. Colton, Eds., *Encclopedia of Biostatistics,* Chichester, Wiley.

Shapiro, S.S. and M.B. Wilk (1965). An analysis of variance test for normality. *Biometrika* **52**: 591–611.

Silverman, B.W. (1986). *Density Estimation in Statistics and Data Analysis.* London, CRC/Chapman & Hall.

Schal,R.R. and F.J. Rohll (1981). *Biometry,* 2nd ed., San Francisco, W.H. Freeman.

Somes, G.W. and K.F. O'Brien (1985). Mantel–Haenszel Statistic. *Encyclopedia of Statistical Sources.* S. Kotz, N.L. Johnson and C. B. Read. New York, Wiley. **5**.

Thall, P.F. and S.C. Vail (1990). Some covariance models for longitudinal count data with overdispersion. *Biometrics* **46**: 657–671.

Therneau, T.M. and P.M. Grambsch (2000). *Modeling Survival Data: Extending the Cox Model.* New York, Springer.

Timm, N.H. (2002). *Applied Multivariate Analysis,* New York, Springer.

Tufte, E.R. (1983). *The Visual Display of Quantitative Information.* Cheshire, CT, Graphics Press.

Vaupel, J.W., K.G. Manton, and E. Stallard (1979). The impact of heterogeneity in individual frailty on the dynamics of mortality. *Demography* **16**: 439–454.

Wantell, D.G. and R. Gray (1987). The numerical approach to classification: a medical application to develop a typoloty of facial pairs. *Statistics in Medicine* **6**: 137–164.

Yates, F. (1982). Regression models for repeated measurements. *Biometrics* **38**: 850–853.

Zeger, S.L. and K.Y. Liang (1986). Longitudinal data analysis for discrete and continuous outcomes. *Biometrics* **42**: 121–130.

Zerbe, G.O. (1979). Randomization analysis of the completely randomized design extended to growth and response curves. *Journal of the American Statistical Association* **74**: 215–221.

Index

C

D

E

F

G

H

I

K

L

M

N

O

P

Q

R

S

T

U